MW01087512

NEUROTICISM

Also Available

Anxiety and Its Disorders: The Nature and Treatment
of Anxiety and Panic, Second Edition
David H. Barlow

Clinical Handbook of Psychological Disorders:
A Step-by-Step Treatment Manual, Sixth Edition
Edited by David H. Barlow

Handbook of Assessment and Treatment Planning
for Psychological Disorders, Third Edition
Edited by Martin M. Antony and David H. Barlow

Neuroticism

A NEW FRAMEWORK
FOR EMOTIONAL DISORDERS
AND THEIR TREATMENT

Shannon Sauer-Zavala

David H. Barlow

THE GUILFORD PRESS
New York London

Copyright © 2021 The Guilford Press
A Division of Guilford Publications, Inc.
370 Seventh Avenue, Suite 1200, New York, NY 10001
www.guilford.com

Printed in the United States of America

This book is printed on acid-free paper.

Last digit is print number: 9 8 7 6 5 4 3 2 1

The authors have checked with sources believed to be reliable in their efforts to provide information that is complete and generally in accord with the standards of practice that are accepted at the time of publication. However, in view of the possibility of human error or changes in behavioral, mental health, or medical sciences, neither the authors, nor the editor and publisher, nor any other party who has been involved in the preparation or publication of this work warrants that the information contained herein is in every respect accurate or complete, and they are not responsible for any errors or omissions or the results obtained from the use of such information. Readers are encouraged to confirm the information contained in this book with other sources.

Library of Congress Cataloging-in-Publication Data is available from the publisher.

ISBN 978-1-4625-4718-0

About the Authors

Shannon Sauer-Zavala, PhD, is Assistant Professor in the Department of Psychology at the University of Kentucky and founding Director of Clinical Services at the University's Clinic for Emotional Health. Her research is focused on exploring emotion-focused mechanisms that maintain psychological symptoms (particularly high-risk symptoms such as suicidal thoughts and behaviors) and using this information to develop more targeted, easily disseminated intervention strategies. Dr. Sauer-Zavala has coauthored over 75 peer-reviewed articles, numerous book chapters, and three books. She is a codeveloper of the Unified Protocol for the Transdiagnostic Treatment of Emotional Disorders.

David H. Barlow, PhD, ABPP, is Professor Emeritus of Psychology and Psychiatry and Founder and Director Emeritus of the Center for Anxiety and Related Disorders at Boston University. Dr. Barlow has published over 650 articles and chapters and over 90 books and clinical manuals, mostly on the nature and treatment of emotional disorders and clinical research methodology. His books and manuals have been translated into more than 20 languages. His numerous awards and citations include psychology's three highest honors: the Distinguished Scientific Award for the Applications of Psychology from the American Psychological Association, the James McKeen Cattell Fellow Award from the Association for Psychological Science, and the Gold Medal Award for Life Achievement in the Practice of Psychology from the American Psychological Foundation.

Preface

Case 1: Worry. Beth has always been a worrier. At present, she describes spending long periods of time (90% of her day) thinking about her finances, her ability to complete her schoolwork, and her health and safety. Her mind often jumps to the worst-case scenario, such as getting evicted for being late on rent, failing out of graduate school, and being attacked while commuting. To cope, Beth often tries to distract herself by surfing the Internet for several hours every evening. This tactic has resulted in putting off a large project that is important for graduating on time. She describes feeling extremely guilty about her lack of progress but still feels paralyzed when she tries to approach the task. Additionally, she engages in checking behaviors (e.g., going to the doctor frequently, looking up symptoms on the Internet), as well as refusing to enter crowded public spaces that she thinks might be more susceptible to terrorist attacks. In addition to her worries, Beth also experiences feelings of restlessness, difficulty concentrating, and muscle tension. She has noticed that she has been more irritable with her friends and family, often snapping at them over minor provocations.

Case 2: Panic. Marty recently had a panic attack (i.e., racing heart rate, shortness of breath, dizziness, a lump in his throat, nausea, and sweating) while driving to work; he immediately pulled to the side of the road and got out of his car. Although he had always been aware of physical sensations (e.g., accelerated heart rate, sweaty palms) during times of stress, he had never experienced anything like this before, and he was terrified that he would lose control of the car. Following this first attack, Marty is now having panic attacks regularly. Most feel like they come "out of the blue," but he is especially likely to have them in situations from which he feels it would be difficult to escape or leave, such as a meeting or social event with friends or driving on the highway. He constantly worries about having another panic attack and has made changes to his behavior in order to prevent them. For example, Marty has stopped driving on the highway. Instead, he has added 30–45 minutes to his commute by taking back roads. In addition, he has started leaving work earlier, in order to avoid rush-hour traffic. He has also begun avoiding other situations, such as airplanes, elevators, stores, shopping malls, theaters, and crowds. Marty has been trying a number of different things to "get rid of" his uncomfortable physical sensations, including relaxation, hypnosis, and even medication that his doctor has prescribed. However, none of these things has helped. Marty can't shake the feeling that there is something wrong with his brain and that he is weak for experiencing these symptoms.

Case 3: Social Isolation. As far back as she can remember, Amira has struggled to make friends. Throughout her schooling, she worried that her classmates would view her as "awkward and weird," so she avoided large social gatherings. Despite these challenges, she developed a few close relationships with friends she had known "forever." However, now that Amira has started college in a new city, she is feeling increasingly alone. She has isolated herself from other students in her dorm because she's afraid they will reject her. She has also held back from asking questions in class because she is worried her teachers will think she is stupid. These difficulties have been weighing on Amira, and she is feeling really down. She feels hopeless to solve her problems and has stopped engaging with her hobbies, such as biking, yoga, and knitting. Amira believes she doesn't deserve to do "fun" things.

Case 4: Impulsivity. Jami began restricting her eating in middle school after starting to socialize with a new friend group. However, following frequent arguments and falling-outs with these individuals, Jami would "lose control" and binge on large quantities of junk food. She described feeling "numb" while eating, though this was typically followed by extreme guilt and behavioral attempts to compensate for the calories she had consumed (i.e., taking laxatives, forcing herself to exercise). This cycle persisted until high school, when Jami began experimenting with cutting herself when she was especially distressed. Like binge eating, she noticed that using a razor blade to cut her thighs helped her calm down whenever she felt angry or insecure in relationships. By college, Jami was cutting regularly and also started to drink alcohol or use marijuana to unwind every evening. After an argument with the person she was dating, which occurred during a particularly stressful final exam period, Jami noticed that she couldn't remember several hours of her evening the following day. Startled by this period of lost time, she went to her university's counseling center, stating that she is unable to control her actions when she feels upset.

How can the problems facing the individuals described above be best understood? Mental health professionals may recognize the symptoms of generalized anxiety disorder in Beth, panic disorder and agoraphobia in Marty, social anxiety disorder and depression in Amira, and binge-eating disorder and borderline personality disorder in Jami.* Although focusing on the differences among these people in terms of discrete diagnostic features is one approach to understanding their difficulties, there are commonalities among these presentations that may offer another path for conceptualizing them. Specifically, Beth, Marty, Amira, and Jami all experience the frequent and intense negative emotions that suggest high levels of neuroticism. At a fundamental level, neuroticism can be thought of as stress reactivity, that is, strong surges of negative emotion in response to both external and internal triggers (Barlow, Ellard, Sauer-Zavala, Bullis, & Carl, 2014a). Anxiety, fear, guilt, anger, and sadness are the discrete states most often referenced with regard to this propensity to experience negative emotions. Additionally, neuroticism is characterized by the perception or sense that the world is a dangerous and threatening place, along with the belief that challenging stressors cannot be managed (Barlow, 2002; Barlow, Sauer-Zavala, Carl, Bullis, & Ellard, 2014b; Clark & Watson, 2008; Eysenck, 1947).

Neuroticism is strongly associated with the development and maintenance of a range of common mental health conditions (Kendler, Neale, Kessler, Heath, & Eaves, 1993; Kendler, Gatz, Gardner, & Pedersen, 2006) and also has implications for physical health, as well as social and occupational functioning (Brickman, Yount, Blaney, Rothberg, & De-Nour, 1996; Lahey, 2009; Shipley, Weiss, Der, Taylor, & Deary, 2007; Smith & MacKenzie, 2006; Suls & Bunde, 2005). Despite the far-reaching consequences of this trait, efforts to intervene in neuroticism directly have rarely been undertaken, with extant treatment approaches focused more narrowly on discrete conditions or difficulties. However, consider addressing neuroticism in the context of care for Beth, Marty, Amira, and Jami. Rather than directly focusing on the symptoms that brought them to treatment, we contend that addressing the risk factors (i.e., the propensity to experience negative emotions) that contribute to the development and maintenance of these difficulties is a more efficient approach. Indeed, targeting neuroticism broadly rather than the discrete symptoms each patient experiences allows for a streamlined approach to address co-occurring emotional problems in the context of a single intervention, benefiting patients like Amira and Jami, who exhibited symptoms of more than one mental disorder.

Additionally, assuming Beth, Marty, Amira, and Jami are treated by the same therapist, this clinician would enjoy increased efficiency by applying a unified, neuroticism-focused approach to all four patients. Indeed, given the far-reaching risk conferred by the neurotic temperament, an intervention

*All case material presented in this book has been disguised to conceal the identities of our patients.

aimed at this trait would likely reduce the time and monetary costs (i.e., buying manuals, attending training workshops) needed for clinicians to prepare for sessions, compared with reviewing all of the disorder-specific interventions relevant to the range of diagnoses in the *Diagnostic and Statistical Manual of Mental Disorders* (DSM-5; American Psychiatric Association, 2013).

OUTLINE OF TOPICS COVERED IN THIS TEXT

Given the public health implications of neuroticism, the purpose of this book is to define the nature of this trait, informed by its historical origins and bolstered by recent empirical work aimed at understanding how neuroticism develops and is maintained, how it is related to psychopathology, how it is assessed and incorporated into nosological schemes, and how it might best be addressed in treatment. Toward this end, in Chapter 1, we expand on the definition of neuroticism provided at the start of this preface, integrating various theoretical perspectives on this trait. Specifically, we discuss how an understanding of neuroticism grew from the study of biologically based temperaments, as well as from more descriptive, lexical taxonomies of personality. After more firmly rooting our definition of neuroticism within historical conceptions of this trait, we then articulate a theory for understanding how neuroticism develops, integrating genetic, neurobiological, and environmental contributions (Chapter 2). Of note, our model for the development of neuroticism (triple vulnerability theory; Barlow, Ellard, et al., 2014a) was previously articulated as an etiological framework for trait anxiety and its disorders (Barlow, 1988, 2002), underscoring the close relationship between the neurotic temperament and psychopathology. In Chapter 3, this relationship is further clarified, as we argue for the existence of a general neurotic syndrome (Andrews, 1990, 1996; Tyrer, 1989) that accounts for the development of many common mental health conditions.

Next, in Chapter 4, we propose a functional model through which high levels of neuroticism develop into various manifestations of emotional disorders (e.g., anxiety, depressive, and related disorders). Then, given the strong associations between neuroticism and psychopathology, we consider how this trait has been incorporated into various systems for classifying mental disorders and advocate for moving beyond descriptive accounts of psychopathology (both categorical and dimensional) in favor of our functional approach (Chapter 5). Indeed, when the processes in this functional model become the focus of treatment, improvements in both trait vulnerabilities (neuroticism) *and* disorder symptoms become possible (Sauer-Zavala et al., 2020). In fact, there is a growing literature to suggest that neuroticism is more malleable than originally believed, and we present specific behavioral strategies for intervening in this trait (Chapter 6).

Finally, though the majority of this book is dedicated to understanding neuroticism as a risk factor for a broad range of psychopathology, other traits warrant discussion, particularly the tendency to experience positive emotions—also known as *extraversion* or *positive affectivity* (Costa & McCrae, 1992). Deficits in positive emotionality have been linked, beyond the contributions of neuroticism, to several conditions (e.g., depression, social anxiety, and agoraphobia; Rosellini, Lawrence, Meyer, & Brown, 2010), whereas maladaptively high levels of positive emotions are associated with mania (Gruber, Johnson, Oveis, & Keltner, 2008). Thus neuroticism alone cannot account for all DSM emotional disorders, and, by expanding our view to consider additional dimensions of personality, a limited number of risk factors may emerge that can become the focus of treatment, instead of their numerous downstream clinical endpoints (i.e., each DSM diagnosis). Chapter 7 first describes the rationale for expanding existing personality-based, dimensional approaches to understanding psychopathology to include the functional processes that account for how traits evolve into disorder symptoms. Neuroticism serves as an example of how research underscoring functional relationships between traits and disorders can inform treatment targets; however, theoretical and empirical data linking additional dimensions of personality to psychopathology are less robust. Existing literature in this area is summarized, along with preliminary suggestions for treatment approaches that map onto these established functional relationships. A dimensional understanding of psychopathology, when linked to clear treatment recommendations based on functional relationships, has the potential to dramatically streamline care for mental disorders, ultimately increasing the likelihood that evidence-based strategies will be employed in routine practice.

Acknowledgments

This book could not have been written without the generous contributions of many individuals. First, we would like to thank our editor, Jim Nageotte, who recognized the importance of organizing our work on this topic into a single volume; we are incredibly proud of the result, which would not exist without his encouragement. A number of additional individuals at The Guilford Press warrant mention. First, thank you to Jane Keislar, who tirelessly fielded questions about obtaining permissions and carried us across the finish line. We also extend our gratitude to Judith Grauman, Anna Brackett, and Liz Geller, who shepherded this project from manuscript to bound book. And thank you also to our copy editor, Elaine Kehoe—your attention to detail is beyond measure. Finally, thank you to Paul Gordon, who provided us with the cover art for this project and was so good natured about our many requests in this area.

In addition, we would like to thank members of our research team— your willingness to engage in discussion on the topics covered helped us refine our thinking. Specifically, thank you to Todd Farchione, Stephanie Jarvi Steele, Elizabeth Eustis, Clair Robbins, Amantia Ametaj, Julianne Wilner Tirpak, Brittany Woods, Andrew Curreri, Maya Nauphal, Nicole Cardona, Stephen Semcho, and Nicole Stumpp. We owe a huge debt of gratitude to Bethany Harris and Lauren Woodard, who were always willing to lend a hand on technically challenging aspects of the book (i.e., formatting figures and tables)—with a smile, no less. Thank you also to Anna Garlock, Alex Urs, Destiney MacLean, and Sohayla Elhusseini for your assistance with references. Finally, thank you to Amanda Tarullo for your generous feedback on Chapter 2, as well as Matthew Southward for help in conceptualizing the intermediary mechanisms described in Chapter 7.

We would also like to acknowledge our families, without whom this project would not have been possible. First, to Jason Zavala, your tireless support and encouragement kept me going. Additionally, to Juan and Dorothy Zavala and Marilyn Matern-Bratz and Dave Bratz, thank you for your willingness to provide child care whenever there was a chapter that needed to be finished (or sanity that needed to be otherwise saved). Thank you to Skylar Zavala, who is responsible for pressuring us to have a first draft of these chapters before she made her debut in this world (and also responsible for making the second draft late!). Thank you also to Fiona Zavala—the pride you take in the fact that your mom "helps people" inspires me to keep doing it. Finally, thank you to Beverly Barlow, who didn't get too mad that David agreed to write another book when he is (supposedly) retired.

Contents

1

Perspectives on Temperament and Personality

Scholars have long sought to understand individual differences, particularly with regard to describing patterns of emotional responding and behavior. Indeed, references to humans' emotional nature are found in the writings of Greek and Roman philosophers, and these early conceptualizations can be traced to modern-day accounts with remarkable continuity. Whereas early perspectives on individual differences in emotional reactivity came from medical or philosophical traditions, psychology became the dominant voice in this conversation around the turn of the 20th century. Within psychology, however, there has been variability in the approach used to characterize an individual's nature. For instance, despite obvious overlap, the research literatures on *temperament* and on *personality* have largely proceeded independently (Rothbart, Ahadi, & Evans, 2000). Personality research has been, for the most part, structural in nature; that is, researchers have primarily focused on creating comprehensive descriptive taxonomies of personality traits and their correlates rather than focusing on etiology. Although this strategy has provided a robust nomological network of relationships between traits and observable phenomena (e.g., behaviors), it has been met with the criticism that "it does not attempt to determine *how* various traits develop and *how* they influence behavior" (Baron, 1998, p. 488). Temperament research, on the other hand, has focused on understanding the biological mechanisms that underlie phenotypic manifestations of traits. The purpose of this chapter is to delineate various historical perspectives on characterizing an individual's disposition, particularly the susceptibility to negative emotions, in order to arrive at a modern consensus on the nature of neuroticism.

ANCIENT CONCEPTIONS OF TEMPERAMENT

Four Humors Theory

The Greek physician Hippocrates (460–370 B.C.E.) is often credited with developing the first biological account to characterize a patient's emotional style. Specifically, according to *The Nature of Man*, a writing now attributed to one of Hippocrates' students, the human body consists of four "humors" (blood, black bile, yellow bile, and phlegm), with good health believed to result from a balance among them (Hippocrates, 1978). Although a full account of the relationship between the humors and temperament was not expressed in the Hippocratic canon, there are passing references to differences in character that may occur from excesses in one humor or another; for example, the tendency to experience negative emotions was associated with heightened levels of black bile (see Digman, 1990). It appears likely that Hippocrates was influenced by the medical tradition at the time, emanating from ancient Egypt or Mesopotamia, referencing humors as the cause of disease (see Flaskerud, 2012). Additionally, principles of Pythagorean philosophy are also incorporated, including emphasis on harmony and balance, along with explicit links between the four humors and other tetradic categories highlighted by these thinkers (e.g., the four seasons, Empedocles' four elements [earth, air, fire, water]; see Stelmack & Stalikas, 1991). In fact, each humor is associated with an element, temperature, and season (see Figure 1.1 later in the chapter). For example, blood, a manifestation of air, is considered warm and moist and predominates in the springtime, whereas black bile is a manifestation of earth and is cold, dry, and associated with autumn. Likewise, yellow bile is hot and dry and is associated with fire and summer, whereas phlegm is cold and wet and is associated with water and winter. It was Galen (131–200 C.E.) who more fully elaborated a theory for how the four humors influence an individual's emotional presentation. In his treatise, *On Temperaments*, Galen indicates that an optimal disposition (Gr. *Eucrasia* = best possible mixture) results from a balance of all four humors:

> The best temperate man is he who in the body seems to be the mean of all extremities. In his soul he is in the middle of boldness and timidity, of negligence and impertinence, of compassion and envy. He is cheerful, affectionate, charitable, and prudent. (Galen, 1938/170 C.E., p. 86)

Indeed, the term *temperament*, still used today to describe one's emotional character, comes from Latin (*temperare*) and literally means to combine or blend in proper proportion. Galen retained Hippocrates' associations between humors and *temperature* (hot, cold, moist, dry), a word with similar etymological roots that may underscore common colloquial interactions between character and climate (e.g., *hot tempered*).

Additionally, Galen assigned temperamental labels, with dispositional descriptors, to each of the four humors. Specifically, *sanguine* was used to categorize individuals dominated by blood (wet and hot) who were prone to cheerfulness and optimism, whereas the term *melancholic* represented those with an excess of black bile (cold and dry) who were likely to exhibit a dour and downcast nature. *Choleric* individuals were associated with greater levels of yellow bile (hot and dry) and were said to be easily emotionally aroused; and, finally, *phlegmatic* types demonstrated detachment and impassivity as a result of excess phlegm (cold and wet). Parallels to neuroticism can be seen in Galen's descriptions of the melancholic temperament:

> The melancholics . . . show fear and depression, discontent with life, and hatred of all people. The desire to die is not common to all, although fear of death is the principal concern of some. A few people are bizarre since they dread and desire death at the same time. As external darkness renders almost all people fearful . . . , the color of the black humor, obscuring the area of thought, brings about the fear. People call this melancholia, indicating by this term that the (black) humor is etiologically responsible. (Siegel, 1973, p. 195)

Of particular note, Galen references a biological basis for temperament (i.e., levels of humors in the body), a perspective that has been carried into the modern conceptions that are described later in this chapter.

The influence of the four-humors theory can be traced well into the Enlightenment, with references to this understanding of temperament attributed to Nicholas Culpepper (an English physician and astronomer working in the 17th century), Immanuel Kant (a German philosopher active in the 18th century), Wilhelm Wundt (a 19th-century German physician often credited as the father of modern psychology), and others (e.g., Steiner, Adler, Kretschmer, and Fromm; see Flaskerud, 2012). For example, in addition to translating Galen's theory for English readers in 1652, Culpepper provided his own well-developed descriptions of each temperament (he referred to them as complexions), along with combinations of all possible pairs (Stelmack & Stalikas, 1991).

Kant also acknowledged a biological basis of temperament with humoral roots but indicated that a psychological meaning of this construct, consisting of feelings and behaviors, also exists; this distinction stems from his belief, described in *Anthropology from a Pragmatic Point of View*, that there are both a corporeal and a spiritual nature of man (Kant, 1974). According to Kant, there may be a causal relationship between one's physical constitution and emotional character, but that understanding biology may be of secondary importance when classifying temperament:

> For in order to correctly assign a man to the title of a particular class, we do not need to know beforehand what chemical composition of the blood entitles

us to name a certain characteristic property of temperament; we need to know, rather, what feelings and inclinations we have observed in him. (Kant, 1974, p. 152)

Kant's work marked a transition from considering temperament as a causal construct, determined by humors with implications for health and behavior, to a more descriptive view of characterizing individual differences—a perspective that bears similarity to modern-day *personality* classification (see the following section "Modern Conceptions of Personality"). He classified Galen's temperaments into categories of "feeling" and "activity," which he further divided into subgroups based on duration. For example, *melancholy* and *sanguine* describe emotional tendencies, with the former characterized by weak and long-lasting emotions and the latter by strong and short-lasting affective states. In contrast, the choleric temperament was associated with intense but short-lasting activity, whereas phlegmatic individuals demonstrated enduring periods of inactivity. Of note, Kant's system emphasized four simple temperaments that could not be combined.

Wundt (1886) is credited with shifting the emphasis of the typology of his predecessors from four independent categories to a two-dimensional system. Specifically, Wundt described two independent dimensions, emotionality and activity, on which an individual could be placed anywhere along a continuum between poles (Stelmack & Stalikas, 1991). Within this system, the degree to which one experiences emotions is rated on a continuous spectrum from unstable (strong emotions) to stable (weak emotions), and one's activity level is rated between poles of unchangeable (low activity) and changeable (high activity). Galen's four temperaments are located in the quadrants formed by each combination of high and low levels on these poles. Wundt's dimensions of emotionality and activity, used in this context to understand Galen's four temperament types, have clear connections to modern-day neuroticism and extraversion, representing a remarkable continuity from ancient humoral theory to today's understanding of temperament. Thus, within this framework, individuals assigned a melancholic temperament would likely be characterized by high neuroticism and low extraversion.

MODERN CONCEPTIONS OF TEMPERAMENT

Indeed, although the specifics differ, modern conceptions of temperament share the belief (with the ancient biological models described previously) that emotions are of the utmost importance to understanding individual differences and that biological factors are responsible for observable characteristics (Clark & Watson, 2008). For example, Gordon Allport (1937) provides a definition of temperament, emphasizing these features, that is still relevant nearly a century later:

> Temperament refers to the characteristic phenomena of an individual's emotional nature, including his susceptibility to emotional stimulation, his customary strength and speed of response, the quality of his prevailing mood, and all peculiarities of fluctuation and intensity of mood these phenomena being regarded as dependent on constitutional makeup and therefore largely hereditary in origin. (p. 54)

This view of temperament was likely influenced by Allport's visit, as a recent college graduate, with Sigmund Freud. In his autobiographical essay in *Pattern and Growth in Personality,* Allport (1961) describes breaking the ice with Freud by recounting an interaction with a boy he met on the train while on his way to Vienna; the child was afraid of getting dirty and refused to sit down near other passengers. Allport reportedly suggested that the boy had learned this dirt phobia from his mother, who appeared to be a neat and overbearing person herself. As the story goes, Freud responded by asking, "And was that little boy you?" Allport was uncomfortable with Freud's attempt to dismiss his observation by assuming that he was describing an unconscious conflict stemming from his own childhood. While Allport never denied that unconscious and historical variables have a role to play in shaping an individual's emotional nature, he found the conscious, observable aspects of experience more compelling for explaining temperament.

Despite agreement that there is a biological basis for the propensity to experience particular emotions, which figures prominently into Allport's definition of temperament, researchers across the 20th century have employed idiosyncratic definitions of this term. These inconsistencies prompted a roundtable discussion at the 1985 meeting of the Society for Research in Child Development titled "What Is Temperament?" followed by a now-seminal article (Goldsmith et al., 1987) summarizing the perspectives of theorists linked to four compelling theories (i.e., Goldsmith, Rothbart, Buss and Plomin, and Thomas and Chess). Rothbart's conception of temperament is quite broad, including emotionality and motor activity, as well as attentional processes that serve to regulate these characteristics (Rothbart & Derryberry, 1981). In contrast, Goldsmith more narrowly focuses attention on emotional experiences, emphasizing dimensions that correspond to discrete emotions (i.e., anger, fear) instead of a single "emotionality dimension" (Goldsmith & Campos, 1982). Buss and Plomin's approach is composed of three dimensions (emotionality, activity, and sociability), which they describe as enduring across age and situation and, arguably most important to their theory, as being genetically mediated (Goldsmith et al., 1987). Finally, Chess and Thomas used data derived from their well-known New York longitudinal study (Thomas & Chess, 1977) to identify three child behavior "types" (i.e., easy, difficult, slow to warm) that they assumed had a biological basis. These perspectives share elements, yet emphasize different features; at the end of the article, the moderator, Robert McCall, attempted to integrate the four approaches into a shared definition:

> Temperament consists of relatively consistent, basic dispositions inherent in the person that underlie and modulate the expression of activity, reactivity, emotionality, and sociability. Major elements of temperament are present early in life, and those elements are likely to be strongly influenced by biological factors. As development proceeds, the expression of temperament increasingly becomes more influenced by experience and context. (Goldsmith et al., 1987, p. 524)

Twenty-five years later, former trainees of McCall's panelists published a follow-up article to reflect on developments in the study of temperament (Shiner et al., 2012). These researchers provide an updated definition, suggesting that "temperament traits are early emerging basic dispositions in the domains of activity, affectivity, attention, and self-regulation, and these dispositions are the product of complex interactions among genetic, biological, and environmental factors across time" (p. 437). Empirical findings challenged some of the assumptions from the 1987 panel, including the notion that temperament is stable; for example, inhibitory systems come online as children age, making them less reactive (Rothbart, 2011), though temperament does appear to become more consistent into adulthood (Roberts & DelVecchio, 2000). Additionally, although current temperament researchers agree with the traits included in the 1987 definition (i.e., activity, reactivity, emotionality, sociability), there is also consensus that important individual-difference dimensions of attention and self-regulation had been left out. It is now recognized that affective and cognitive systems are highly integrated systems (e.g., Forgas, 2008) and that processes typically considered cognitive in nature (attention, executive control) can fall within the purview of temperament. Finally, early conceptions of temperament assumed that biology exerted a stronger effect early in life and that the environment became more influential over time; however, as temperament research has matured, it has become clear that interactions between biological and environmental contributions are much more complex and interactive (see Chapter 2 for a detailed account of the biological and environmental contributions to neuroticism).

Of note, the dimensions that emerge in attempts to define temperament in the child development literature appear to overlap with structural models of personality (that were mostly derived from the study of adults) described later in this chapter (e.g., negative emotionality and reactivity correspond to neuroticism, positive emotionality and activity correspond to extraversion, sociability to agreeableness, and self-regulation to conscientiousness). Staying within the broader temperament tradition, various influential researchers have described the tendency to experience negative emotions specifically. Additionally, their theories go beyond lip service to the notion that this trait is biologically based by including more fleshed-out biological models that mediate its expression.

Hans Eysenck

The label *neuroticism* was first used by Eysenck (1947), who drew inspiration from the early DSM category of neurosis, representing what we now consider anxiety, depressive, and related disorders. Eysenck proposed that neuroticism, on a continuum with emotional stability, is marked by a low tolerance for stress or aversive stimuli and that individuals with high levels of this trait are at increased risk for a diagnosis of neurosis. Although Eysenck regretted employing a term with Freudian roots, noting that "it would no doubt be preferable in some ways to use a more neutral kind of label" (1947, p. 49), he felt it was more important to emphasize the robust relationship between personality and psychopathology. Despite this, he also made it clear that "some so called 'neurotic' inmates (of a hospital) show very little evidence of the 'neurotic constitution' and would likely be situated rather towards the normal end of the distribution" (1947, p. 48), theorizing that individuals without this temperamental vulnerability would have to be subjected to extreme hardship to trigger neurosis. Of course, Eysenck's view is consistent with the prevailing diathesis–stress model (Meehl, 1962), in which those who are more temperamentally vulnerable may develop psychopathology without much provocation, whereas those lower in neuroticism would require a high degree of environmental stress.

In addition to neuroticism, Eysenck's (1947, 1967) conception of temperament also originally included a dimension to characterize an individual's willingness to engage with their environment,* referred to as extraversion (on a continuum with introversion); individuals high on this trait approach life with energy, enthusiasm, and cheerfulness. When crossed, these two dimensions resemble the four Greek temperaments articulated by Galen (melancholic, choleric, phlegmatic, sanguine) and reinforced by Wundt (described earlier in this chapter; see Figure 1.1), underscoring remarkable continuity in how theorists understand individual differences. Eysenck's

---

A note about language: In this book, we use "they/them/their" when referring to a single individual. We have made this choice to be inclusive of readers who do not identify with masculine or feminine pronouns.

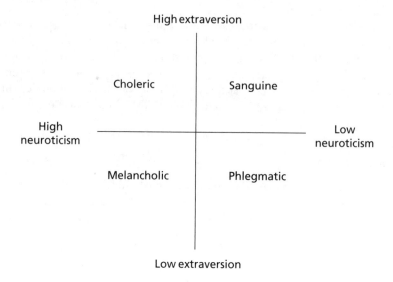

FIGURE 1.1. Hippocrates' humors expressed as modern dimensions of temperament.

early work grew into the well-known Big Three model (Eysenck & Eysenck, 1975), which added the third temperamental dimension of psychoticism (i.e., disinhibition) versus constraint. The pioneering efforts of Eysenck and colleagues indeed influenced psychologists for decades to come; for example, Tellegen (1985) proposed three similar factors (i.e., negative emotionality, positive emotionality, and disinhibition), as did Watson and Clark (1993; i.e., negative temperament, positive temperament, and constraint).

Eysenck's greatest contribution to the study of temperament, however, is arguably his emphasis on understanding the biological bases of his traits. He contends that "the field of personality is not an isolated island, lying far from other more civilized countries and continents; personality interacts constantly and inevitably with experimental psychology, pharmacology, and neurology" (1967, p. xi). Although this view of the relationship between personality and physiology is commonplace today, Eysenck is credited as a forerunner of this approach. He was heavily influenced by Pavlovian principles of learning, describing neuroticism as fundamentally a strong drive to avoid situations that may produce negative emotions and conducting a series of experimental studies to test this theory (see Eysenck, 1967). Eysenck (1961, 1981) also relates this tendency to become emotionally aroused to neural structures, articulating that neuroticism is associated with a lower threshold for activation, along with overarousal, of the limbic system.

Jeffery Gray

Jeffery Gray, a student of Eysenck's at the Institute of Psychiatry in London, proposed his own account of the tendency to experience negative emotions, particularly anxiety. Specifically, Gray (1970) described flaws in Eysenck's (1967) theoretical understanding of how readily individuals at extreme temperamental poles (i.e., neurotic vs. stable, introverted vs. extroverted) form conditioned reflexes related to perceived threat. He rotated Eysenck's axes of neuroticism and extraversion 30 degrees and labeled his dimensions *anxiety* and *impulsivity*; *anxiety* roughly corresponds to high levels of neuroticism and low levels of extraversion in Eysenck's model, whereas *impulsivity* relates to high neuroticism and high extraversion. Gray further articulated a neural structure to account for these dimensions, which he referred to as the *behavioral inhibition system* (BIS) and the *behavioral activation system* (BAS; Gray, 1982). The BIS is described as responding to imminent punishment or frustration, novel stimuli, and innate sources of fear (e.g., snakes, spiders, heights) with the inhibition of ongoing behavior, increased attention to environmental stimuli, and increased arousal. In contrast, the BAS is sensitive to signals of reward and nonpunishment and increases the probability of approach behavior. Gray also proposed the fight–flight system (FFS), which involves defensive aggression (i.e., fight) and/or unconditioned escape behavior (i.e., flight) in response to unconditioned punishment, such as pain, and unconditioned frustrative nonrewards (Gray & McNaughton, 1996). As such, the FFS may represent a biological vulnerability to the distinct emotion of fear/panic specifically, as opposed to anxiety more generally (Barlow et al., 2014b).

Fifteen years later, Gray and McNaughton (1996) presented a revised theory, clarifying the stimuli to which each system (i.e., BIS, BAS, FFS) responds. Similar to the original model, the BAS remains responsive to all positively valenced (unconditioned and conditioned) stimuli. They added freezing reactions to the fight-or-flight responses that were previously described as occurring in the presence of unavoidable threat, and thus they renamed the FFS the *fight/flight/freeze system* (FFFS); this system is thought to mediate reactions to all aversive stimuli. Finally, the BIS was no longer described as mounting responses to conditioned aversive stimuli but as instead associated with resolution of conflict in situations in which both the BAS and FFFS have been activated. If reward outweighs threat, the BIS will resolve the conflict by engaging the BAS and inhibiting the FFFS, resulting in approach. If threat outweighs reward, the BIS will further activate the FFFS and inhibit the BAS, resulting in avoidance.

Subsequently, at Eysenck's invitation and with feedback from Gray on drafts of their manuscript, Matthews and Gilliland (1999) reviewed the literature supporting these two alternative models of personality structure and neural underpinnings. They concluded that there is clear support for the Eysenck theory in the context of certain paradigms. Specifically, there is evidence for Eysenck's conception of emotional arousal as a moderator of learning; indeed, individuals high in neuroticism demonstrate conditioned avoidance of aversive stimuli more quickly than those who are emotionally stable, but only in emotionally arousing situations. In other settings, this theory fails to explain empirical data adequately, especially in studies of subjective response, attention, and performance. Similarly, Matthews and Gilliland suggest that Gray's theory has advanced research by stimulating interest in understanding personality effects via motivational variables. They contend that Gray may provide a better explanation for certain data, such as instrumental conditioning to reward stimuli and the positive affectivity of extraverts. Overall, however, there is little evidence that Gray's personality axes are generally more predictive of physiological reactions and learning criteria than Eysenck's original dimensions. Nonetheless, these theorists (and empiricists) pioneered the modern study of temperament by connecting observable behavioral features to neural functioning, which prompted decades of fruitful research.

Jerome Kagan

In another trait theory focused explicitly on children, Kagan (1989) examined toddlers' approach and withdrawal behavior and created temperamental profiles to characterize extreme manifestations of these phenomena. Specifically, he noted that, in the context of an unfamiliar setting, "some children consistently become quiet, vigilant, and restrained while they assess the situation and their resources before acting, [whereas] others act with spontaneity, as though the distinctions between familiar and novel situations were of minimal psychological consequence" (Kagan, 1989, p. 10). Kagan and colleagues described the more withdrawn children as "behaviorally inhibited" and, complementarily, the more sociable youth were considered "uninhibited" (Kagan, Reznick, & Snidman, 1988). This definition of behavioral inhibition is similar to Gray's (1982) and also shares commonalities with Rothbart's conception of reactivity (Rothbart & Derryberry, 1981); indeed, Rothbart's reactivity refers to physiological and behavioral responses to sensory stimuli and, in the context of behavioral inhibition, includes the disposition to express particular discrete emotions to novel or unfamiliar situations. Additionally, Kagan's use of "types" (i.e., inhibited, uninhibited) resembles the categorical approach employed by Thomas and Chess (1977) described above.

Kagan was heavily influenced by his contemporaries studying behavioral neuroscience, particularly the research of LeDoux and Davis (e.g., Davis, 1986; LeDoux, Iwata, Cicchetti, & Reis, 1988); he sought to connect his behavioral observations to the underlying biology of behavioral inhibition. Specifically, LeDoux and Davis (in independent labs) described the amygdala as the brain structure responsible for fear conditioning and the potentiation of fear behaviors (Davis, 1992; LeDoux et al., 1988), which was, at the time, quite cutting edge. Kagan viewed his work as overlapping with that of these neuroscientists and suggested that individual differences in behavioral inhibition were the result of an overactive amygdala. Indeed, Kagan and colleagues had collected psychophysiological data, including increased salivary cortisol levels and muscle tension, greater pupil dilation, and elevated urinary catecholamine levels (Davis, 1986), to support the notion that behaviorally inhibited children exhibit an enhanced fear response to novelty and unfamiliarity. This attempt to bridge the behavior–neuroscience gap came at a time when the work of Davis and LeDoux was receiving widespread attention, and it facilitated a broader discussion of the ways in which the interplay of biology and behavior could be understood in the context of child development (Fox, Henderson, Marshall, Nichols, & Ghera, 2005).

Compared to the work of Eysenck and Gray, Kagan's work on behavioral inhibition was inherently developmental in approach and theory. Kagan found that, although children develop a greater repertoire of behaviors in response to novel social situations, there was significant preservation of individual differences in inhibition across time. In other words, behaviorally inhibited children displayed marked continuity in their distinctive pattern of responding to unfamiliar social and nonsocial stimuli as they moved through childhood. Moreover, whereas Eysenck and Gray were more concerned with understanding the neurobiological underpinnings of the experience of emotion/reactivity for its own sake, Kagan's behavioral inhibition was explicitly linked to developmental consequences, specifically the emergence of anxiety, depressive, and related disorders (Biederman et al., 1993; Hirshfeld et al., 1992), a topic we return to later in the chapter (see the section on public health implications).

Achenbach, Clark, and Watson: Using Psychopathology to Understand Temperament

Several prominent researchers have taken a different approach to understanding temperament. Instead of identifying individual differences in emotional responding in adults (Eysenck and Gray) and children (Kagan) and subsequently relating these differences to the emergence of psychopathology, other groups have started with mental disorders in an attempt to better understand the temperamental characteristics that define them. For example, in his groundbreaking factor analytic work, Thomas Achenbach (1966) found that anxiety, depressive, obsessive, phobic, and somatic complaints were associated with a higher order factor that closely aligned with Eysenck's conception of neuroticism. He used the term *internalizing* to define this factor, describing it as the propensity to focus distress inward. Like the term *neuroticism, internalizing* has its roots in psychoanalytic traditions, though Achenbach notes that this "label is not intended to carry dynamic implications . . . it means only that [internalizing] symptoms describe problems with the self" (p. 10). In addition, in Achenbach's factor analysis, aggressive and delinquent behavior loaded onto an *externalizing* factor (denoting problems with the environment that most closely align with Eysenck's psychoticism dimension).

Achenbach's internalizing–externalizing factors have remained in favor with researchers interested in empirically derived, higher order representations of adult psychopathology (see Kotov et al., 2017). Krueger (1999) was the first to apply factor analytic approaches to adult epidemiological data and replicate the two-factor latent structure of mental disorders consistent with Achenbach's original formulation. Since then, many high-quality studies, using large-scale epidemiological data and interview-based measures of psychiatric diagnoses, have found this internalizing–externalizing solution across samples of adolescent and adult participants from multiple countries and cultures (see reviews by Carragher, Krueger, Eaton, & Slade, 2015; Krueger & Eaton, 2015). Though the primary concern of this empirical approach has been to classify psychopathology, internalizing is all but isomorphic with neuroticism (Griffith et al., 2010), and elevated neuroticism has been shown to be a core and central feature of internalizing psychopathology (Beauchaine & McNulty, 2013).

Additionally, in one of the best-known modern conceptualizations of temperament, Clark and Watson (1991) also describe neuroticism (they refer to this construct as *negative affectivity*) and indicate that their thinking was heavily influenced by Eysenck and Gray (Clark & Watson, 2008), as well as their mentor Auke Tellegen, who described a three-factor model of personality (negative emotionality, positive emotionality, and constraint; Tellegen, 1985). Similar to Achenbach (1966), they propose a model of psychopathology (not personality) to explain the features of anxiety and depression, though Clark and Watson (1991) explicitly describe the factors in their tripartite theory as temperamental vulnerabilities. In this conception, negative affectivity refers to the pervasive predisposition to experience negative emotions and subsumes a broad range of negative mood states, including fear, anxiety, hostility, scorn, and disgust (Watson & Clark, 1984). In contrast, positive affectivity is a dimension reflecting one's level of pleasurable engagement with the environment and corresponds to Eysenck's extroversion. High positive affectivity reflects the specific states of enthusiasm, energy level, mental alertness, interest, joy, and determination, whereas low levels of this temperament are best defined by descriptors reflecting lethargy and fatigue. Despite the appearance of being opposite poles on a single dimension, negative affectivity and positive affectivity are independent. Interestingly, states of sadness and loneliness also have relatively strong loadings on both the high end of negative affectivity and the low end of positive affectivity (Watson & Tellegen, 1985).

Summary

Taken together, these lines of temperament research have focused on relating an individual's emotional nature to its biological underpinnings, and early theorists, such as Eysenck and Gray, paved the way for contemporary researchers. In particular, our own views of neuroticism have been heavily influenced by the tradition of understanding temperament. In order to explain the origins of anxiety disorders specifically, Barlow (1988), working around the same time as Kagan, Clark, and Watson, proposed biological and environmental contributions to *trait anxiety*—the propensity to experience anxious states (in contrast to discrete anxiety experiences). In our evolving view, this theory, described in detail in Chapter 2, has broader implications beyond anxiety, extending to the tendency to experience the full range of negative emotions. While recognizing that a variety of terms have been employed (i.e., *behavioral inhibition, negative affectivity, reactivity*), we adopted the term *neuroticism* given (1) its historical significance as the first label for this disposition (Eysenck's) in the modern study of temperament and (2) the semantic connection to psychopathology (i.e., neuroses), along with the fact that (3) *neuroticism* is the term employed in the leading structural theory of personality (i.e., the five-factor model, described in detail below). We use a fairly broad definition of this trait, describing it as the tendency to experience frequent and intense negative emotions, such as anxiety, fear, irritability, anger, or sadness, in response to various sources of stress. As with earlier thinkers, we also include cognitive components to our definition, such as the pervasive perception that the world is a dangerous and threatening place, along with beliefs about one's inability to manage or cope with challenging events. This cognitive component is often manifested in terms of heightened focus on criticism, either self-generated or from others, as confirming a general sense of inadequacy and perceptions of lack of control over salient events, including intense emotional experiences (Barlow, 2002; Clark & Watson, 2008; Eysenck, 1947; Goldberg et al., 1986). Of note, some authors (e.g., Lilienfeld, 2020) have referred to this broad construct reflecting both propensity for negative emotions and the cognitive vulnerabilities that increase their likelihood as *negative emotionality*. Finally, consistent with the temperament tradition, a developmental argument is made such that early experiences (e.g., negative life experiences, parenting messages) interact with biological vulnerabilities to maintain and exacerbate negative emotions (Barlow et al., 2014a).

HISTORICAL CONCEPTIONS OF PERSONALITY

In contrast to etiological models proposed in the temperament literature, characterizing an individual's *personality* became another approach to understanding individual differences. Allport (1937) defined personality as "the dynamic organization within the individual of those psychophysical systems that determine his unique adjustment to his environment" (p. 48). He further described a personality *trait* as "a neuropsychic structure having the capacity to render many stimuli functionally equivalent and to initiate and guide equivalent (meaningfully consistent) forms of adaptive and expressive behavior" (Allport, 1961, p. 347).

An operational definition of personality for psychologists interested in classifying individual differences was considered necessary to distinguish emerging empirical pursuits from lay conceptions (referred to as *character* or *personality* interchangeably) and case study approaches popular in psychiatry and psychoanalysis (Barenbaum & Winter, 2008). Specifically, the rapid societal changes in the early 20th century (e.g., industrialization, urbanization, immigration) led to concerns of depersonalization and prompted Americans to emphasize the cultivation of a distinct personality (see Susman, 1979). Magazine articles and biographies describing unique personal stories were dubbed "the literature of personality" (Johnston, 1927, p. 34). In addition to popular press stories aimed at lay Americans, personality also became the province of psychiatry; this discipline primarily employed case studies of patients to inform theories on personality development. These early understandings of personality converged when Freud graced the cover of *Time* magazine in 1924 (Fancher, 2000).

Freudian Perspectives on Personality Development

With regard to the case-study approach to psychopathology and personality in the medical specialty of psychiatry, psychodynamic perspectives, based largely on the unconscious, predominated. *Psychodynamic* is an umbrella term used to refer to Freud's psychoanalysis, along with subsequent adaptations that may not incorporate all of his more controversial theories. Psychodynamic approaches to personality emphasize the importance of unconscious cognitive, affective, and motivational processes and may also include some of the following components: compromises among competing psychological tendencies that may be negotiated unconsciously; defense and self-deception; the influence of the past, directly or combined with genetic predispositions; and the enduring effects of interpersonal patterns laid down in childhood (Fancher, 2000).

Based on his data, consisting of a collection of free associations and patterns of transference observed from his patients, Freud articulated several theoretical models of the mind to account for personality features and clinical phenomena. First, he forwarded his *topographic model,* in which he organized mental processes into conscious (presently on one's mind), preconscious (of which one is not currently aware but can readily pull into awareness), and unconscious (actively kept out of awareness due to their content) thoughts (Freud, 1900/1953a). Freud assumed these mental processes required energy and that, when certain thoughts are held in the unconscious, this energy is displaced and is likely to be expressed in another form that may not be under one's control (e.g., as symptom, dream, joke, slip of the tongue, or behavior). The contents of one's unconscious may be determined by conflicts among the components of Freud's (1933/1964) *structural model*: id, ego, and superego. The id is considered the basis of sexual and aggressive energy and is largely held in the unconscious, emerging as illogical, associative, or wishful thinking. The superego is one's conscience and is established via identification with parental figures or social groups at large. The ego is tasked with balancing reality with the demands of desire (id) and morality (superego).

Conflicts between the search for pleasure and internalized views of virtue may be rooted in problems moving through the developmental stages articulated in Freud's "Three Essays on the Theory of Sexuality" (Freud, 1905/1953b): oral, anal, phallic, latency, and genital. In the oral stage, associated with dependency, children explore the world with their mouths and experience gratification and social connection by doing so. The anal stage typically takes place during toddlerhood and is a period of differentiation from caregivers characterized by experimentation with compliance and defiance; the child associates the anus with pleasurable excitation and, according to Freud, the chief area of conflict with parents occurs during toilet training. During the phallic stage, children discover their genitals and masturbation, and this period is associated with identification with the same-sex parent, Oedipal conflicts, and an expanding social network. In the latency stage, sexual impulses undergo repression, and the child continues to identify with significant others, learning culturally acceptable limitations on sex and aggression. Finally, in the genital stage, genital sex becomes the primary end of sexual activity, and the individual is capable of maintaining mature relationships with others. Freud is clear that his *development model* relates not only to sexual development but also to the emergence of one's personality. Indeed, a central theme across all of Freud's models is the notion that one's mind is always in conflict and that the specific nature of these discrepancies, shaped by early experiences, determines one's thoughts, feelings, and behaviors (or personality).

Not unlike temperament researchers (i.e., Achenbach, Clark, and

Watson) who drew their understanding of individual differences from study-ing psychopathology, Freud also explicitly connected personality and mental disorders. Freud used the term *neurosis* to refer to instances in which "the ego has lost the capacity to allocate the [id] in some way" (Freud, 1920/1968, p. 315). This designation was originally coined by Scottish physician William Cullen to describe physical symptoms without an obvious medical cause (see Bailey, 1927); indeed, Freud viewed these symptoms as resulting from the failure of the ego to contain the increased insistence of the id, noting that, in many cases, the symptoms experienced are as bad as or worse than the conflict they were designed to replace. Though the symptom is a substitute for the instinctual impulse, it is thought to be so reduced, displaced, and distorted that it looks more like a compulsion or even an illness than a gratifi-cation of the id's desire. Of course, Freud's neuroses are more closely linked with psychopathology than with the personality trait neuroticism; indeed, neurosis was an early category in the *Diagnostic and Statistical Manual of Mental Disorders* (DSM-I; American Psychiatric Association, 1952) that referred to chronic, interfering distress that occurred in the absence of delu-sions or hallucinations (see Chapter 5 for more information on neurosis, neuroticism, and nosology). It is, however, worth noting that Eysenck drew inspiration from this Freudian label when he coined the term *neuroticism*, noting that individuals with neuroses would likely exhibit high levels of the biologically based tendency to experience negative emotions.

Additional Psychodynamic Perspectives on Personality Development

Within the psychodynamic tradition, Freud's accounts of the nature of one's thoughts, feelings, and behaviors have gradually fallen out of favor. Theorists began to question whether observed individual differences could accurately be reduced to sexual and aggressive impulses and whether other motives (e.g., relatedness to others, success, self-esteem) may paint a more complete picture of the human condition. For example, object relations theory is a well-known and influential modernization of classical analytic perspectives and posits that the primary human need, beginning in infancy, is related-ness to others; in this view, early childhood experiences are important for how individuals view themselves (self-representations) and others (object representations) and shape enduring patterns of interpersonal functioning, along with the cognitive and emotional processes that mediate them (see Greenberg & Mitchell, 1983; Scharf & Scharf, 1998). Contemporary rela-tional theories (see Mitchell & Aron, 1999) continue to emphasize the impor-tance of the internalization of interpersonal interactions, arguing that the building blocks of personality are the ideas and images the child forms of the self and significant others. These accounts of personality are supported by Bowlby's (1969, 1973, 1982) work on attachment, which has amassed considerable empirical evidence to suggest that early relational disruptions can have lasting effects.

Perhaps the most well-known figure in the object relations tradition is Kernberg (1975, 1984), who articulated a model of personality organization stipulating that normal personality is on a continuum with pathology—no doubt influenced by his work with patients. For example, Kernberg suggests that people with normal personality organization, as well as those on the neurotic spectrum, are able to form stable representations of themselves and can experience successful relationships. In contrast, those with borderline personality organization exhibit difficulty maintaining consistent views of themselves and others, leading to severe disruptions in interpersonal functioning. These levels of personality organization are thought to result from progression, or lack thereof, through Kernberg's developmental stages, in which children learn to differentiate themselves from their caregivers (infancy; disruption linked to psychotic functioning), to evaluate objects and events as good or bad based on affective valence (toddlerhood; disruption linked to borderline functioning), and to develop a mature understanding of situations and relationships that allows for ambivalent feelings (early childhood; linked to the capacity for healthy functioning). Here, the emphasis on understanding one's personality remains firmly associated with early interpersonal events and their effect on subsequent functioning.

Other perspectives, rather than specifying a primary drive (e.g., Freud's sexual urges, attachment), have implicated affect as the foremost motivational mechanism in humans, through which these other, more specific drives manifest (Pervin, 1982; Sandler & Sandler, 1978; Watson & Clark, 1984; Westen, Weinberger, & Bradley, 2007). Indeed, humans, like most animals, are driven toward pleasure and away from pain; in other words, people seek to approach actions and objects that elicit positive feelings and are drawn to avoid those associated with negative feelings. Of course, in keeping with the psychodynamic tradition, these motives need not be conscious, and behavior is thought to be influenced by multiple (sometimes contradictory) emotional inputs. This view draws a strong parallel to the seemingly unrelated biologically based accounts of activation and inhibition that are closely linked to neuroticism and extraversion (see Gray, 1982; Gray & McNaughton, 1996, discussed earlier in this chapter), as well as with the empirical evidence suggesting that positive and negative affectivity are independent dimensions (Clark & Watson, 1991; Clark, 2005). These unconscious, emotion-mediated motivations endure, over time resembling the characteristic thoughts, feelings, and behaviors that represent an individual's personality.

MODERN CONCEPTIONS OF PERSONALITY

In the 1920s and 1930s, psychologists sought to distance themselves from both popular literature on personality and its study in other disciplines (Barenbaum & Winter, 2008). Case-study approaches, employed by psychodynamically oriented psychiatrists, were considered "old-fashioned and unscientific" (Hale, 1971, p. 115), and they were eschewed in favor of psychometric and statistical studies of groups using paper-and-pencil tests (e.g., Young, 1928). In contrast with the temperament literature, which viewed individual differences as a biologically based phenomenon, much of the research on understanding personality has historically been concerned with using personality instruments to create a comprehensive descriptive taxonomy. Here, the goal was to reduce various ways of thinking, feeling, and behaving to a manageable number of dimensions, with little attention paid to etiological origins of these dimensions within what became known as the *structural* tradition.

As a starting point for developing personality inventories, several influential psychologists have identified linguistic tendencies (i.e., the words people use to describe themselves and others) as a promising source of attributes for cataloguing individual differences (Digman, 1997). Indeed, the *lexical hypothesis* states that the most socially relevant and salient personality characteristics are encoded in natural language (John, Naumann, & Soto, 2008).

Personality research has focused on creating a comprehensive taxonomy.

Following Baumgarten's (1933) study in the German language, Allport and Odbert (1936) conducted a seminal lexical investigation of personality terms in an unabridged English dictionary. They selected all the terms that could be used to "distinguish the behavior of one human from that of another" (Allport & Odbert, 1936, p. 24). This process resulted in more than 18,000 words, described by the authors as a "lexical nightmare" that would keep psychologists "at work for a lifetime" (p. 25, vi). They attempted to classify these words into four major categories: (1) personality traits (e.g., *sociable, aggressive, fearful*), (2) temporary states, moods, and activities (e.g., *afraid, rejoicing, elated*), (3) evaluative judgments (e.g., *excellent, worthy, average*), and (4) physical characteristics, capacities, and talents. These linguistic groupings are clearly overlapping to some degree, particularly as distinctions among them were not empirically identified (Chaplin, John, & Goldberg, 1988).

Cattell (1943) expanded on Allport and Odbert's (1936) work by attempting to further refine the 4,500 terms that fell within the personality-trait category. Using both semantic and empirical clustering procedures, Cattell reduced these trait words to 35 variables, eliminating more than 99% of the original terms; this work was necessitated by the fact that early factor analysis was prohibitively costly and complex with a large number of variables. Next, using this smaller set of 35 variables, Cattell conducted several oblique factor analyses (i.e., allowing for correlated factors) and concluded that he had identified 12 factors. Unfortunately, researchers interested in replicating Cattell's work were not able to confirm his proposed factors and have concluded that clerical errors may have influenced his findings (see Digman & Takemoto-Chock, 1981)—understandable given the complexity of this work at that time.

Despite these difficulties in interpretation, Cattell's pioneering work prompted others to explore the dimensional structure of trait ratings. First, Fiske (1949) factor analyzed self-, peer-, and therapist ratings on 22 of Cattell's variables and found a five-factor structure. To clarify these factors, Tupes and Christal (1961) reanalyzed correlation matrices of eight samples and found "five relatively strong factors and nothing more of any consequence" (p. 14). This five-factor structure has been replicated in Cattel's original 35-variable dataset by several other groups (e.g., Borgatta, 1964; Digman & Takemoto-Chock, 1981; Norman, 1963). These factors were initially labeled (I) Extraversion or Surgency (talkative, assertive, energetic); (II) Agreeableness (good-natured, cooperative, and trustful); (III) Conscientiousness (orderly, responsible, dependable); (IV) Emotional Stability (calm, not neurotic, not easily upset; on a continuum with neuroticism); and (V) Culture (intellectual, polished, independent minded).

These same factors have been reproduced many times in English-language studies across different types of samples, raters, and methodological strategies (e.g., Botwin & Buss, 1989; Conley, 1985; Digman & Inouye, 1986; Goldberg, 1981, 1990; John, 1990; McCrae & Costa, 1985; de Raad, Mulder, Kloosterman, & Hofstee, 1988). Further generalization (or lack thereof) across languages provides additional important information regarding the nature of personality. Specifically, replication across cultures suggests that there is a universal taxonomy for individual differences and that it is consistent with the evolutionary-based perspective that the characteristics most important for survival are innate (Buss, 1996; Hogan, 1982). In contrast, if cross-cultural research reveals dimensions that are unique to particular context, there may be evidence that personality is, to some degree, socially constructed (Mischel & Peake, 1982). With regard to Germanic languages, the same five factors have emerged in studies conducted in Dutch (e.g., de Raad, Perugini, Hrebickova, & Szarota, 1998b) and German (Ostendorf, 1990). Evaluating evidence for these five factors in non-Western languages is a bit more complex; however, dimensions similar to these have been found in Chinese (Yang & Bond, 1990), Czech (Hrebickova & Ostendorf, 1995), Greek (Saucier, Georgiades, Tsouasis, & Goldberg, 2005), Hebrew (Almagor, Tellegen, & Waller, 1995), Hungarian (Szirmak & de Raad, 1994), Italian (de Raad, di Blas, & Perugini, 1998a), Polish (Szarota, 1995), Russian (Shmelyov

& Pokhil'ko, 1993), Spanish (Benet-Martinez & Waller, 1997), Filipino Taga-
log (Church & Katigbak, 1989) and Turkish (Somer & Goldberg, 1999). These
consistently replicated factors became known as the *Big Five*, a term coined
by Goldberg (1981) to reflect their broad nature.

RECONCILING DIVISIONS BETWEEN TEMPERAMENT AND PERSONALITY

The Big Five structure initially drew ire from senior researchers, including
Eysenck (1992, 1997), who felt that there was a lack of precision with regard
to which five traits were included in this structure. It is true that various
research groups have assumed different labels for these dimensions (despite
similar factor content). Of course, this same criticism can be lobbied against
temperament researchers who have also used diverse labels to refer to essentially the same traits (i.e., neuroticism, behavioral inhibition, internalizing;
see the section "Modern Conceptions of Temperament" in this chapter).

Despite initial divisions, much of the disagreement between temperament and structural personality researchers has been resolved through the
gradual understanding that descriptive traits essentially represent psychobiological dimensions of temperament (Clark & Watson, 2008). With regard
to concerns that these traditions characterize individual differences using
divergent numbers of traits, research has emerged to suggest that temperament or personality traits can be arranged hierarchically; thus emphasizing
different broad domains does not represent a fundamental incompatibility in
approach. For example, at its higher order level, personality can be understood by two superfactors (alpha and beta; Digman, 1997). One step down
in the hierarchy, alpha can be broken down into neuroticism/negative emotionality and disinhibition (beta represents positive emotionality), reflecting Eysenck's Big Three model (Eysenck & Eysenck, 1975). The Big Five
emerges when beta is disaggregated into separate extraversion and openness
domains and disinhibition is further split into disagreeable disinhibition (i.e.,
inability to regulate undesirable interpersonal behaviors; on a continuum
with Big Five agreeableness) and unconscientious disinhibition (i.e., inability
to regulate orderly, planning behaviors; on a continuum with conscientiousness). These broad traits can also be subdivided into more specific facets
(e.g., neuroticism/negative emotionality becomes anxiety, hostility, depression; Costa & McCrae, 1992). In sum, competing perspectives on the nature
of personality/temperament (e.g., Big Two, Big Three, Big Five) can all be
organized within a common hierarchical structure, and all levels of abstrac-
tion (i.e., facet-level analysis) are necessary to characterize an individual's
disposition in a comprehensive way (Clark & Watson, 2008). Indeed, when
scales that were developed by temperament researchers (i.e., Buss & Plomin,

1975; Strelau, Angleitner, Bantelmann, & Ruch, 1990) were factor analyzed, the domains revealed were essentially isomorphic with the Big Five (Angleitner & Ostendorf, 1994; McCrae & Costa, 2003; Strelau & Zawadzki, 1995). Additionally, there has a been an influx of research in recent years linking phenotypic Big Five traits to their genetic underpinnings (e.g., Bouchard & Loehlin, 2001; Loehlin, McCrae, & Costa, 1998). Historically, there was relatively less pushback on the assumption that the Big Five neuroticism and extraversion were related to similar temperament domains given their clear relevance for emotions and early work suggesting that they are indeed heritable (Eaves, Eysenck, & Martin, 1989). Additionally, the fact that all five traits are reproduced across cultures and languages (as described above) indicated that these dimensions must have heritable underpinnings (McCrae, Costa, & Martin, 2005). Additionally, the same factors have also been found in well-validated observer ratings of chimpanzees (King & Figueredo, 1997), suggesting that human and primate personality factors may have common evolutionary precursors. Finally, by the end of the 20th century, there was solid evidence from twin and adoption studies that each Big Five trait was heritable (e.g., Jang, McCrae, Angleitner, Riemann, & Livesley, 1998), with early estimates suggesting that more than two-thirds of the variance in each factor is accounted for by genetic influences (Bouchard & Loehlin, 2001; Riemann, Angleitner, & Strelau, 1997). Thus it was beginning to be difficult to empirically distinguish adult temperament from personality.

Additionally, as technology has gotten more sophisticated, there has been an explosion of research linking Big Five personality traits to individual differences in brain structures and functions using electroencephalograms (EEG), positron emission tomography (PET), and functional magnetic resonance imaging (fMRI). Additionally, developments in molecular biology and genetics have made it possible to identify common variations in genes that are related to personality traits. Moreover, these genetic variations are being mapped onto brain circuits by combining molecular genetics with noninvasive brain imaging (see Drabant et al., 2006). Although it is beyond the scope of this book to review the body of work relating all five traits to their genetic and neural underpinnings (for thorough treatment of this topic, see Anokhin, 2016; Canli, 2008), we do describe these relationships for neuroticism in Chapter 2. Suffice it to say, however, that the convergence of temperament and personality research has

Traits have a biological basis and are important mediators of behavior.

resulted in the consensus that traits indeed have a biological basis and can be considered important mediators of behavior, rather than simply descriptive summaries. Most relevant for the present context, neuroticism-like constructs feature prominently in both lexically derived personality research and biologically based studies of temperament, underscoring the relevance of this trait for how we understand human nature.

WHY STUDY TEMPERAMENT/PERSONALITY? THE PUBLIC HEALTH IMPLICATIONS OF NEUROTICISM

It is clear that understanding the differences that characterize individuals has been of universal interest for millennia, observed in writings from medical practice in ancient Mesopotamia to magazine articles for laypeople in the 1900s and beyond. Modern theoretical and empirical study of these individual differences (i.e., personality/temperament) has largely been conducted by psychologists. As described previously, temperament researchers have focused on elucidating the biological underpinnings that lead to the propensity to experience negative and positive emotions, whereas personality researchers have prioritized understanding the empirical structure of how people describe themselves and others (arriving at five broad dimensions on which individuals can vary). Once the structure and putative biological underpinnings of these traits (e.g., neuroticism, extraversion) were established, researchers naturally turned their attention to the real-world implications of their work, including repercussions for health.

Neuroticism—the tendency to experience negative emotions along with the perception that the world is a threatening place that cannot be managed—features prominently in both temperament and personality-based conceptions of individual differences. Regardless of the tradition in which it is studied, this trait has a strong impact on public health (see Cuijpers et al., 2010; Lahey, 2009). Indeed, neuroticism, more than other individual-difference variables, is associated with and predicts a wide range of mental and physical disorders, comorbidity among them, and the frequency of health service use. Given that developing a full understanding of the nature and origins of neuroticism has strong implications for quality of life, it is no surprise that this trait has been the focus of intense empirical investigation, summarized below.

Neuroticism is associated with a wide range of mental and physical disorders.

Neuroticism and Psychopathology

Neuroticism is strongly associated with a range of common mental health conditions (Clark, Watson, & Mineka, 1994; Khan, Jacobson, Gardner, Prescott, & Kendler, 2005; Krueger & Markon, 2011; Sher & Trull, 1994; Watson & Clark, 1994b). Indeed, in a meta-analysis using 33 population-based samples, Malouff, Thorsteinsson, Rooke, and Schutte (2007) found large associations between neuroticism and traditional "Axis I" disorders, including mood, anxiety, and somatoform disorders, schizophrenia, and eating disorders. Studies conducted after this meta-analysis continue to support the strong link between neuroticism and a range of common psychiatric diagnoses (e.g., Brown & Barlow, 2009; Chien, Ko, & Wu, 2007; Khan et al., 2005; Merino, Senra, & Ferreiro, 2016; Weinstock & Whisman, 2006; Zinbarg et al., 2016). Additionally, neuroticism is also robustly related to drug and alcohol abuse (e.g., Kornør & Nordvik, 2007; Malouff, Thorsteinsson, & Schutte, 2006, 2007; Rogers et al., 2019; Sher & Trull, 1994)

The neurotic temperament has also been consistently linked to personality disorders—a fact that is, perhaps, unsurprising given the name of this class of conditions (Clarkin, Hull, Cantor, & Sanderson, 1993; Costa & Widiger, 2002; Henry et al., 2001; Koenigsberg et al., 2001; Krueger & Markon, 2011; Larstone, Jang, Livesley, Vernon, & Wolf, 2002; Putnam & Silk, 2005; Samuel & Widiger, 2008; Saulsman & Page, 2004; Trull & Sher, 1994; Watson & Clark, 1994b). For example, in a meta-analytic investigation, Saulsman and Page (2004) found moderate associations between this trait and borderline, avoidant, and dependent personality disorders and smaller relationships between schizotypal, paranoid, and antisocial personality disorders. The magnitude of these effects suggests that the propensity to experience negative emotions may have more relevance for some personality disorders but may have less of an impact on others that are characterized by dysfunction in other domains (low extraversion, low agreeableness, low conscientiousness).

Neuroticism also significantly contributes to the co-occurrence of mental disorders; in fact, the highest levels of this trait are observed when these conditions are co-occurring (Putnam & Silk, 2005). In our own work studying the latent structure of emotional disorders (e.g., Brown, Chorpita, & Barlow, 1998; Zinbarg & Barlow, 1996), we have also found significant relationships between high-order temperamental factors (neuroticism and extraversion) and DSM disorders. For example, Brown and colleagues (1998) demonstrated significant paths from a latent neuroticism factor to factors representing each of five DSM disorders included in the study (social anxiety disorder, panic disorder, generalized anxiety disorder, obsessive–compulsive disorder, and depression). In this model, extraversion uniquely predicted only depression and social anxiety disorder (see also Brown & McNiff, 2009). In a recent update to this work, Rosellini et al. (2010) found that agoraphobia (but not panic disorder) was associated with high neuroticism and low extraversion, providing support for the change in DSM-5 separating agoraphobia from panic disorder as a distinct diagnosis (American Psychiatric Association, 2013).

These findings on latent structure have been extended by our research team (Brown, 2007; Brown & Barlow, 2009) and others (e.g., Griffith et al.,

2010; Kessler et al., 2011). Specifically, in one study, neuroticism accounted for 20–45% of the comorbidity among internalizing disorders (i.e., major depression, generalized anxiety disorder, panic disorder, and phobias), and 19–88% of the comorbidity between internalizing and externalizing disorders (i.e., substance dependence, antisocial personality disorders, conduct disorders; Kessler et al., 2011). Similarly, Griffith et al. (2010), studying a large sample of ethnically diverse adolescents, found that a single internalizing factor was represented in lifetime diagnoses of mood and anxiety disorders, suggesting that neuroticism may be the core of "internalizing" disorders. Relatedly, Krueger (1999) found, using factor analysis, that the variance in seven anxiety and mood disorders can be accounted for by the higher order dimension of internalizing/neuroticism. In sum, virtually all the considerable covariance among latent variables corresponding to the DSM constructs of depression, social anxiety disorder, generalized anxiety disorder (GAD), obsessive–compulsive disorder (OCD), and panic disorder have been explained by the higher order dimension of neuroticism (and, to a lesser degree, extraversion).

Individuals with comorbid mental disorders are at an increased risk for experiencing more severe and impairing symptoms and are more likely to seek costly mental health services (Kessler, Chiu, Demler, & Walters, 2005). Neuroticism is associated with greater use of both specific mental health services and primary care services for mental health problems, and this remains true even after controlling for the number of comorbid mental disorders (Jylhä & Isometsä, 2006; ten Have, Oldehinkel, Vollebergh, & Ormel, 2005). Additionally, among those with common mental health diagnoses, higher levels of neuroticism predict a more chronic course of illness and a worse prognosis (Clark et al., 1994). Finally, the tendency to experience negative emotions predicts the subsequent recurrence of depressive episodes (Kendler et al., 1993; Kendler et al., 2006) and suicide risk (Fergusson, Woodward, & Horwood, 2000) following a first depressive episode.

Physical Health

The public health implications of neuroticism extend beyond its robust associations with mental disorders to also confer risk for physical disorders. Costa and McCrae (1987) report that individuals high in neuroticism are more likely to express unfounded medical complaints, as well as to seek services following substantial worry (Goubert, Crombez, & Van Damme, 2004). These medical claims do not result in diagnoses, but they still result in patient suffering and costly health service use, underscoring the public health burden of this trait. However, in addition to unnecessary treatment seeking, substantial evidence also supports the association between neuroticism and objective measures of health (Brickman et al., 1996; Lahey, 2009; Shipley et al., 2007; Smith & MacKenzie, 2006; Suls & Bunde, 2005). One approach to connecting neuroticism to physical health problems has been to conclude that a higher prevalence of medical conditions in individuals with mental disorders (which are themselves strongly linked with neuroticism) is evidence for this link (Currie & Wang, 2005; Robles, Glaser, & Kiecolt-Glaser, 2005; Sareen, Cox, Clara, & Asmundson, 2005; Watkins et al., 2006). For example, depression and anxiety disorders are associated with disrupted immune functioning (Maier & Watkins, 1998; Pace et al., 2006; Robles et al., 2005), abnormalities in cardiac functioning (Barger & Sydeman, 2005), and increased mortality among individuals with other risk factors for cardiac disease (Penninx et al., 2001; Robles et al., 2005). Of course, this literature only provides indirect evidence of the association between neuroticism and physical health problems.

But direct evidence relating these variables is increasingly available. For example, neuroticism itself is associated with a range of physical impairments, including cardiovascular disease (Suls & Bunde, 2005), atopic eczema (Buske-Kirschbaum, Geiben, & Hellhammer, 2001), asthma (Huovinen, Kaprio, & Koskenvuo, 2001), and irritable bowel syndrome (Spiller, 2007). Relationships between neuroticism and these conditions are significant, even when controlling for depression and other risk factors such as social support (Bouhuys, Flentge, Oldehinkel, & van den Berg, 2004; Russo et al., 1997). The fact that neuroticism has been associated with both mental and physical disorders has been described as particularly important for public health (Lahey, 2009), as comorbidity among medical conditions and mental disorders has been linked to more complicated health problems, greater need for health services, and significantly poorer outcomes (Baune, Adrian, & Jacobi, 2007; McCaffery et al., 2006).

As with mental disorders, higher levels of neuroticism are associated with poorer outcomes for medical conditions. Indeed, each increase of 1 standard deviation in neuroticism was associated with 10% greater mortality from cardiovascular disease, even when controlling for age, sex, socioeconomic status, smoking or alcohol consumption, physical activity, and initial health (Shipley et al., 2007). Similar results were also found in longitudinal studies that included large samples of older adults (Wilson, de Leon, Bennett, Bienias, & Evans, 2004; Wilson et al., 2005). Additionally, neuroticism strongly predicts deterioration among patients with type 1 diabetes (Brickman et al., 1996). With regard to cancer, a 25-year longitudinal study revealed that those deemed high in neuroticism had a 130% greater death rate than those who were low in neuroticism (Nakaya et al., 2006). Proposed mechanisms underscoring this risk include the trait's influence on health-related daily habits and medical practices, such as diet changes, exercise, and medication compliance (Suls & Bunde, 2005). Taken together, neuroticism is associated with an increased likelihood of experiencing physical health problems, greater co-occurrence of physical and mental disorders, and a worse prognosis for those suffering.

Economic Costs of Neuroticism

Finally, the economic burden associated with neuroticism is estimated to exceed the cost attributed to common mental and physical disorders. Data drawn from baseline (N = 7,076) and follow-up (N = 5,618) waves of the Netherlands Mental Health Survey and Incidence Study (NEMESIS; Bijl, van Zessen, Ravelli, de Rijk, & Langendoen, 1998) explored relationships between neuroticism and the costs purported to be associated with it. The study defined three categories of costs, including direct medical expenses (i.e., costs incurred by the mental health care sector in the Netherlands), direct nonmedical costs (e.g., out-of-pocket costs such as travel expenses and parking), and indirect nonmedical costs (e.g., the cost of production loss due to absenteeism). They also used these data to estimate per capita costs for individuals grouped in the highest quartile of survey respondents on neuroticism scores. Results suggest that costs associated with neuroticism for the top 25% highest scorers amount to almost $1.4 billion per 1 million inhabitants. In addition to neuroticism and health service use, NEMESIS also tracked diagnostic status for mental and physical health. This allowed Cuijpers et al. (2010) to determine that the economic burden of neuroticism is almost 2.5 times higher than for mood disorders (approximately $600 million per 1 million inhabitants) and, surprisingly, amounts to nearly two-thirds the expense of all somatic (physical) disorders. These results suggest that the effect of neuroticism on mental health care and population health far exceeds the cost of common mental disorders.

CONCLUSIONS

Neuroticism is clearly a public health liability in its own right, given its strong association with a range of mental and medical health conditions. Thus it is no surprise that the propensity to experience negative emotions has been the subject of intense theorizing for millennia. Of course, the trait-like susceptibility for distress has carried many names over the years, from neuroticism to internalizing and behavioral inhibition to negative affectivity. Current evidence now suggests that these constructs are largely synonymous and isomorphic (Brown, Chorpita, & Barlow, 1998; Brown, 2007; Brown & Barlow, 2009). Similarly, recent literature suggests that there is limited empirical basis for differentiating between "neuroticism" derived from personality and from temperament-based traditions, as the lexically generated traits have now been related to the same biological underpinnings denoted in temperament-based approaches. In order to take advantage of the vast literatures related to both areas of research, the terms *temperament* and *personality research* are used interchangeably throughout this book. Additionally, for parsimony, the tendency to experience negative emotions is generally referred to as *neuroticism*, though investigators in the studies cited may have used another label to describe this trait.

2

Triple Vulnerability Theory and the Origins of Neuroticism

As we reviewed in the previous chapter, ancient Greek physicians were speculating on the origins of an individual's emotional nature as early as 460 B.C.E. They, of course, focused on the four "humors," determining that excesses or deficiencies in blood, black bile, yellow bile, and phlegm were likely causes of one's emotional style. For example, they determined that a melancholic or gloomy temperament resulted from high levels of black bile.

Earlier, we defined the neurotic temperament as the tendency to experience frequent and intense negative emotions in response to various sources of stress. It is also widely accepted that beyond exaggerated negative emotionality, neurotic temperament (or neuroticism) is characterized by the pervasive perception that the world is a dangerous and threatening place, along with beliefs about one's inability to manage or cope with challenging events, including intense emotionality itself (Barlow, 2002; Barlow et al., 2014b; Clark & Watson, 2008; Eysenck, 1947; Goldberg, 1993). In some ways, neuroticism can be conceived as stress reactivity—that is, increased arousal of negative valence in response to both external and internal sources of stress and associated with a perception of an inability to manage or control these strong emotional reactions.

Neuroticism is the tendency to experience negative emotions coupled with the perception that the world is a dangerous place.

In this chapter, we integrate genetic, neurobiological, and environmental contributions to this trait to articulate a theory of the development of neuroticism. Because neuroticism and psychopathology, particularly emotional disorders, are strongly related (see Chapter 3), an increased understanding of how neuroticism develops should have implications for both treatment and prevention of common conditions such as anxiety and depressive disorders (Barlow et al., 2014b). This strategy of identifying core, risk-conferring processes, such as temperamental vulnerabilities, is consistent with the National Institute of Mental Health's (NIMH) Research Domain Criteria (RDoC) initiative with its focus on looking beyond diagnoses to identify underlying mechanisms implicated in the development and maintenance of symptoms across a range of disorders (Insel, 2010). This approach is also consistent with other emerging quantitative approaches to classifying psychopathology, such as the hierarchical taxonomy of psychopathology (HiTOP; Kotov et al., 2017), in which overarching higher order factors such as "internalizing" (i.e., neuroticism) subsume most symptoms of the emotional disorders. As such, neuroticism itself becomes a valid target for treatment, and understanding its origins provides a framework for how this might happen.

TRIPLE VULNERABILITY THEORY

We submit that "triple vulnerability theory" (Barlow, 1991, 2002), originally proposed to describe the emergence of anxiety and depressive disorders, actually best depicts the development of neuroticism itself, in turn conveying risk for the onset of emotional disorders. A visual depiction of how our revised conception of the triple vulnerabilities accounts for this development can be seen in Figure 2.1. Specifically, triple vulnerability theory describes three separate but interacting "diatheses" (Barlow, 1988, 2000; Brown & Naragon-Gainey, 2013). These include the following:

1. A general biological (heritable) vulnerability.
2. A general psychological vulnerability consisting of a heightened sense of unpredictability and uncontrollability and associated changes in brain function resulting from early adverse experience.
3. A more specific psychological vulnerability, also largely learned, accounting for why one particular emotional disorder may emerge instead of another.

It now seems clear that the two generalized vulnerabilities identified in triple vulnerability theory, interacting with stress, dynamically contribute to the development and expression of neuroticism itself (Brown & Barlow, 2009; Suárez, Bennett, Goldstein, & Barlow, 2009). Indeed, we hypothesize that these two generalized vulnerabilities function as direct risk factors for the development of this trait, which in turn mediates risk for the development of anxiety, mood, and related emotional disorders, as described in subsequent chapters. The third vulnerability pertaining to the development of specific emotional disorders is explicated in some detail in Chapter 4.

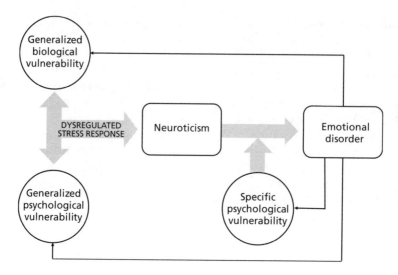

FIGURE 2.1. The development of neuroticism. From Barlow, Ellard, Sauer-Zavala, Bullis, and Carl (2014a). Copyright © 2014 Sage Publications. Reprinted with permission.

GENERALIZED BIOLOGICAL VULNERABILITY

Genetic and neurobiological contributions to personality traits or temperament styles have long been recognized (Barlow, 2000). As noted previously, the triple vulnerability framework was originally explored to account for the development of trait anxiety and emotional disorders, and a genetic link to these conditions has been well established in both family and twin studies (e.g., Hettema, Neale, & Kendler, 2001; Skre, Onstad, Torgersen, Lygren, & Kringlen, 1993). Over the decades, behavioral geneticists have also explored the genetic contributions to neuroticism itself, and there is strong evidence to suggest that this trait is also heritable. Indeed, estimates suggest that genetic contributions constitute between 40 and 60% of the variance in the expression of this temperament (e.g., Bouchard & Loehlin, 2001; Clark et al., 1994; Kendler, Prescott, Myers, & Neale, 2003). These data are derived primarily from self-report personality measures in twins, with results consistently showing that genetics accounts for nearly half of the variance in predicting phenotypic expressions of personality, that shared environmental effects (such as parental socioeconomic status and religious traditions) predict very little, and that nonshared environmental effects (e.g., different teachers, leisure activities, different kinds of life events) account for the remaining variance (Turkheimer, 2000).

Genome-wide association studies across large samples of individuals that aim to identify genetic markers for anxiety disorders and anxiety-related traits, including neuroticism, have begun to point to several candidate genes that seem to be associated with some risk. However, these candidate genes have historically been difficult to replicate and, in some cases, are poorly understood (Howe et al., 2016; Smith et al., 2016; Weber et al., 2016). Recent work, however, has demonstrated that the influence of genetic contributions to neuroticism is stronger for younger individuals, whereas the environment appears to exert more influence with increasing age (Laceulle, Ormel, Aggen, Neale, & Kendler, 2013). In one study, Kendler and Myers (2010) noted that phenotypic continuity in personality was the result of cumulative environmental effects, underscoring the importance of interactions between genetically mediated physiology and the environment (described in detail below; e.g., Craske et al., 2017).

In view of these findings, what may be a more productive research strategy than attempting to identify genetic risk markers in isolation is to search for genetic influences at the neural systems level, looking specifically at activity and interconnectivity of brain regions strongly associated with both emotional disorders and neuroticism (Barlow et al., 2014a; Craske et al., 2017). Genetically mediated neuroticism has been linked to heightened reactivity in emotion-generating structures in the brain, most notably amygdala hyperexcitability, coupled with reduced or inefficient inhibitory control by prefrontal structures (Craske et al., 2017; Keightley et al., 2003; Shackman et al., 2016; Stein, Simmons, Feinstein, & Paulus, 2007; Westlye, Bjørnebekk, Grydeland, Fjell, & Walhovd, 2011).

More specifically, heightened amygdala responses are associated with a functional polymorphism in the promoter region (5-HTTPR) of the serotonin transporter gene; that is, the presence of the s/s genotype (presence of two short alleles) is linked to increased amygdala response to emotional stimuli (Drabant et al., 2012; Lonsdorf et al., 2011; Munafò, Brown, & Hariri, 2008). This genotype is also characterized by reductions in functional connectivity between the amygdala and the ventromedial prefrontal cortex (vmPFC), which seems to function to inhibit excessive amygdala response (Pezawas et al., 2005). The presence of this s/s allele functional polymorphism has independently been found to be associated with neuroticism (Lesch et al., 1996; Montag, Basten, Stelzel, Fiebach, & Reuter, 2010; Stein, Campbell-Sills, & Gelernter, 2009) and has also been linked with the development of psychopathology following life stressors (Caspi et al., 2003; Owens, Stevenson, Hadwin, & Norgate, 2012). These results are still tentative, as large-scale studies have yielded mixed results or have failed to replicate these findings (Terracciano et al., 2009a). Nevertheless, the studies described above suggest that one pathway to the development of neuroticism may consist of a genetically mediated increased tendency to react to aversive or potentially threatening stimuli and a reduced ability to normalize this activation once the threat diminishes. Importantly, the hyperexcitability of neural circuits in response to stress and fear seen in neuroticism results not only from genetic factors or biological predispositions but also from stressful or traumatic experiences during critical stages of development (Barlow et al., 2014a; Gunnar & Quevedo, 2007; Lanius, Frewen, Vermetten, & Yehuda, 2010; Rosen & Schulkin, 1998; Shackman et al., 2016). That is, early adversity contributes to the stress response that forms the basis of the neurotic phenotype. Of course, physiological reactivity to stressors (e.g., heightened arousal) is not in and of itself a marker of neuroticism. Arousal responses in ordinary circumstances represent an adaptive capability that enables the individual to mount the necessary and context-appropriate behavioral response to adversity. Our own view and those of others suggest that it is the combination of heightened physiological reactivity with a psychological perception of the unpredictability or uncontrollability of the stressor that leads to the development of negative emotionality or neuroticism (e.g., Barlow, 2002; Koolhaas et al., 2011; Shackman et al., 2016).

GENERALIZED PSYCHOLOGICAL VULNERABILITY

The second component of triple vulnerability theory is a generalized psychological vulnerability, which can be characterized as a pervasive sense of unpredictability and uncontrollability in relation to life events and a perceived inability to cope with negative outcomes from challenging circumstances (Barlow, 2000, 2002). Much of the research on this topic to date has focused on examining relationships between these constructs and the development of specific emotional disorders. However, recent work highlighting the role of neuroticism as a latent factor underlying these disorders leads us to hypothesize that experiences with unpredictability and uncontrollability are important factors in the development of neuroticism itself.

Basic Animal Research: The Effects of Uncontrollability and Unpredictability

Findings from studies employing laboratory paradigms with animals suggest that severe and chronic negative emotionality can be experimentally induced. For over 70 years, investigators such as Pavlov (1927), Masserman (1943), Liddell (1949), and Gantt (1942) have produced behavior characterized by extreme agitation, restlessness, distractibility, hypersensitivity, increased autonomic responding, muscle tension, and interference with ongoing performance. In fact, these states were commonly termed *experimental neurosis*. Procedures to induce this behavior in animals included the punishment of appetitive responses, long periods of restraint and monotony, the introduction of extremely difficult discriminations that are required to obtain food, and the presentation of insoluble problems, accompanied by the punishment of mistakes. In an important early review, Mineka and Kihlstrom (1978) suggested that, across these studies with different methodologies, the cause of ongoing negative emotions in these animals was that "environmental events of vital importance to the organism [became] unpredictable, uncontrollable, or both" (p. 257).

On the contrary, aversive events of substantial intensity or duration will be better tolerated (with marked individual differences) if they occur predictably and if the organism at least perceives that some control over these events is possible. The *lack of predictability* of these "stressful" events seems to lead to animal manifestations of chronic anxiety and/or depression (Mineka & Kihlstrom, 1978; Seligman, 1975). Indeed, Amat and colleagues (2005) found that certain areas of the rat brain (in this study, the infralimbic and prelimbic regions of the vmPFC) detect whether a stressor is under an organism's control and suggest that the presence of a sense of control may inhibit stress-induced neural activity (for comprehensive reviews, see Gunnar & Fisher, 2006; Levine, 2005).

The effects of a sense of control on behavioral and physiological outcomes have also been examined in appetitive-oriented situations. In infant rhesus monkeys, Roma, Champoux, and Suomi (2006) attempted to replicate earlier experiments (i.e., Insel, Scanlan, Champoux, & Suomi, 1988; Mineka, Gunnar, & Champoux, 1986) illustrating the causal relationship between controllability of appetitive stimuli and adaptive responses to novel situations. The authors gathered physiological data (salivary cortisol) to shed light on the impact of controllable versus uncontrollable stress on hypothalamic–pituitary–adrenocortical (HPA) axis regulation in early development. Results indicated that "master" monkeys (reared in conditions that allowed control over food availability through lever pressing) were significantly more active and exhibited reduced cortisol reactivity in response to novel stimuli relative to their "yoked" counterparts (with noncontingent, or no, control over access to food), even though both groups were provided with equal portions of food. These findings suggest that environmental control in infancy results in increased competence, which in turn buffers stress reactivity. When taken together, these studies demonstrate the negative influence of experiences with uncontrollability in the early environment. In addition, whereas experimental neurosis paradigms suggest the importance of control over aversive stimuli, this evidence suggests that control over appetitive stimuli may be equally important in the development of mastery and competence in response to stressful situations. This finding underscores the centrality of a sense of control, rather than the particular experiences that are associated with it.

This concept is also illustrated in studies of cortisol reactivity among dominant and subordinate baboons (Sapolsky, 1990; Sapolsky, Alberts, & Altmann, 1997; Sapolsky & Ray, 1989). In early studies, investigators examined levels of cortisol in these animals as a function of their social rank and discovered that dominant males have lower resting levels of cortisol than subordinate males. However, when some "emergency" occurs, levels of cortisol rise more quickly in the dominant males than in their subordinate counterparts. Cortisol, of course, is the final step in a cascade of hormone secretion that begins with the limbic system during periods of stress or anxiety. Furthermore, the hippocampus, a brain structure implicated in the formation of emotion-related memories, is very responsive to corticosteroids. When stimulated by these hormones during HPA axis activity, the hippocampus contributes to a down-regulation of the stress response, thereby articulating the close link between the limbic system and various parts of the HPA axis. When produced chronically, cortisol can have damaging effects on a variety of physiological systems, ultimately causing damage to the hippocampus and the immune system. This damage to the hippocampus after a period of chronic stress may then lead to reduced negative feedback sensitivity, to chronic secretion of stress hormones, and ultimately to physical disease and death.

Thus it seems that Sapolsky's subordinate baboons are caught in a perpetual state of scanning for danger, probably as a function of perceived lack of control over their condition, resulting in chronic arousal and reduced reactivity (autonomic restriction) to actual stressors. In later studies, Sapolsky and colleagues (Sapolsky, 1990, 2005; Sapolsky, Romero, & Munck, 2000) found that those baboons whose ranking within the social hierarchy was either uncertain or under challenge actually exhibited the highest levels of chronic cortisol output, indicating that even life at the top of the social hierarchy does not always provide a stress-mitigating sense of control. High cortisol concentrations were not associated with instability of interactions with the population as a whole but were associated with the degree of instability of interactions between males close in rank, probably because this instability had greater potential consequences for social status and was more unpredictable in outcome (Gesquiere et al., 2011; Sapolsky et al., 2000; Sapolsky, 1992).

Studies of the relationship between early experiences and corticotropin-releasing factor (CRF) in macaques also point to important implications about the impact of unpredictability and uncontrollability (Coplan, Paunica, & Rosenblum, 2004). In several early studies, Coplan and colleagues (Coplan et al., 1996; Coplan et al., 1998) evaluated the development of negative emotionality among infant bonnet macaques whose nursing mothers were subjected to three different conditions related to foraging for food. These different conditions led to differential interactions with their infants. Findings revealed that infants with mothers who were exposed to a condition of unpredictability in food availability exhibited heightened anxiety-like behavior during development, as well as substantially increased behavioral inhibition to a variety of novel and anxiety-producing contexts relative to infants of mothers exposed to high or low, but predictable, food availability (Coplan, Rosenblum, & Gorman, 1995). Of more importance, CRF levels in the cerebrospinal fluid of these monkeys were persistently elevated (Coplan et al., 1996), which correlated with increased levels of serotonin and dopamine metabolites (Coplan et al., 1998); these changes persisted into adulthood (Coplan et al., 2004). Much as in the Roma et al. (2006) study described above, Coplan's body of work suggests that elevated levels of stress hormones were not a result of lack of food in and of itself, but rather of the unpredictable nature of the food supply, and that this tendency was passed on to the next generation.

Coplan et al. (1998) concluded that increasing adversity during early childhood results in enhanced CRF activity, which in turn causes alteration in other systems underlying the adult expression of stress and negative emotions. Behaviors associated with the variable-foraging-demand condition included inconsistent, erratic, and dismissive behaviors on the part of the mother—behaviors likely to result in diminished maternal attachment. Furthermore, the results seemed due to the unpredictability of this condition, as adult mothers in a predictable high-foraging-demand condition did not exhibit elevated CRF concentrations. Thus Coplan et al. (1998) suppose, as do others (e.g., Nemcroff, 2004; Gunnar & Fisher, 2006; Ladd et al., 2000; Levine, 2005), that adverse early experience—in combination, of course, with a genetic predisposition—creates a neurobiological diathesis. This diathesis becomes activated in later life by the experience of additional stressful life events or other triggers, completing the diathesis–stress model of the development of neuroticism.

Finally, some recent findings from cross-fostering studies in rhesus monkeys have important implications for the contribution of parenting styles to a generalized psychological vulnerability to develop the neurotic temperament. In these studies, Suomi and colleagues (Suomi, 1999, 2000) experimented with a particularly emotional and stress-reactive group of young monkeys by cross-fostering them to nonreactive mothers. Reactive young animals that were raised by calm mothers for the first 6 months of their lives were able to overcome their biological propensity to respond emotionally. These animals developed normally, demonstrating the kinds of social competence characteristic of nonreactive animals. Furthermore, these changes in their "temperaments" seemed to be enduring, in that they, in turn, raised their own offspring in a nonreactive and calm manner, much to the benefit of their offspring—reflecting a process known as nongenetic inheritance of behavior (Dick, 2011). On the other hand, infants with the same biological vulnerability raised by emotional and stress-reactive mothers retained their emotionality, perhaps because they developed a synergistic psychological vulnerability accompanying their genetic loading. Recent findings indicate that specific early learning experiences actually alter gene expression through epigenetic mechanisms, such as DNA methylation of specific promoter genes, in a way that produces permanent changes (e.g., Cameron et al., 2005; Mill, 2011; Rutter, 2010; Rutter, Moffitt, & Caspi, 2006). These findings, of course, have implications for the prevention of neuroticism, although we are still a long way from understanding how this process might work in humans. A discussion of the effects of parenting styles on the development of anxiety in humans is provided later in the chapter.

Moreover, findings from the animal laboratories have important implications for the relationship between experiences with unpredictability and uncontrollability and the development of anxiety and other negative emotions, such as fear and panic. For example, monkeys evidenced more extreme fear (alarm or panic) when confronted with a potentially life-threatening situation if they had previously experienced unpredictability or uncontrollability over important life events, even positive events (Mineka et al., 1986; Roma et al., 2006).

In summary, the evidence indicates that in animals, at least, early stress—particularly uncontrollable and/or unpredictable life events—leads to increased HPA axis response, negative emotionality, and alarm reactions. Instillation of a sense of mastery or control during development seems to protect against the likelihood of a lifetime of easily triggered negative emotions. The development of coping responses that imply a sense of control (whether real or apparent) buffers negative emotionality as well (Coplan et al., 1996; Suomi, 1986). With this suggestive evidence in mind, it becomes possible to examine findings on the etiology of human negative emotions and, perhaps, neuroticism.

Basic Human Research

Research exploring the constructs of unpredictability and uncontrollability in humans and their potential relationship to the development of emotional disorders and neuroticism more generally has been ongoing in diverse and often unrelated contexts. In this section, we briefly summarize research on locus of control and attributional style, along with research on parenting styles emanating mostly from attachment theory. Also considered is relevant developmental research, as well as more recent findings focused on neuroendocrinology.

Locus of Control and Attributional Style

Evaluation of the role of control in humans has led to the development of constructs such as *locus of control* and *attributional style*. Rotter (1966) suggested that one's "locus of control" could be rated along a dimension of internal to external causality, with external locus of control representing less personal agency or a diminished sense of control. Rotter also developed an instrument to measure perception of control (Rotter, 1966). These ideas sparked the development of other psychometrically sound questionnaires to measure these constructs, including the Nowicki–Strickland Locus of Control Scale (Barlow, Chorpita, & Turovsky, 1995; Nowicki & Strickland, 1973) and the Anxiety Control Questionnaire (Brown, White, Forsyth, & Barlow, 2004; Rapee, Craske, Brown, & Barlow, 1996). Findings using these measures suggest that low perceived control acts as a diathesis or vulnerability to the experience of negative emotional states and is associated with elevated scores on neuroticism scales (Bentley et al., 2013; Gallagher, Bentley, & Barlow, 2014; McCauley, Mitchell, Burke, & Moss, 1988; Nunn, 1988; Siegel & Griffin, 1984; Skinner, Chapman, & Baltes, 1988; Weisz & Stipek, 1982; White, Brown, Somers, & Barlow, 2006; Wiersma et al., 2011). Elaborating further on these findings, a meta-analysis of over 100 independent studies comprising 8,251 individuals found that experiences with uncontrollable stressors led to both higher and less variable levels of daily cortisol output relative to stressors that were more controllable or predictable (Miller, Chen, & Zhou, 2007), mirroring findings with animals reviewed earlier in the chapter.

The importance of a sense of control in the experience of negative emotions is also supported by studies of cognitive styles. Again, findings indicate that a negative attributional style in which one tends to attribute negative events to global, stable, and internal reasons is associated with anxiety (Chorpita, Brown, & Barlow, 1998b; Cole, Peeke, Martin, Truglio, & Seroczynski, 1998) and depression (Nolen-Hoeksema, Girgus, & Seligman, 1992). A 5-year longitudinal study (Alloy et al., 2012) investigated the interrelationships among children's experience of depressive symptoms, negative life events, explanatory style, and helplessness behaviors in social and achievement situations. The results revealed that early in childhood, negative events, but not explanatory style, predicted depressive symptoms; later in childhood, a pessimistic explanatory style emerged as a significant predictor of depressive symptoms, alone and in conjunction with negative events. When children suffered periods of depression, their explanatory styles not only deteriorated but remained pessimistic even after their depression subsided, presumably putting them at risk for future episodes of depression. Some children seem repeatedly prone to depressive symptoms over periods of at least 2 years. Children with depression consistently showed helpless behaviors in social and achievement settings (Alloy et al., 2012; Luten, Ralph, & Mineka, 1997).

Taking a closer look at studies leading to these conclusions reveals a progression of ideas on the nature and function of cognitive vulnerabilities, from specific factors to indicators of a more generalized psychological vulnerability. In 1978, Abramson, Seligman, and Teasdale reformulated

Seligman's theory of learned helplessness, suggesting that the relationship between negative life events and learned helplessness is *moderated* by one's attributional style. That is, the experience of negative events is not sufficient to develop helplessness. Rather, negative life events are most likely to lead to learned helplessness when a person makes internal, global, and stable attributions regarding negative events. Abramson, Metalsky, and Alloy (1989) modified this theory to further emphasize the role of hopelessness, rather than helplessness, as more specific to depression. They suggested that, for many forms of depression, attributions play a causal role only when they contribute to a sense of hopelessness in which individuals believe they will never gain any influence over important events in their world. Helplessness, in their view, is more relevant to anxiety.

Nolen-Hoeksema and colleagues (1992) provided important information regarding the development and subsequent effects of cognitive response styles in childhood and early adolescence. In this 5-year longitudinal study, the authors found that, in early childhood, negative life events rather than control cognitions or explanatory style were the best predictors of depression. They also found that the presence of depression in early childhood led to a deterioration of explanatory style. Specifically, children who experienced depression at a young age developed an increased tendency to make internal, stable, and global attributions for negative life events and to make external, unstable, and specific attributions for positive events. This pessimistic explanatory style was found to predict a recurrence of depression in later childhood, with negative life events predicting the specific time at which relapse occurred. In other words, there is a suggestion that cognitive style comes to *moderate* negative life events and depression in older children. The results of this study suggest that adult models of depression (e.g., Abramson et al., 1978) may apply only to older children. The data indicate that by early adolescence, certain cognitive response styles develop. Indeed, maladaptive cognitive response styles (which may result from childhood depression, early negative life events, or a combination) serve as a psychological vulnerability or diathesis; thus, when faced with negative life events, adolescents with such cognitive styles seem to be at a greater risk of developing depression.

There is also evidence to suggest that anxiety is the first consequence of this negative cognitive style traditionally associated with depression. Results from a prospective longitudinal study of anxiety and depression among children (Sapolsky, Romero, & Munck, 2000; Sapolsky, 1990) clearly supported the temporal hypothesis that anxiety leads to depression in children and adolescents. In fact, this finding had been repeatedly obtained in prior studies, albeit with less satisfactory methodologies (Hershberg, Carlson, Cantwell, & Strober, 1982; Kovacs, Gatsonis, Paulauskas, & Richards, 1989; Orvaschel, Lewinsohn, & Seeley, 1995).

However, Luten and colleagues (1997) reported that a pessimistic attributional style was related more strongly to underlying negative affect or neuroticism than to anxiety or depression specifically. They also suggest that a generalized psychological vulnerability—as represented by a pessimistic attributional style reflecting a sense of uncontrollability—may lead initially to anxiety, followed by depression. Finally Alloy et al. (2012), examining multiple putative cognitive vulnerabilities for depression, found that negative inferential style, rumination, negative self-referent information processing, and hopelessness were all associated with later depressive symptoms and diagnoses, as well as anxiety symptoms and diagnosis, with only hopelessness showing any specificity for depression. These studies again point to the role of these vulnerabilities as reflecting a sense of uncontrollability associated with the development of neuroticism itself.

Parenting Styles and Perceptions of Control

Studies on early environment and the role of parenting styles also shed some light on the possible origins of the sense of control in children. Shear (1991) noted that, from an early age, human infants exert control over their environment through their effects on caregivers. When caregivers or parents are insensitive to the child's expressive, exploratory, and independent behaviors, the child is at risk of developing inhibition and a sense of uncontrollability over their world, which may contribute to the development of negative emotionality more generally (Hane, Henderson, Reeb-Sutherland, & Fox, 2010; Williams et al., 2009).

Accordingly, parenting styles and family characteristics have been linked to the development of a sense of control (Chorpita & Barlow, 1998; McLeod, Wood, & Weisz, 2007; Schneewind, 1995; van der Bruggen, Stams, & Bögels, 2008), as well as to the development of anxiety and depression (Eun, Paksarian, He, & Merikangas, 2018; Rubin, Coplan, & Bowker, 2009), and this finding seems generalizable across cultures (e.g., Ghazwani, Khalil, & Ahmed, 2016). Consistent with attachment theory (Bowlby, 1980; Thompson, 1998), specific parenting dimensions that facilitate or inhibit the development of a sense of control in children have been described as (1) warmth or sensitivity, consistency, and contingency and (2) encouragement of autonomy and absence of intrusion or an overcontrolling style (Barlow, 2002). Both parental dimensions (warmth, consistency, and contingency on the one hand, and encouraging autonomy on the other) appear to provide opportunities for a child to experience control over reinforcing events in early development, through social contingency and mastery of the environment. Over time, such experiences can become part of the child's stored (learned) information and contribute to a generalized sense of control (e.g., Carton & Nowicki, 1994). In a longitudinal study, results revealed that low maternal responsiveness during infancy (suggesting that nurturing responses are not contingent upon infant communication, e.g., crying) was associated with children reporting a less well-developed perceived sense of control over their environment at age 11 (Dan, Sagi-Schwartz, Bar-haim, & Eshel, 2011).

In the context of positive attachment, promotion of independence also enhances the child's sense of self-efficacy and ability to cope with life events (Barlow, 2002; Bowlby, 1980; Chorpita, 2001; Thompson, 1998). In contrast, intrusive and controlling parenting behaviors (so-called "helicopter" parenting) tend to decrease a child's perception of control (Chorpita & Barlow, 1998).

Several studies have implicated the same two dimensions of parenting behavior in the development of anxiety and depression, more specifically. Siqueland, Kendall, and Steinberg (1996), for example, assessed families, with and without children, who had anxiety disorders in order to examine differences in family interactions. Ratings by independent observers during a videotaped interaction task indicated that parents of children with anxiety disorders gave their children less psychological autonomy than did parents of children without anxiety disorders. In addition, children with anxiety disorders rated their parents as less accepting than did children without anxiety. Hudson and Rapee (2002) also found that mothers of children with anxiety were more intrusive in their interactions with those children and their siblings than mothers of children without anxiety. Taken together, these studies provide evidence that overcontrolling, intrusive parenting styles are associated with anxiety disorders in children, and similar parenting styles have been linked to depression (Ingram & Ritter, 2000; Reiss et al., 1995), suggesting that these styles may be associated more generally with negative emotionality.

Perceived Control and the Development of Neuroticism

Although the majority of research in this area has focused on the relationships between parenting styles and the development of anxiety (Hudson & Rapee, 2002; Rubin et al., 2009; van der Bruggen et al., 2008) and depression (Ingram & Ritter, 2000; Reiss et al., 1995), there is evidence that parenting styles moderate the effects of early vulnerabilities on stress reactivity and emotionality more generally (Barlow et al., 1995; Chorpita & Barlow, 1998; Suárez et al., 2009). It is generally accepted that negative life events interact with preexisting generalized biological and psychological vulnerabilities to result in emotional disorders early on. Chorpita and colleagues (1998b) utilized a cross-sectional design to evaluate this "diathesis–stress" model of the development of anxiety. The major hypothesis was that an overcontrolling family environment that fosters diminished personal control should, in fact, produce a sense of uncontrollability, as reflected in a more external locus of control. This external locus of control should, in turn, contribute to increased neuroticism and ultimately to clinical symptoms. Based on evidence from childhood depression studies, the role of attributional style as a mediator in the model was also evaluated.

Compared with a number of alternatives, the best fit for the data is the model that depicts a diminished sense of personal control (external locus of control) functioning as a mediator between a family environment that fosters less autonomy and subsequent negative affect and clinical symptoms. These findings once again suggest that a family environment characterized by limited opportunity for personal control is associated with subsequent higher levels of neuroticism, as well as anxiety symptoms. Interestingly, perceived control in the children appears to be a more robust mediator between family environment and the development of symptoms than attributional style.

In summary, there is evidence supporting a model of the development of negative emotionality characterized by a generalized psychological vulnerability (or sense of relative uncontrollability) as a mediator between salient events and anxiety or depression early in development. Interestingly, and as noted above, this *mediational* model in early childhood contrasts with a *moderational* model that seems to operate for late childhood and adulthood (Chorpita, 2001; Chorpita et al., 1998b; Cole & Turner, 1993; Nolen-Hoeksema et al., 1992). An important developmental progression in the formulation of this vulnerability can be derived from these findings. That is, the environment may help to foster a (cognitive) template, with early experience contributing to the formation of a vulnerability (i.e., mediational model). Later in development, this vulnerability may then begin to operate as an amplifier for environmental events (i.e., moderational model). Data support this moderational role in patients with panic disorder; specifically, anxiety was positively associated with agoraphobia severity, but this relationship was moderated by perceived control such that this association was stronger in patients with low perceived control (White et al., 2006).

In another study, Hedley, Hoffart, and Sexton (2001) evaluated the relationships between perceived control, anxiety sensitivity, and the presence of avoidance and catastrophic thoughts. Support for triple vulnerability theory was based on the finding that beliefs about losing control predicted a fear of bodily sensations, which, in turn, predicted the presence of avoidance and catastrophic thoughts about physical and social harm. This model fit the data better than (1) a cognitive model, in which it was hypothesized that catastrophic beliefs would lead to both anxiety about body sensations and avoidance, and (2) a behavioral model, in which the anxiety about bodily sensations was thought to lead to catastrophic beliefs and avoidance.

On the other hand, in a test of the moderational versus mediational role of perceived control in the relationship between family functioning and anxiety, Ballash, Pemble, Usui, Buckley, and Woodruff-Borden (2006) found support for only the mediating effects of perceived control using the Anxiety

Control Questionnaire in a nonclinical sample of young adults. Results showed that while family communication and general family functioning directly predicted anxiety, other variables (i.e., affective involvement, behavioral control, and family communication) were also predictive of a perceived lack of control, which in turn (indirectly) predicted increased anxiety. Limitations of the study included the exclusion of a clinical sample and a limited age range among participants (ages 18–25). Also, in an application of the triple vulnerability model to social anxiety using structural equation modeling, Hofmann (2005) found that the relationship between catastrophic thinking (the estimated cost of negative events) and anxiety among patients with social anxiety disorder was mediated by the participants' perceptions of control. A moderational model was not tested.

Neuroendocrine Function

Earlier in this chapter, we reviewed the relation between early experiences and HPA axis functioning in animals and the likelihood that HPA axis functioning mediates, to some extent, genetic influences on the development and maintenance of anxiety. There is even evidence for the effects of prenatal stress on the child's neuroendocrine functioning and subsequent development of anxiety and depression (Hentges, Graham, Plamondon, Tough, & Madigan, 2019). Several studies have examined the profound effect of early stressful experiences and neuroendocrine function (typically associated with anxiety and depression) as evidenced by elevated basal cortisol levels in humans. For example, Gunnar, Larson, Hertsgaard, Harris, and Brodersen (1992) demonstrated that 9-month-old infants showed an elevated cortisol response when separated from their mothers but that this effect was eliminated when an infant was accompanied by a highly responsive versus a less responsive caregiver.

Granger, Weisz, and Kauneckis (1994) specifically examined the effects of a sense of control, as well as of current behavioral and emotional problems, on cortisol levels in children as a function of a parent–child conflict task. They found that children with higher neuroendocrine activation were more socially withdrawn and socially anxious, had more social problems, and perceived themselves as having less personal control over the outcomes of their lives. They also tended to perceive social outcomes as being less contingent on their actions in general than did low reactors. Although the findings are correlational, they suggest that children with a lower sense of control during parent–child conflict may evidence exaggerated HPA axis reactivity in the face of stressors.

In a review of the literature to that point, Gunnar and Fisher (2006) summarized accumulating evidence for the influence of social regulation of cortisol levels in early human development and described possible mechanisms at work in this relationship. Although this brief description oversimplifies their detailed account, the authors noted that, early in life, cortisol activity is sensitive to social regulation. In a child provided with sensitive and responsive caregiving, high cortisol responsivity diminishes, and it becomes more difficult to provoke increases in cortisol. These children, in turn, learn that attachment behaviors and distress reactions will result in helpful responses from caregivers. When exposed to lesser levels of responsive care, cortisol levels increase, particularly among temperamentally vulnerable children (those who are easily angered and frustrated, or anxious and fearful). The authors further suggest that abusive and neglectful care will hurt an individual's ability to respond to threat in a healthy physiological manner and ultimately affect their viability. Furthermore, unlike rodents for whom these influences on the developing brain are only operative for a week or two after birth, in humans this vulnerability seems to last throughout childhood (Gunnar & Fisher, 2006).

These studies, then, create an important link between the effects of early stressful experiences (particularly those associated with intrusive, controlling parenting styles) and the development of a generalized psychological vulnerability (manifested as diminished control cognitions). This vulnerability, in turn, directly influences the expression of clinical and neurobiological correlates of neuroticism in both humans and animals.

Generalized Psychological Vulnerability: Conclusions

Earlier in this chapter, we reviewed genetic influences on the development and maintenance of neuroticism. We discussed important characteristics associated with negative emotionality, such as increased psychological arousal and tendencies toward temperamental inhibition and/or low positive affect. Evidence suggests that a reciprocal relationship exists between an inherited tendency to be "nervous," "emotional," or "inhibited" and important environmental factors (such as exposure to early adverse events and inconsistent or overcontrolling parenting styles), which, in turn, lead to the development of an overall diminished sense of control.

Although genetic factors contribute to the development of temperaments such as neuroticism, the evidence reviewed earlier supports the notion that neurobiological processes underlying negative emotionality that may emerge from this biological (genetic) diathesis seem to be influenced substantially by early psychological processes, thus contributing to a generalized psychological vulnerability. In this sense, early experiences with controllability and predictability, based in large part (but not exclusively) on interactions with caregivers:

contributes to something of a psychological template, which at some point becomes relatively fixed and diathetic. Stated another way, this psychological dimension of a sense of control is possibly a mediator between stressful experience and anxiety, and over time this sense becomes a somewhat stable moderator of the expression of anxiety. . . . (Chorpita & Barlow, 1998, p. 16)

This relationship also reflects current thinking on gene–environment interaction (Rutter et al., 2006).

In summary, findings from a number of areas of research, including both animal and human studies, support the key role of a sense of unpredictability and uncontrollability in the development of trait anxiety or neuroticism. A diminished sense of predictability and controllability appears to adversely affect stress hormone functioning in children, which in turn is associated with persistent state of negative emotionality (or neuroticism). Early adversity and parenting behaviors have been shown to influence children's perceptions of control and associated cognitive styles, thereby increasing either their risk or resilience to stress. Rather than conferring direct risk for the development of specific anxiety or depressive disorders, these environmental variables may moderate risk for a persistent state of negative emotionality or neuroticism, which in turn increases the probability of developing anxiety and mood disorders.

Early adversity influences children's cognitive styles, affecting their resilience to stress.

INTERACTIONS BETWEEN GENERAL BIOLOGICAL AND PSYCHOLOGICAL VULNERABILITIES

Nevertheless, the relationship between general biological and psychological vulnerabilities and the development of neuroticism or temperament more generally cannot be characterized as cause and effect. Rather than a static, one-directional relationship, it is more accurate to conceptualize a dynamic, interacting relationship among these constructs (Brown & Rosellini, 2011; Shackman et al., 2016). In this regard, environmental stressors interact with biological vulnerabilities described earlier in a bidirectional manner to influence dispositional levels of neuroticism. So an individual with a genetic predisposition toward greater reactivity to stress may be more susceptible to the detrimental impact of stress and trauma. This detrimental effect would be reflected in a decreased capacity to cope and greater negative impact as a result of such stressors. Further, whereas genetic factors may predispose a lowered threshold for reactivity at the neural level (e.g., greater limbic reactivity), repeated exposure to stressful environmental contexts may potentiate these responses through a process of "sensitization" (Charney, Deutch,

Krystal, Southwick, & Davis, 1993; Figueiredo, Bodie, Tauchi, Dolgas, & Herman, 2003; Rosen & Schulkin, 1998; Shackman et al., 2016). Long-term potentiation of fear circuitry through repeated activation sensitizes this system, leading to hypervigilance and greater reactivity to threat (Lanius et al., 2010). Repeated or prolonged exposure to stressors also produces a "kindling" effect, whereby neural reactivity to stress-related stimuli becomes more diffuse and widespread (Gelowitz & Kokkinidis, 1999).

This kindling effect sets in motion a series of additional steps, including the expression of immediate-early genes in limbic structures (Campeau et al., 1997; Shin, McNamara, Morgan, Curran, & Cohen, 1990). Immediate-early genes (IEGs) are genes whose transcription is activated by extracellular stimuli rapidly (within minutes) and transiently (Sheng & Greenberg, 1990). IEGs encode transcription factors that influence gene expression and neuronal plasticity, leading to long-term alterations in neuronal functioning. Thus the expression of IEGs through neuronal kindling can have long-lasting effects on brain organization and functioning, resulting in enduring phenotypic changes in response to stimuli (Anacker et al., 2016; Pérez-Cadahía, Drobic, & Davie, 2011). It is also possible that early prolonged stress interacts with the immune system, contributing to possible inflammatory underpinnings discovered to be associated with emotional disorders (Hostinar, Nusslock, & Miller, 2018). In other words, these variables play a crucial role in brain development across the lifespan. But how do psychological and environmental factors contribute to these processes?

HPA Axis as a Model of Biological/Psychological/Environmental Interactions

Developmental scientists have produced robust evidence that repeated exposure to stress, particularly during early experience, is linked to molecular and morphological changes in brain circuits that mediate stress responses. These changes are, in turn, associated with exaggerated responses to subsequent threatening or fearful stimuli (Cowen, 2010; Rosen & Schulkin, 1998; Tafet & Bernardini, 2003). In particular, associations between chronic stress and aberrant functioning of the HPA axis modulating acute stress responses have been well established, as mentioned briefly above (Essex et al., 2011; Gillespie, Phifer, Bradley, & Ressler, 2009; Gunnar & Quevedo, 2007; Heim & Nemeroff, 1999; Miller et al., 2007; Sapolsky et al., 2000). These findings represent a cogent model to illustrate the interactions between environmental, psychological, and biological factors in the development of neuroticism. Therefore, at this point, it is useful to describe these interactions in some detail.

Repeated exposure to stress can lead to exaggerated neurological responses to threatening stimuli.

A major function of the HPA axis is to regulate the body's reaction to stress by mounting an appropriate behavioral response through the secretion of stress hormones (glucocorticoids). Cortisol, which has been studied extensively, functions to modulate the body's response to threat through its influence on widespread bodily systems, including cardiovascular, digestive, and immunological systems, as well as key neural systems influencing learning, memory, emotion, and attentional control (Hostinar et al., 2018; Radley, 2012; Sapolsky et al., 2000). When functioning adaptively, the output of cortisol is regulated through a negative feedback loop to the hippocampus. Specifically, the production of this hormone is suppressed once excess levels are detected, thereby maintaining adaptive allostasis. But, as noted briefly earlier, excessive secretion of cortisol and other stress hormones under conditions of chronic stress may "overwhelm" this system, leaving the stress responses activated without capacity to down-regulate the cascade of cortisol (Gunnar & Quevedo, 2007; Shackman et al., 2016). Evidence suggests that the inability to inhibit the production of these hormones may be due to the fact that, at high levels, they become neurotoxins that destroy the very brain structures (e.g., hippocampus) that activate suppression. This system failure also has the effect of preventing adequate neurogenesis in the hippocampus (Conrad, 2008; Magariños & McEwen, 1995; Zeev-Wolf, Levy, Goldstein, Zagoory-Sharon, & Feldman, 2019). Moving beyond this particular finding, it now seems that chronic stress may have more wide-ranging effects on brain development, leading to chronically impaired coordination across brain regions (Zeev-Wolf et al., 2019).

Effects of Stress-Related Changes in Neural Function

Important for this chapter is the conclusion that stress-related alterations in neural network structure and function may underlie much of the vulnerability for pathology seen across emotional disorders. As noted earlier, neuroticism has been linked to heightened limbic reactivity and deficient cortical down-regulation of limbic activation, representing the neurobiological correlate of emotion dysregulation (Keightley et al., 2003; Stein et al., 2007; Westlye et al., 2011). To take one example, stress-related reductions in hippocampal neurogenesis have recently been linked to the overgeneralization of fear in emotional disorders. Deficient neurogenesis is associated with impairments in the ability of hippocampal structures to encode distinct memory traces, a process referred to as *pattern separation* (Deng, Aimone, & Gage, 2010; Tronel et al., 2012). Pattern separation during memory encoding is crucial to the ability to distinguish between similar sensory inputs and contexts so that information specific to a stimulus or context can be retrieved. Impairments in pattern separation during memory encoding can lead to information about two distinct yet similar stimuli being encoded and retrieved as indistinguishable from one another. Impaired pattern separation is likely the mechanism underlying the overgeneralization of fear across multiple contexts (e.g., fear triggered by the sudden sound of gunfire in a war zone or at a shooting range; Kheirbek, Klemenhagen, Sahay, & Hen, 2012; Sahay et al., 2011).

Effects of Chronic Stress and HPA-Axis Dysfunction across the Lifespan

Interesting and useful lines of research are beginning to focus on the long-term effects of chronic stress and HPA axis dysfunction on patterns of neural organization and function. For example, Burghy and colleagues (2012) found that exposure to early life stress was associated with higher cortisol levels during the school-age years, which, in turn, led to lower resting state functional connectivity between the amygdala and vmPFC at age 18. As noted earlier, the amygdala–vmPFC pathway is a critical cortico-limbic pathway for the regulation of fear and anxiety (Delgado, Nearing, LeDoux, & Phelps, 2008; Milad et al., 2007; Ochsner, Bunge, Gross, & Gabrieli, 2002; Ochsner et al., 2004; Phelps, Delgado, Nearing, & LeDoux, 2004). Thus this study provides preliminary empirical evidence for a developmental sequence wherein early exposure to chronic stress and associated HPA axis functioning affects later brain development and organization in neural regions key to the adaptive regulation of emotions, particularly negative emotions (Merz et al., 2019).

Indeed, the impact of chronic stress and trauma on HPA axis functioning seems to be far-reaching across the lifespan. Early disruptions in the parent–child relationships described above (one early source of a sense of uncontrollability) result in higher cortisol levels by preschool age, and these higher levels, in turn, predicted increased behavioral and emotional problems by school age (Essex, Klein, Cho, & Kalin, 2002). Relative to securely attached infants, infants with a disorganized attachment status show elevated cortisol levels during separation from their primary caregivers, as well as slow return to baseline cortisol levels after being reunited (Hertsgaard, Gunnar, Erickson, & Nachmias, 1995). Multiple investigations have linked early life stress, childhood maltreatment, or childhood physical or sexual trauma to elevated cerebrospinal fluid concentrations of corticotropin-releasing hormone (CRH; Cicchetti & Rogosch, 2001; Gunnar & Quevedo, 2007; Heim & Nemeroff, 1999; Rogosch, Dackis, & Cicchetti, 2011).

These relationships are also moderated to some extent by individual differences in caregivers, as well as in children themselves. For example, Tarullo, St. John, and Meyer (2017) found that mothers with higher levels of hair cortisol, reflective of chronic biological stress, were more intrusive in their parenting style, and this intrusiveness moderated the links between maternal cortisol and cortisol in young children. Thus chronic physiological stress in mothers may up-regulate an infant's HPA function. Also, not all children are equally vulnerable, and child emotion regulation and reactivity seem to affect sensitivity to environmental risks. For example, Kao, Tuladhar, Meyer, and Tarullo (2019) found that emotional reactivity in preschoolers moderated links between risk factors (such as parental sensitivity) and child levels of cortisol such that children with lower emotional reactivity were buffered from the impact of these environmental/parenting risks on their own HPA function.

Drilling down further into hypothetical mechanisms for these effects, Heim and Nemeroff (1999) suggest that early traumatic experiences may lead to an initial sensitization of the stress hormone system, leading to increased CRH secretion, followed by eventual blunted adrenocorticotropic hormone (ACTH) secretion in an attempt to down-regulate excessive CRH. They suggest that this aberrant function of the HPA axis is responsible for a vulnerability to experience frequent, strong negative emotions.

Hyper- versus Hypocortisolism and Neuroticism

Thus far we have highlighted the association between chronic stress, neuroticism, and elevated levels of circulating cortisol, but contradictory evidence exists, in which both hypercortisolemia and lower levels of cortisol (*hypo*cortisolemia) are associated with neuroticism and depression (for a review, see Blaisdell, Imhof, & Fisher, 2019). This evidence has led to some confusion in the literature regarding the role of HPA dysfunction in neuroticism. For example, in one study, higher scores on the personality dimension of neuroticism were associated with *blunted* cortisol responses to stress in women (Oswald et al., 2006), and, in a second study, findings revealed lower ACTH and cortisol output in individuals with high negative emotionality relative to individuals with low negative emotionality (Jezova, Makatsori, Duncko, Moncek, & Jakubek, 2004). However, Duncko and colleagues (Duncko, Makatsori, Fickova, Selko, & Jezova, 2006) found evidence to suggest that neuroticism is not associated with a consistently elevated or diminished responsiveness of HPA axis functioning. Rather, individuals high in neuroticism evidence alterations in the coordination of neuroendocrine responses to stress (Doane et al., 2013). These findings are consistent with conceptualizations of stress reactivity that suggest that it is not the overall magnitude of the response to stimuli that constitutes a stress response, but rather the ability to recover to baseline following exposure to stress (Koolhaas et al., 2011).

Miller and colleagues (2007) found evidence to support the co-occurrence of both hyper- and hypocortisolism related to chronic stress, trauma, anxiety, and depression in the meta-analysis of over 100 studies mentioned earlier in this chapter. They increased our understanding of some of the inconsistencies of varying cortisol levels of neuroticism by identifying several factors that mediated cortisol output, including time since the onset of the chronic stressor, the specific type of chronic stressor, and the controllability of the stressor. First, time since the onset of the stressor was negatively correlated with HPA axis reactivity, such that immediately present stressors elicited significantly higher daily cortisol output, whereas more distant trauma elicited significantly lower morning cortisol output. These findings are consistent with hypotheses suggesting initial sensitization of stress responses followed by eventual blunting of responses when the individual reaches allostatic load, a conclusion recently supported by results from Kaess, Whittle, O'Brien-Simpson, Allen, and Simmons (2018). Second, stressors that involve threats to physical integrity or stressors that are perceived as uncontrollable elicit a high and flat diurnal pattern of cortisol output, characterized by lower-than-normal morning output, higher-than-normal afternoon and evening output, and greater overall daily output volume. This finding suggests that measures of cortisol output are dependent upon (1) the proximity of the stressor, (2) the type of stressor, and (3) the time of day in which measurements of cortisol output are taken. Blunted or hyporeactive responses of stress hormones may also represent avoidant processing of stress-related cues (Duncko et al., 2006). A confirmatory factor analysis of cortisol output in posttraumatic stress disorder found blunted cortisol levels to be independently related to severity of trauma-related numbing symptoms, suggestive of avoidant processing (Horn, Pietrzak, Corsi-Travali, & Neumeister, 2014). Future research is needed to clarify this relationship.

CONCLUSIONS

Evidence reviewed in this chapter suggests that the origins of neuroticism may arise out of a combination of genetic factors, which predispose the individual to greater reactivity to threat or stress, coupled with early environmental experiences of chronic stress or trauma or parenting styles that decrease a sense of control and blunt the development of resilience. These factors are consistent with the triple vulnerability theory's general biological and psychological risk factors. The combination of genetic factors and early adverse experiences emanating from a number of sources sensitizes key circuits within the brain in response to acute stress, leading to altered stress reactivity. This process, in turn, affects neural development and organization, with long-term effects on the way individuals process and respond to threat-related information, both of which are defining characteristics of neuroticism.

There has long been a suspicion, which has waxed and waned over the years, that research on the nature and origins of neuroticism would reveal important information on the nature and origins of emotional disorders. But accounts of this relationship have taken many different forms over the decades, based on differing theoretical perspectives, many of them nonempirical. In the next chapter, we attempt an integration of these two traditions.

3

Integrating Temperament into the Study of Emotional Disorders

During the last two decades of the twentieth century, the study of temperament and personality proceeded largely independently from research on anxiety, depressive, and related disorders. Now that we have explicated our theory of the origins of neuroticism, the temperamental tendency to experience negative emotions, it is necessary to take a step back to outline the developments in clinical science that resulted in a new and more empirical focus on incorporating temperamental constructs into any consideration of the nature, classification, and treatment of emotional disorders (See Bullis, Boettcher, Sauer-Zavala, Franchione, & Barlow, 2019).

EVIDENCE-BASED TREATMENTS AND THE DSM

Prior to 1980, the emergence of anxiety and depressive disorders, along with other related conditions, was generally accounted for by widely accepted but empirically unsubstantiated theories of personality development, and these conditions were classified very broadly under the umbrella term *neurosis*. Then two advances in clinical science profoundly changed the landscape of how the development and treatment of these emotional disorders were viewed. First, methods of scientific verification were enhanced during the 1970s and 1980s, resulting in an ability to determine, in an objective fashion, the efficacy of psychological and pharmacological interventions for these conditions. This was accomplished primarily by the refinement and increasing sophistication of clinical trial methodology, including the introduction of rigorous, cost-effective single-case experimental designs capable of establishing the efficacy of interventions for individual patients, that could then be replicated in additional cases (Barlow, Nock, & Hersen, 2009; Barlow & Hersen, 1984). Also, clinical scientists began to realize, based partly on the pioneering work of Hans Strupp (1973), that successfully evaluating interventions required defining their therapeutic procedures sufficiently such that other clinicians could deliver these treatments in the manner in which they were intended, albeit with flexible adaptations for particular patients or other local circumstances. Thus detailed individual therapeutic protocols began to appear, each targeting specific forms of psychopathology, particularly anxiety and depressive disorders.

Indeed, results from the clinical trials during that era began to show efficacy of both psychological and pharmacological treatments tailored to various specific disorders (e.g., phobic disorders, depression; cf. Barlow & Hersen, 1984). These positive outcomes in treating discrete disorders with manualized protocols, accompanied by a growing mandate for evidence-based practice by heath care policymakers and third-party payers (Baker, 2001; Barlow, 1996, 2004; Sackett, Strauss, Richardson, Rosenberg, & Haynes, 2000), began to undermine the credibility of the more traditional broad-based, but nonspecific, treatment approaches focused on problems with personality development more generally.

A second influence, perhaps having an even greater impact on the shift away from personality-based conceptions of psychopathology and treatment, was the appearance of the third edition of the *Diagnostic and Statistical Manual of Mental Disorders* (DSM-III; American Psychiatric Association, 1980) in 1980. In this revolutionary approach to diagnosis, global conceptions of psychopathology based on unsubstantiated theories (i.e., neuroses) were eschewed in favor of an atheoretical, empirically derived taxonomy focused on observable presenting problems. Thus individuals who had received a diagnosis of neurosis during the preceding years of the 20th century were now classified more narrowly into specific anxiety, depressive, dissociative, and related disorder categories. See Chapter 5 in this volume for detailed treatment of the evolution of the DSM system.

The impact of this development is hard to imagine 40 years later, but suffice it to say that the "death of neurosis" (Barlow, 1982) was extremely contentious, provoking outrage in some circles; indeed, this controversy played out not only in scholarly outlets such as journals and professional meetings, but also in the popular press. Nevertheless, the result was a completely transformed nosological system consisting of narrowly construed and thinly sliced definitional criteria for psychopathology that, for the first time, made possible operational definitions of behavioral disorders. Thus clinical investigators were better able to identify dependent variables in clinical trials (the disorders) in a reliable fashion. This development complemented the increasing specificity of independent variables in clinical trials research, the psychological interventions that had also been operationalized into fairly detailed guidelines or manuals, as noted above (e.g., Barlow, 1985, 2004). These advances in clinical science led to an explosion of efficacy trials testing discrete interventions for each DSM-III disorder during the 1990s, with strong support from funding agencies around the world. As a result, a new gold standard for psychological care, evidence-based interventions for narrowly defined conditions, emerged that, in turn, had broad impact on mental health policy, service delivery, and funding (Barlow, 2004; Barlow, Bullis, Comer, & Ametaj, 2013; McHugh & Barlow, 2010).

However, even during that era, with its focus on discrete disorders, clinicians and investigators recognized phenomena that were common across large classes of mental illness and began focusing once again, but with more experimental rigor, on features characterizing psychopathology more generally (Barlow, 1988). An age-old tension exists in the science of classification of mental disorders between researchers who came to be called "splitters," advocating the advantages of narrowly defined slices of psychopathology, and those called "lumpers," who found more value in drilling down to common underlying factors among disorders (Brown & Barlow, 2005, 2009). The rationale among "lumpers" was that ensuring adequate reliability of diagnostic categories might have been achieved at the expense of validity, in that DSM-III and its successive iterations were overemphasizing categories that are minor variations of a broader underlying syndrome. (See Chapter 5, this volume, for a description of prominent proposals for the classification of mental disorders that highlight shared features across disorders rather than emphasizing differences.)

COMMONALITIES ACROSS DIAGNOSES: ANXIETY AND FEAR/PANIC

With the development and embrace of DSM-III, it was no longer acceptable to use *neurosis* as an umbrella term for similar conditions (Barlow, 1982). And yet the apparent shared features of these conditions prompted a closer examination of commonalities across disorders along the traditional neurotic spectrum. One parallel across the anxiety disorders was the presence of similar affective states, including anxiety, fear, and the newly introduced (in 1980) phenomenon of panic, which were explored with more objective, experimental rigor.

Fear/Panic

In the mid- to late 1980s, it became clear that the constructs of anxiety and fear, terms that had previously been used interchangeably, actually refer to different emotional states. Both of these states occur across all emotional disorders, and each plays a unique role in the origins and presentations of them (Barlow, 1988). By the 1990s, it had also become widely accepted that the newly recognized phenomenon of panic attacks encompassed the well-known fight-or-flight component of fear, albeit occurring at inappropriate times (i.e., when there was nothing to be afraid of; Barlow, 1988; Barlow et al., 1985; Cannon, 1929). Two primary types of evidence supported this distinction between anxiety and fear/panic, which was to become increasingly important in the conceptions of psychopathology that would ultimately inform nosology and etiology of emotional disorders (Bouton, 2005; Bouton, Mineka, & Barlow, 2001).

First, outpatient reports of anxiety and mood symptoms subjected to quantitative analyses seemed to clearly differentiate a state of fear or panic, characterized by high autonomic arousal, from a more general state of apprehension, tension, and worry, which seemed to fit better with conceptions of anxiety (Brown, Chorpita, & Barlow, 1998). Anxiety in this context was best described as trait anxiety (Barlow, 1988; Cattell, 1962), although the important distinction between trait and state anxiety was not always made clear at that time. Second, findings from behavioral neuroscience research, mostly from the animal laboratories, distinguished anxiety and fear at neural and behavioral levels. For example, a number of investigators demonstrated that lesions of the amygdala eliminate fear conditioning in rats but do not eliminate behavioral manifestations of anxiety in these animals (Fanselow, 1994; LeDoux, 1996). On the other hand, different investigators (e.g., Davis, Walker, & Lee, 1997) suggested that lesions in the bed nucleus of the stria terminalis (BNST), with downstream effects on the CRF system, eliminate anxious responding in the form of well-established behavioral measures of anxiety without affecting fear conditioning.

Thus evidence from both outpatient clinical samples and basic neuroscience (see Barlow, 2002; Suárez et al., 2009) converge to underscore the distinction between fear and anxiety. In short, fear arises when danger is perceived as actual and present; anxiety represents a focus on the possibility of future threat accompanied by a sense of one's inability to predict, control, or obtain desired outcomes if these negative events unfolded. If one were to put anxiety into words, one might say, "That terrible event could happen again, and I might not be able to deal with it, but I've got to be ready to try." The behavior driven by these emotions also differs. Fear activates immediate escape behaviors or (if escape is impossible) attack directed at the source of threat—better known as the fight–flight response. LeDoux (1996) even established one fear circuit that directly bypasses the cortex (the high road) for a direct connection from the retina to the emotional brain (the low road), which makes possible the activation of the fight–flight response before the organism is even aware of the nature of the danger—a useful evolutionary adaptation. Anxiety, on the other hand, is more associated with the behavioral action tendency that Jeffrey Gray had called "stop, look, and listen" (sometimes called *freezing*), reflecting a state of heightened vigilance and apprehension as the organism prepares to cope with future threat (Gray, 1982; Gray & McNaughton, 1995).

Despite narrow conceptions of panic attacks as restricted to panic disorder, panic proved to be ubiquitous across anxiety disorders (Barlow & Craske, 1988; Barlow, 2002) and came to play an important role in new conceptions of the etiology of emotional disorders and the relation of emotional disorders to temperament. But we also recognized that an even more common thread running through anxiety and related disorders is, of course, the emotion of anxiety itself, although not the vaguely conceptualized construct from prior decades.

Chronic (Trait) Anxiety

During the 1980s and 1990s, conceptions of anxiety, now research-based, broadened and deepened to describe a unique but coherent cognitive-affective structure within a defensive motivational system (Barlow, 2000, 2002; Lang, 1979, 1985). As noted previously, anxiety was clearly distinguished from the emotion of fear, reflecting a sense of uncontrollability focused on the possibility of future threat, danger, or other potentially negative events. This perception of uncontrollability could also be described as a state of helplessness in which the organism struggles to plan effectively for dealing with what seems like overwhelming stress with little confidence in a successful outcome (i.e., limited self-efficacy). Associated with this negative affective state is a distinct physiological component that seems best described as a substrate of readiness to prepare the organism to counteract future challenges. Research at that time linked the somatic aspect of anxiety to activation of distinct brain circuits, including the CRF system and, more importantly, Gray's BIS (Chorpita & Barlow, 1998; Gray & McNaughton, 1995). Once again, the characteristic behavioral profile associated with this state is best described as reflecting vigilance or an expectation of danger in the surrounding environment, along with an ongoing effort to prepare for additional threats. Thus trait anxiety came to be typified by persistent central nervous system tension and arousal, as well as autonomic inflexibility (Thayer, Friedman, & Borkovec, 1996), which seemed to reflect the consequences of a state of perpetual readiness to confront threat or danger, real or imagined. A description of trait anxiety as then conceptualized is presented in Figure 3.1. This is an illustration of the process of chronic trait anxiety, and not a description of the etiology of anxiety or emotional disorders.

It also became clear that conscious evaluation was not necessary for this process to occur. That is, the triggers could be "implicit" in that individuals often experience anxiety with little awareness of cues that may prompt

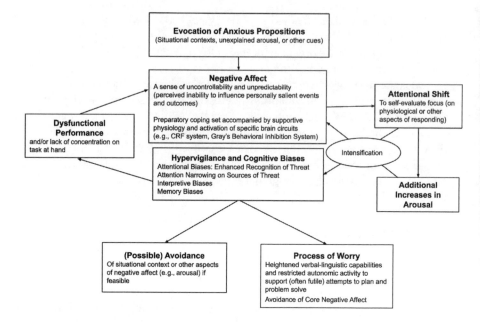

FIGURE 3.1. The nature of anxious apprehension. From Barlow (2002). Copyright © 2002 The Guilford Press. Reprinted with permission.

this emotional state. Indeed, implicit cues in emotional reactivity have come to be foundational in studies of emotion and psychopathology (LeDoux, 1996; Öhman, Flykt, & Lundqvist, 2000). This is, perhaps, most evident in the addictions (Wiers & Stacy, 2013) and posttraumatic stress disorder (PTSD; Lindgren, Kaysen, Werntz, Gasser, & Teachman, 2013), but it also is observed across the emotional disorders.

Another important area of study in that era focused on attentional shifts during the experience of anxiety. Although it had been well known that attentional focus on potentially threatening cues increases during anxiety (and fear), it also became clear that attention can shift to a hyperfocus inward, resulting in a characteristically critical, irrational, and inaccurate evaluation of the self. Indeed, studies of patients indicated that attention often rapidly shifts in its focus from the potentially threatening stimulus to the inadequate capacity of the individual to deal with the threat. Increasing self-focused attention was further found to increase arousal and negative affect in a feedback loop leading to increased intensity of the emotion (Barlow et al., 1995; Barlow, 1988, 2002).

Narrowing of attention, along with the activation of interpretive biases or *schemas* related to a sense of uncontrollability, leads to distorted information processing of internal and external cues. This narrow and intense focus on threatening cues and self-evaluation disrupts concentration and performance in the moment, potentially fulfilling an expectation of inadequate functioning, as best demonstrated in the case of sexual dysfunction (Barlow, 1986). Briefly, research during the 1980s demonstrated that, contrary to the theories of Masters and Johnson (1966), it was not anxious arousal that interfered with sexual response (erectile adequacy in males, lubrication in females) but rather a distracting internal focus on possible inadequate responding and its consequences. Thus the individual is literally "distracted" from processing sexual cues that would ordinarily result in adequate sexual arousal (Barlow, 1986, 2002; Cranston-Cuebas & Barlow, 1990; Wiegel, Scepkowski, & Barlow, 2007). What also became clear during that period is that, although anxiety is normal and can be adaptive even at intense levels when it occurs periodically in response to real challenges or threats, what most defines pathological trait anxiety is intensity, chronicity, and a consistent interference with performance, engagement, and adaptive functioning. Affect intensity was found to significantly predict the perceived intensity of panic-relevant physical (e.g., breathlessness, smothering sensations) and cognitive (e.g., fear of going crazy) symptoms, but not objective physiological arousal (e.g., heart rate), following a hyperventilation physiological challenge test (Vujanovic et al., 2006). Most likely this finding reflects the attention narrowing onto somatic cues mentioned earlier.

Anxiety-Driven Emotion-Regulation Strategies

As a negative affect state, intense anxiety feels uncomfortable and, for some, intolerable. As this research unfolded, it seemed that there were at least two primary consequences of the process of chronic or trait anxiety that develop as one attempts to cope with anxiety and its triggers, as depicted in Figure 3.1. First, a propensity to avoid entering a state of anxiety is constantly present. This tendency becomes more prominent, noticeable, and interfering as the intensity of the anxiety increases and the cues or context that evoke the anxiety are more relevant and specific. Of course, as anxiety becomes more severe and generalizes to many different cues or contexts, overt behavioral avoidance (e.g., completely avoiding crowded places) may not be an available coping strategy, leading to the development of equally maladaptive, yet more subtle, cognitive or behavioral avoidance (e.g., engagement in rituals or superstitious behaviors, attachment to objects or persons who offer an illusory sense of safety).

The second consequence of trait anxiety noted at that time was the development of chronic worry that can be difficult to control at more severe levels (Borkovec, 1994; Borkovec, Alcaine, & Behar, 2004; Borkovec & Inz, 1990; Brown, Dowdall, Côté, & Barlow, 1994c). Borkovec and colleagues pointed out that this worry process could be best understood as another unsuccessful attempt to cope with (regulate) the unpleasant affective and physical experience of anxiety by activating brain functions that tend to suppress pure (negative) affective experience. As with anxiety itself, the process of worry is not always maladaptive and interfering; in some cases, it is warranted and even adaptive until it becomes frequent, intense, unproductive (in that one does not achieve a rational plan or solution to the challenge or threat), and uncontrollable. Indeed, the "uncontrollability" of worry became the defining diagnostic criteria for GAD in DSM-IV (American Psychiatric Association, 1994).

Of course, the fact that the constructs of anxiety (and fear/panic) were common across anxiety and related disorders was not thought to be particularly significant in terms of predictive validity among nosologists constructing various iterations of the DSM. Rather, specific symptomatic presentations—such as perceptual derealization, phobic avoidance of blood, sensitivity to social evaluation, intrusive thoughts, flashbacks of traumatic experiences, cognitive rituals, and psychomotor retardation, among other symptoms—continued to be the basis for categorical classification through DSM-IV (and DSM-5). And yet all of these diverse phenomena are included under the more encompassing general classification of anxiety or mood disorders.

COMORBIDITY

Earlier we reviewed the ubiquity of the constructs of anxiety and fear (panic) across the emotional disorders. Other approaches to phenomenology and nosology have supported additional phenotypic similarities across the anxiety and depressive disorders, including studies describing high rates of comorbidity among common conditions.

Brown, Barlow, and Liebowitz (1994b), upon reflecting on one particular condition, GAD, noted, during the creation of DSM-IV, the extremely high rates of comorbidity of additional anxiety and mood disorders accompanying GAD and suggested that this disorder may be better conceptualized as a vulnerability to developing more diagnoses. Other evidence supported this suggestion, including the earlier age of onset for this condition than for other anxiety and mood disorders, with other comorbid presentations developing later. Thus Brown and colleagues (1994b) went on to say that contemporary classification systems may be "erroneously distinguishing phenomena on the basis of differing manifestations of a common pathophysiology" (p. 1278). They cited a study largely overlooked at the time in the context of psychopathology and classification, reporting that anxiety and mood disorders seemed to respond in a very similar fashion to antidepressant medication (Hudson &

Pope, 1990), a distinct departure from the orthodoxy of the day that different DSM disorders had not only different phenotypes but also different pathophysiology and would require unique pharmacological treatments. Moving beyond the diagnosis of GAD, it became increasingly clear that the constructs of anxiety and depression, in general, were more closely related than previously thought. Data from a number of studies conducted during that period supported this contention. For example, one of our early large-scale diagnostic reliability studies of anxiety and depressive disorder criteria in DSM-IV included a sample of 1,127 patients presenting at the Center for Anxiety and Related Disorders at Boston University (CARD) and looked at the presence of disorders over a lifetime. We found that major depression was by far the most common additional diagnosis in patients with a principal anxiety disorder of any type (Brown, Campbell, Lehman, Grisham, & Mancill, 2001a; Brown, Di Nardo, Lehman, & Campbell, 2001b). Another interesting finding was the relative infrequency of cases presenting with a mood disorder without current or past anxiety disorders (cf. Mineka, Watson, & Clark, 1998). Specifically, in our study mentioned above, of the 670 patients who had a lifetime diagnosis of major depression or dysthymia, only 5% ($n = 33$) did not have a current or past anxiety disorder. Also, in a large majority of cases, anxiety disorders were most likely to precede rather than follow the onset of mood disorders, particularly in cases of major depressive disorder. These findings were consistent with psychometric studies of anxiety and depression that reported very high correlations among prominent self-report measures or clinical rating scales of the two constructs (Zinbarg & Barlow, 1996).

It was also notable that, when groups of patients with anxiety disorders could be differentiated from those with depressive disorders, it was depressive signs and symptoms and not anxious signs and symptoms that best discriminated these groups. That is, almost all patients with depression are anxious, but not all patients with anxiety are depressed. Specific symptoms that do seem to discriminate individuals with depression from those with anxiety could be characterized under the heading of low positive affect, or anhedonia, as reflected in loss of pleasurable engagement. Along with cognitive and motor slowing, these symptoms are often referred to as the classic "melancholic" cluster (Rush & Weissenburger, 1994).

When lifetime rates of comorbidity are considered across the full range of anxiety and depressive disorders, co-occurrence of these common mental disorders is even more striking (e.g., Allen et al., 2010; Brown et al., 2001a; Kessler et al., 1996, 1998, 2003, 2008). In the study of 1,127 patients mentioned previously, 55% of patients with a principal anxiety disorder had at least one additional anxiety or depressive disorder at the time of assessment. This rate increased to 76% when lifetime diagnoses were examined (Brown et al., 2001a). Although the principal diagnostic categories of PTSD and

GAD were associated with the highest comorbidity rates, substantial comorbidity was associated with all disorders. To take one example, of 324 patients diagnosed with DSM-IV panic disorder, 60% met criteria for an additional anxiety or mood disorder, breaking down to 47% with an additional anxiety disorder and 33% with an additional mood disorder. When lifetime diagnoses are considered, the percentages rise to 77% experiencing any comorbid anxiety or mood disorder, breaking down to 56% for an additional anxiety disorder and 60% for a mood disorder. Relatedly, Merikangas and colleagues (2003) followed almost 500 individuals for 15 years and found that relatively few people suffer from a specific anxiety or depressive disorder alone; when patients did meet criteria for a single disorder at one point in time, an additional anxiety or depressive episode disorder almost always emerged at a later time.

These summaries are most likely conservative due to artifactual constraints that were present in DSM-IV, constraints that continue in DSM-5, such as the nature of inclusion–exclusion criteria used. For instance, when adhering strictly to DSM-IV diagnostic rules, the comorbidity between dysthymia and GAD was 5%. However, when we suspend the hierarchical rule that GAD should not be assigned when occurring exclusively during a course of a mood disorder, the comorbidity estimate increases to 90%. These data also ignore the presence of subthreshold symptoms that did not meet diagnostic thresholds for one disorder or another.

Thus it began to be clear that anxiety and depressive disorders might be variable manifestations of a more fundamental common diathesis (Barlow, 1991; Gray & MacNaughton, 1995). Indeed, there was emerging evidence to suggest that the origins of sadness and depressive disorders may also be similar to the origins of anxiety and anxiety disorders in that both states may arise out of a common set of vulnerabilities: a shared generalized psychological vulnerability emerging from early experiences and instilling a sense of uncontrollability (accompanied by a heritable disposition to experience negative affect, as reviewed in Chapter 2). Supporting this view, Alloy, Kelly, Mineka, and Clements (1990) referred to depression emerging out of a state of anxiety as "hopelessness depression." In this conception, depression would reflect an extreme vulnerability to experiences of unpredictability and uncontrollability and would be dependent on the extent of one's psychological vulnerability, the severity of the current stressor, and the coping mechanisms at one's disposal. In more recent research, temperamental variables (neuroticism and extraversion), as well as trait anxiety, remained stable over time, and depression emerged episodically out of these traits (Prenoveau et al., 2011).

> *Depressive disorders and anxiety disorders may both arise out of early experiences instilling a sense of uncontrollability.*

BROAD IMPACT OF PSYCHOLOGICAL TREATMENTS

In addition to common phenotypic presentations (i.e., the occurrence of anxiety, panic, and sadness across conditions) and high rates of comorbidity among anxiety and depressive disorders, broad response to specific treatment also points to important similarities in these conditions. Specifically, psychological treatments for a given anxiety disorder often produce improvement in additional comorbid anxiety or depressive disorders that are not explicitly addressed by the intervention (Allen et al., 2010; Borkovec, Abel, & Newman, 1995; Brown, Antony, & Barlow, 1995; Tsao, Lewin, & Craske, 1998; Tsao, Mystkowski, Zucker, & Craske, 2002). Early on, we examined the course of additional diagnoses in a sample of 126 patients who were being treated for panic disorder at our Center (Brown et al., 1995). A significant pre- to posttreatment decline in overall comorbidity was noted (40% to 17%, respectively). More recently, we examined effects on comorbidity across 179 adults seeking outpatient treatment at our Center. Patients were randomized to receive either a transdiagnostic cognitive-behavioral protocol that addresses emotional disorders generally (Barlow et al., 2017a, 2017b) or established single-disorder protocols that target specific diagnoses, such as panic disorder (Steele et al., 2018). The principal (most severe) diagnoses in this study were panic disorder, social anxiety disorder, OCD, and GAD. In both treatment conditions, participants' mean number of comorbid diagnoses dropped significantly from baseline to posttreatment and from baseline to the 12-month follow-up assessment. Interestingly, changes were particularly robust in terms of comorbid GAD, social anxiety disorder, and depression, in addition to any changes in the principal (most severe) diagnosis.

A COMMON NEUROBIOLOGICAL SYNDROME

There are a number of possible explanations for high rates of comorbidity and overlapping treatment response. We have reviewed these explanations extensively elsewhere (Brown & Barlow, 2002, 2009). One possibility is overlapping definitional criteria; that is, the criteria sets defining one disorder often are similar to criteria sets defining other disorders, even if they are considered distinct disorders. Another possibility is that disorders are sequentially related, such that the features of one disorder (e.g., social anxiety disorder) act as risk factors for another disorder (e.g., depression). However, a more intriguing explanation, noted above, is that these patterns of comorbidity reflect the existence of a higher order factor, such as trait anxiety or neuroticism, with implications for both classification and treatment of common mental health conditions. If this is true (and the thesis of this book supposes it is), then the mix of symptoms that define emotional disorders (e.g., panic attacks, anhedonia, dissociative symptoms) can be understood as variations in the manifestation of a broader syndrome. These findings could suggest (but do not prove) that treatments, when successful, are targeting "core" features of emotional disorders. Also, the fact that a wide range of emotional disorders (e.g., major depressive disorder, OCD, panic disorder) respond approximately equivalently to antidepressant medications, including selective serotonin reuptake inhibitors (SSRIs), has also been interpreted by some as indicating that these medications may be targeting shared features of these disorders (e.g., Gorman, 2007; Hudson & Pope, 1990).

Indeed, recent research from affective neuroscience suggests the existence of common neurobiological patterns across emotional disorders. Specifically, research among individuals with anxiety and related disorders suggests that hyperexcitability of limbic structures, along with limited inhibitory control by cortical structures, may be one explanation for the increased negative emotionality among individuals with such diagnoses (Etkin & Wager, 2007; Mayberg et al., 1999; Porto et al., 2009; Shin & Liberzon, 2010). Thus increased "bottom up" processing through amygdala overactivation, coupled with inefficient or deregulated cortical inhibition of amygdala responses, is found across a number of emotional disorders, including social anxiety disorder (Lorberbaum et al., 2004; Phan, Fitzgerald, Nathan, & Tancer, 2006; Tillfors, Furmark, Marteinsdottir, & Fredrikson, 2002), PTSD (Shin et al., 2005), GAD (Ellard, 2013; Etkin, Prater, Hoeft, Menon, & Schatzberg, 2010; Hoehn-Saric, Schlund, & Wong, 2004; Paulesu et al., 2010), specific phobia (Paquette et al., 2003; Straube, Mentzel, & Miltner, 2006), and depression. Indeed, a recent meta-analysis of 367 functional imaging studies across 4,500 patients with various mood, anxiety, and trauma-based disorders strongly supported transdiagnostic deficits in cortical inhibitory control (Janiri et al., 2020). This same neurobiological pattern of amygdala overactivation has also been found in individuals high in the personality dimension of neuroticism itself (Keightley et al., 2003). Of course, discrete DSM diagnoses have also been associated with several unique and idiosyncratic neurobiological factors (Blair et al., 2008; Chorpita, Albano, & Barlow, 1998a), but it seems likely that the increasingly robust neurobiological syndrome reviewed above may be a more fundamental characteristic of emotional disorders.

THE LATENT STRUCTURE OF EMOTIONAL DISORDERS

In addition to these three phenotypic commonalities among emotional disorders (anxiety, panic, and sadness), sophisticated quantitative studies have shed some light on the structure and nature of these disorders. At the heart of this line of inquiry is a focus on traits or temperaments.

Traits and Temperament: A Brief Review

The study of traits, personality, and temperament has been ongoing for decades, as outlined in Chapter 1, despite a relative lack of influence on nosological schemes for anxiety and related emotional disorders. This may be because the focus of personality research mostly fell within normal samples rather than psychopathological samples that included individuals with emotional disorders. To review briefly, major personality conceptualizations such as the Big Three (Eysenck & Eysenck, 1975; Tellegen, 1985; Watson & Clark, 1993) and Big Five (Digman, 1990; John, 1990; McCrae & Costa, 1987) prominently feature neuroticism and extraversion, despite disagreement on additional traits (e.g., constraint in the Big Three and agreeableness, openness, and conscientiousness in the Big Five) and different methods of formulation.

Many of these investigators have also been interested in the neurobiological basis for such traits as one approach to better understanding the structure of personality. Hans Eysenck, whose influential theory (1961, 1981) led to the development of the Big Three, was first to explicate the traits of neuroticism and extraversion and their characteristics and relationships. He based his theory on variations in levels of cortical activation and autonomic nervous system reactivity, suggesting that extraversion/positive emotion is associated with moderate levels of arousal, whereas neuroticism/negative emotion is associated with under- or overarousal. Decades later, following up on this influential theoretical position, investigators began to examine the relationship of traits such as neuroticism (and extraversion) to the development and course of psychopathology, such as anxiety and related negative emotions (Clark & Watson, 2008). For example, Gershuny and Sher (1998) found, in a sample of 466 young adults, that the combination of high neuroticism and low extraversion at Time 1 seemed to play an important and predisposing role in the emergence of clinical levels of anxiety assessed 4 years later.

Further bolstering the importance of neuroticism and extraversion in the experience of clinical levels of negative emotions, albeit utilizing data largely from animal labs, Jeffrey Gray (1982; Gray & McNaughton, 1995) described a similar trait theory and its neurobiological correlates that map onto Eysenck's traits: the BIS, the behavioral activation system (BAS), and the fight–flight system (FFS). In Gray's theory, the biological basis for anxiety is the BIS's (over)reaction to either novel signals or punishment with exaggerated inhibition. High levels on Gray's BIS roughly relate to elevated levels of neuroticism and low levels of extraversion in Eysenck's model, and elevations in the BAS roughly correspond to high extraversion and low neuroticism (Barlow, 2002). The FFS involves unconditioned escape behavior (i.e., flight) and/or defensive aggression (i.e., fight) in response to unconditioned punishment, such as pain, and unconditioned frustrative nonrewards (Gray, 1991; Gray & McNaughton, 1995). As such, the FFS would seem to represent a biological vulnerability to the distinct emotion of fear/panic specifically, as opposed to anxiety more generally.

In another trait theory, Kagan (1989, 1994) examined children's approach and withdrawal behavior and characterized a profile he also termed *behavioral inhibition*. Kagan's (1989) definition of behavioral inhibition is similar to Gray's (1982) in that it involves a low threshold for limbic arousal and uncertainty regarding unfamiliar events, and he considered this stable profile to be a temperament, which he suggested is clearly heritable (Robinson, Kagan, Reznick, & Corley, 1992). This temperament showed marked physiological characteristics, including increased salivary cortisol levels and muscle tension, greater pupil dilation, and elevated urinary catecholamine levels, and children with this profile were at risk for the subsequent development of anxiety disorders (Biederman et al., 1993; Hirshfeld et al., 1992). However, only 30% of individuals who clearly met criteria for behavioral inhibition as young children went on to develop anxiety disorders (Biederman et al., 1990), and this temperament appeared to be somewhat malleable, which suggests that environmental factors are also important determinants in the expression of this temperament and possibly subsequent anxiety (Kagan & Snidman, 1991). These findings support the notion of a "constraining" biological vulnerability (in contrast to a "determining" role of temperament) in the development of anxiety in adolescence and adulthood, a theme to which we return when we discuss treatment in subsequent chapters.

The Relationship between Temperament and Emotional Disorders

In the 1990s, we began to explore further the discrepant views of emotional disorders from the perspectives of "splitters" versus "lumpers," mentioned earlier. To accomplish this, we investigated the latent structure of anxiety and mood disorders (Brown et al., 1998; Zinbarg & Barlow, 1996), following in the footsteps of other investigators who were working along similar lines at the time (e.g., Clark & Watson, 1991; Clark, 2005; Tellegen, 1985; Watson, 2005). The basic finding, from a sample of 350 patients with DSM-IV anxiety and mood disorders, was that the data confirmed a hierarchical model of anxiety and mood disorders, with negative affectivity or behavioral inhibition (terms we used at the time) representing a higher order factor common to anxiety and depressive disorders and lower order factors contributing to the unique DSM definitions of specific disorders (Brown et al., 1998). This model, presented in Figure 3.2, illustrated that anxiety and mood disorders are closely related, with a substantial contribution from the higher order factor of negative affectivity.

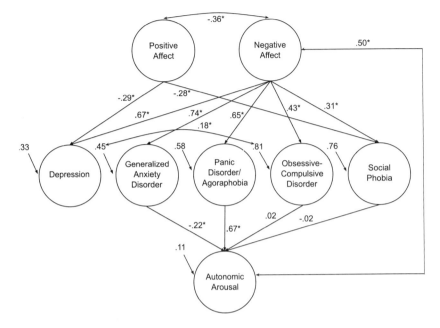

FIGURE 3.2. Structural model of the interrelationships of DSM-IV disorder constructs and negative affect, positive affect, and autonomic arousal. Completely standardized estimates are shown (path coefficients with asterisks are statistically significant, $p > .01$). Structural relationships among dimensions of the DSM-IV anxiety and mood disorders and dimensions of negative affect, positive affect, and autonomic arousal. From Brown, Chorpita, and Barlow (1998). Copyright © 1998 American Psychological Association. Reprinted with permission.

Positive affectivity (extraversion) also contributed to this model. Specifically, low positive affect constituted an important facet of depression and social anxiety disorder (Brown & McNiff, 2009). This finding was mostly consistent with a reformulation of Clark and Watson's hierarchical model (Mineka et al., 1998). Later investigations also discovered that low positive affect was a characteristic of agoraphobia (in addition to depression and social anxiety disorder) when this phenotypic presentation was split from panic disorder in DSM-5 (Rosellini, Lawrence, Meyer, & Brown, 2010). Anxious arousal, which formed the third part of the tripartite model in Clark and Watson's conceptions (1991), was now identified as a separate lower order factor closely associated with panic attacks that contributed to the disorders in an expected fashion, with particularly high loadings on, for example, panic disorder. GAD and depression, consistent with research reported earlier, were very closely related, with high contributions from negative affectivity as reflected in the highest zero-order correlations found in the model: 0.67 between negative affect and depression and 0.74 between negative affect and GAD. This high correlation with GAD further supported notions of GAD as a "basic" disorder, or even perhaps a vulnerability (Barlow, Brown, & Craske, 1994).

These initial findings on latent structure were extended by our research team (Brown, 2007; Brown & Barlow, 2009) and others (e.g., Griffith et al., 2010; Kessler et al., 2011; Kotov et al., 2011). For example, Griffith et al. (2010), studying a large sample of ethnically diverse adolescents and including both self-report and peer report measures of neuroticism, found that a single internalizing factor was common to lifetime diagnoses of mood and anxiety disorders and that this internalizing factor was all but isomorphic with measures of neuroticism. Noting the marked similarity to earlier findings utilizing somewhat different terminology, such as negative affect or behavioral inhibition (e.g., Brown et al., 1998), Griffith and colleagues (2010) suggested that these results provide further evidence that neuroticism itself may be at the core of "internalizing" disorders. Hong, Lee, Tsai, and Tan (2017) picked up a very similar internalizing factor "pervaded with a sense of uncontrollability and vulnerability" (p. 299) as early as age 7 that remained stable through childhood and predicted internalizing symptoms. Krueger (1999) also found that the variance in seven anxiety and mood disorders could be accounted for by the higher order dimension of "internalizing"/neuroticism.

Recent Updates

In recent years, research on a hierarchical structure of emotional disorders has broadened and deepened. To take just a few examples, Zinbarg et al. (2016), in an important prospective study, reported that neuroticism predicted initial onsets of anxiety and unipolar mood disorders and, to a somewhat lesser extent, substance use disorders in a sample of high school students over a period of 3 years. Conway, Craske, Zinbarg, and Mineka (2016), in a similar fashion, found that negative temperament was a robust predictor of both new onsets and recurrences of internalizing disorders. Naragon-Gainey, Gallagher, and Brown (2013) ruled out the potentially confounding effect of mood-state distortion in accounting for these findings, strongly suggesting that the contribution of temperament in the prediction of anxiety and related disorders could not be accounted for by variability in mood during periodic assessments. Brown and Rosellini (2011) also examined the contribution of chronic stress to the influence of temperament on the course of emotional disorders and found that chronic stress moderated this relationship, adding another important element to conceptions of emotional disorders.

Finally, several groups of investigators have used sophisticated analytical procedures and broadened the scope to include hierarchical structural analysis of almost all behavioral disorders. Prominent among these are

Lahey, Krueger, Rathouz, Waldman, and Zald (2017), who found evidence for a general factor of psychopathology, referred to as the p factor, that is largely contributory to the full range of psychopathology. They also demonstrate that this factor is closely related to neuroticism, suggesting that this trait makes some contribution to all psychopathology, not just the emotional disorders. The strong overlap of the p factor with neuroticism has now been replicated in children (Brandes, Herzhoff, Smack, & Tackett, 2019). Other investigators (Oltmanns, Smith, Oltmanns, & Widiger, 2018) suggest that this general p factor may simply be tapping into level of impairment rather than representing a different higher order construct that is broader than neuroticism. These efforts will undoubtedly increase our understanding of psychopathology and have substantial implications for assessment and treatment in the years to come.

Perhaps the most significant advance in this area has been the development of the HiTOP, an empirical quantitative approach to the classification of psychopathology (Kotov et al., 2017). This approach ignores artificial categorical boundaries and began by assembling a comprehensive list of symptoms from all emotional disorders to quantitatively determine the most homogeneous components or sets of symptoms. These components are then sorted into empirically derived syndromes, which are, in turn, grouped under higher order factors. Consistent with research summarized above, all emotional disorders fall under a superordinate factor termed *Internalizing*. Also, three subfactors emerged, replicating previous research, that have been termed *Distress, Fear,* and, somewhat counterintuitively, *OCD/Mania* (Waszczuk, Kotov, Ruggero, Gamez, & Watson, 2017). As noted previously in this chapter, fear and distress seem to correspond to fear/panic and anxiety in our original conceptions.

In any case, although the "key features" of the DSM anxiety and depressive disorders (i.e., the specific symptoms used to discriminate among diagnoses) cannot be collapsed indiscriminately into higher order temperamental dimensions, it seemed safe to conclude, based on studies previously reviewed in this chapter, that what is common outweighs what is not and that these disorders need to be conceptualized in a hierarchical fashion. Summarizing these studies, virtually all the considerable covariance among latent variables corresponding to the DSM constructs of emotional disorders can be accounted for by higher order dimensions.

What is common outweighs what is not.

A NEW FOCUS ON NEUROTICISM

Of course, even when it was less in vogue, some investigators had remained more interested in the possibility of broader underlying syndromes for the variety of specific emotional disorders. For example, Andrews (1990, 1996) and Tyrer (1989) each considered the evidence for the existence of a "general neurotic syndrome" to be stronger and more parsimonious in classifying emotional disorders than individual narrow categories defined by specific symptom presentations. Even earlier, Achenbach, working mostly with children, had identified broad, higher order dimensions of psychopathology that he termed *internalizing* and *externalizing* factors, with the internalizing factor notably encompassing anxiety and depressive symptoms (Achenbach, 1966; Achenbach & Edelbrock, 1978). Now, a substantial literature has accumulated underscoring the roles of these constructs in accounting for the onset, overlap, and maintenance of anxiety, depressive, and related disorders, much as predicted by Tyrer, Andrews, and Achenbach (Brown et al., 1998; Brown, 2007; Brown & Barlow, 2002, 2009; Chorpita et al., 1998a; Gershuny & Sher, 1998; Griffith et al., 2010; Kasch, Rottenberg, Arnow, & Gotlib, 2002; Kessler et al., 2011; Krueger, 1999; Watson, Clark, & Carey, 1988; Watson et al., 1995).

Thus it was becoming clearer during the late 1990s, spilling over into the 21st century, that drilling down into the nature of the coherent cognitive-affective structure of trait anxiety revealed the trait or temperamental nature of this construct. Indeed, various research groups studying the latent structure of anxiety and depressive disorders in both adult and child clinical samples uncovered higher order dimensions that appeared to reflect the temperamental tendency to experience negative emotions. These dimensions carried various labels, including *negative affect, behavioral inhibition, trait anxiety, internalizing, harm avoidance,* and, more recently, *dispositional negativity* (Shackman et al., 2016), all of which are closely related to if not synonymous with *neuroticism*. Also, *positive affect, behavioral activation,* or *externalizing* appeared as alternate terms for *extraversion*. We have chosen to call the first dimension *neuroticism*, the oldest term for this trait (Eysenck, 1947) and the most widely used (e.g., Cuijpers et al., 2010; Lahey, 2009). This new focus on neuroticism, we believe, is likely to lead to a more rich and fruitful perspective on the origins, nature, and treatment of emotional disorders (Barlow et al., 2014b; Brown & Barlow, 2009; Campbell-Sills, Liverant, & Brown, 2004).

AVERSIVE REACTIVITY TO EMOTIONS: A BRIDGE FROM TEMPERAMENT TO DISORDER

Early in this chapter, we discussed the growing concern during the 1990s with splitting diagnostic definitions of emotional disorders into ever narrower slices of psychopathology. We then reviewed the beginnings of research and conceptualizations focused on phenomena that were common across emotional disorders and the emerging consensus that the DSM taxonomy may well be overemphasizing categories that are minor variations of a broader underlying syndrome. Referring back to Figure 3.1, we now believe that the process originally conceptualized as trait anxiety can be broadened to represent neuroticism itself. To briefly review, at the core of neuroticism is the experience of intense and frequent negative emotionality, accompanied by a sense of uncontrollability and unpredictability over stressful or challenging events. This sense of limited control could be described as a perceived inability to influence personally salient events and outcomes, along with a preparatory coping set accompanied by supportive physiology. The sense of uncontrollability, of course, drives an aversion or negative reaction to the experience of an event, including the emotional experience itself (Izard, 1971; Tomkins, 1962). These perceptions are an integral component of the neurotic temperament and, as noted earlier and elaborated on later (see Chapter 4), it is negative reactivity to emotions, rather than the discrete emotional experience itself, that contributes to the development and maintenance of pathology (Barlow, 1988, 1991; Bullis et al., 2019).

As part of that process, we also described two "consequences," represented in Figure 3.1, that develop as one attempts to cope with anxiety (neuroticism) and its triggers. The first is a tendency to down-regulate negative affect and its associated sense of uncontrollability through avoidant behavior that becomes more prominent as the affect increases in intensity; the second is the development of chronic "worry" or repetitive but unproductive negative cognitive activity. Recently, repetitive negative thinking has been shown once again to be transdiagnostically central to anxiety and mood disorders in a sophisticated network analysis (Everaert & Joormann, 2019). The function of this verbal-linguistic activity has also been traditionally described as avoidance or down-regulation of the experience of intense negative affect (Barlow, 2002; Borkovec, 1994).

For the past 20 years, research on constructs found transdiagnostically across the emotional disorders, such as avoidance and worry, that function to regulate emotion has greatly expanded, necessitating further additions and refinements to Figure 3.1. Most of these constructs were originally considered and continue to be conceived as only narrowly associated with one DSM disorder or another; others could be considered more sophisticated elaborations of broad concepts outlined in Figure 3.1. These constructs include those that reflect aversive reactivity to emotional experiences (i.e., anxiety sensitivity, experiential avoidance, intolerance of uncertainty, distress intolerance) and related avoidant coping (e.g., overt situational avoidance, subtle forms of avoidance and safety behaviors, deficits in emotional clarity, emotion/thought suppression, perfectionism, and repetitive negative cognitive activity, which includes both worry and rumination). These constructs, and their functional relationship to both the maintenance of neuroticism and the development of emotional disorders, are reviewed in Chapter 4.

In considering these phenomena more recently, questions began to arise concerning their relationship to well-established temperaments, particularly neuroticism on the one hand and emotional disorders on the other. For example, Paulus, Talkovsky, Heggeness, and Norton (2015) evaluated the relationship of negative affectivity to what they called *transdiagnostic risk factors*, specifically anxiety sensitivity and intolerance of uncertainty, in a proposed hierarchical model using structural equation modeling. They found that these constructs added some information, particularly in the relationship between negative affect and panic disorder for anxiety sensitivity and negative affect and intolerance of uncertainty for several disorders, compared with models without these transdiagnostic risk factors. In each example, though, negative affect alone accounted for most of the variance.

In another example, Naragon-Gainey and Watson (2018), highly respected theorists in the area of temperament, affect, and emotional disorders, chose to describe a subset of the phenomenon mentioned above—specifically, anxiety sensitivity, intolerance of uncertainty, perfectionism, and experiential avoidance—as "social-cognitive vulnerabilities." They noted that these vulnerabilities describe "individual differences in thoughts, emotional experiences, and behaviors that are hypothesized to be related to the onset and/or maintenance of internalizing symptoms, such as anxiety and depression" (p. 143). They also note, as we did earlier, that several of these vulnerabilities arose in the context of theorizing and some experimental work looking at predisposing diatheses for single DSM disorders. For example, anxiety sensitivity is still thought to be primarily a risk factor for panic disorder (e.g., Reiss & McNally, 1985; Reiss, Peterson, Gursky, & McNally, 1986), and both worry and intolerance of uncertainty are thought to be closely related to the onset of GAD (Barlow, Blanchard, Vermilyea, Vermilyea, & DiNardo, 1986; Dugas, Gagnon, Ladouceur, & Freeston, 1998). Naragon-Gainey and Watson (2018) then go on to review a substantial body of literature demonstrating that the four vulnerabilities they focused on were all primarily associated with neuroticism more generally, a finding also reported by Hong and Cheung (2015), but that at least some of the vulnerabilities accounted for a small amount of additional variance beyond the temperament of neuroticism when describing at least some emotional disorders, although not all.

Interestingly, in a paper published a few months later, Naragon-Gainey, McMahon, and Park (2018) changed the label of these same vulnerabilities to "affect-laden clinical traits" and then described these constructs as more "proximal individual differences that can better describe who is likely to develop which specific symptoms beyond the broad risk conferred by affective traits" (p. 1177). While admitting that these traits were largely indistinguishable from neuroticism in their previous study, they point out that there is still some evidence for incremental validity in predicting specific disorders and that these traits comprise more proximal and convenient targets for treatment. This distinction mirrors to some extent the "splitting versus lumping" controversy that has so permeated classification of mental disorders; that is, the initial tendency is to associate one construct or "clinical trait" with one disorder, whereas further analysis reveals not only more general transdiagnostic characteristics but also that these traits are, for the most part, an integral part of neuroticism itself. Of course, as suggested by Naragon-Gainey et al. (2018), this does not mitigate their utility. Indeed, a number of these "clinical traits" have already been targeted in a transdiagnostic treatment for emotional disorders (Barlow et al., 2011, 2017a).

Indeed, in a conceptual paper offering a uniform definition of emotional disorders with accompanying criteria reflecting this definition, we suggest that each of these constructs represents negative reactivity to intense emotional experience, which is then accompanied by a range of cognitive and behavioral strategies to down-regulate negative affect (Barlow et al., 2014b; Bullis et al., 2019). These clinical traits, presented in Figure 3.3 and reviewed in Chapter 4, fall under the broad heading of negative reactivity to emotional experience, often leading to related cognitive and behavioral strategies to down-regulate negative affect, which we refer to as *avoidant emotional behaviors*. This functional relationship, negative avoidant reactivity and resulting temporary down-regulation of negative affect, forms the important bridge between neuroticism and the common core of emotional disorders.

CONCLUSIONS

Overall, the findings reviewed in this chapter suggest that individuals with emotional disorders experience strong negative emotions with frequency and evaluate these experiences as aversive. Because of these negative reactions to their emotions, they are more likely to engage in strategies to down-regulate their emotional experiences, and these strategies, in turn, paradoxically increase the frequency and intensity of negative emotions through a negative reinforcement mechanism. We suggest that this functional relationship, driven by neuroticism, is at the core of disorders of emotion. This relationship, and the evidence supporting it, are reviewed in considerably more detail in Chapter 4.

Thus the study of temperament and personality on the one hand and the psychopathology of emotional disorders on the other, which were largely

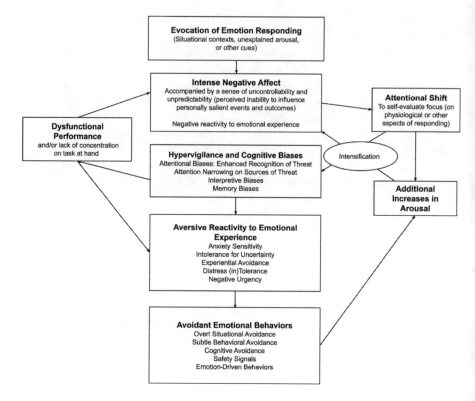

FIGURE 3.3. The process of neuroticism.

unrelated to each other during the last decades of the 20th century, would now seem to be inextricably interrelated. Indeed, at the core of disorders of emotion are relatively stable patterns of temperament, particularly but not limited to neuroticism and extraversion, and advances in our understanding of emotional disorders cannot proceed without a deeper focus on temperamental contributions.

4

Neuroticism
and a Functional Understanding
of Emotional Disorders

motional disorder is a term that has been used to group anxiety, depressive, and related disorders, such as somatoform
and dissociative disorders (Barlow, 1991; Barlow et al., 2014b). As noted in
previous chapters, despite the field's emphasis on identifying characteristics
that differentiate similar conditions, there is ample evidence that shared features across these disorders may outweigh diagnostic differences. Using a
descriptive term such as *emotional disorder* connotes that diagnoses under
this umbrella are characterized by a number of shared emotional disturbances. Indeed, these difficulties appear to be closely linked to neuroticism
itself. The purpose of this chapter is to present a functional understanding of
emotional disorders and their connection to temperamental vulnerabilities,
specifically neuroticism. Additionally, we explicitly relate this functional
model of emotional disorders to the triple vulnerability theory of neuroticism described in Chapter 2.

Not all individuals who experience a high degree of negative affect will
suffer from anxiety or depressive disorders. To better understand how these
difficulties develop, we have articulated a functional model of emotional disorders characterizing the process through which the neurotic temperament
evolves into the distress and interference associated with a broad range of
DSM disorder symptoms (Barlow et al., 2014b; Bullis et al., 2019; Sauer-
Zavala & Barlow, 2014). Specifically, as summarized at the end of the previous chapter, emotional disorders result from three interacting components:
(1) the trait-like tendency to experience negative emotions, (2) aversive reactions to these emotional experiences when they occur, and (3) subsequent
attempts to suppress or otherwise avoid them. Although avoidant strategies

may be effective in the short term, there is compelling evidence to suggest that suppressed emotions return with greater frequency and intensity (Wegner et al., 1987). Indeed, this emotionally avoidant cycle that increases the frequency of negative emotions is responsible for maintaining the neurotic temperament (i.e., frequent, intense negative emotions; Sauer-Zavala et al., 2020), along with symptoms of various mental health disorders (Purdon, 1999). In the following section, we articulate the empirical and clinical evidence suggesting that this functional model can account for symptoms of a variety of disorders, with a particular focus on diagnoses that fall within the traditional neurotic spectrum (e.g., anxiety and depressive disorders).

EMOTIONAL DISORDERS ARE CHARACTERIZED BY FREQUENT AND STRONG NEGATIVE EMOTIONS

Individuals with these common mental disorders experience high levels of negative affect (e.g., Brown & Barlow, 2009) that occur more frequently and intensely than in healthy individuals (Campbell-Sills, Barlow, Brown, & Hofmann, 2006; Mennin, Heimberg, Turk, & Fresco, 2005). As described in detail in Chapter 2, individuals with emotional disorders have an inherited biological predisposition to experience negative emotions (Bouchard & Loehlin, 2001; Clark et al., 1994; Kendler et al., 2003) that is further sensitized by stressful environmental inputs (Barlow et al., 2014a; Gunnar & Quevedo, 2007; Lanius, Frewen, Vermetten, & Yehuda, 2010; Rosen & Schulkin, 1998; Shackman et al., 2016). Additionally, as detailed in Chapter 3, the negative affectivity is strongly linked to the onset and maintenance of emotional disorders (Brown et al., 1998; Gershuny & Sher, 1998). Indeed, there is ample evidence supporting the notion that the propensity to experience negative emotions is a high-order risk factor accounting for the covariance among DSM emotional-disorder constructs (Brown, 2007; Brown & Barlow, 2002, 2009; Brown et al., 1998; Chorpita et al., 1998a; Gershuny & Sher, 1998; Griffith et al., 2010; Kasch et al., 2002; Kessler et al., 2011; Krueger, 1999; Watson et al., 1988). However, beyond the experience of negative emotions itself, the way in which individuals respond to negative affect when it occurs is also important not only for the development of subsequent emotional disorders but also for maintenance of this trait.

EMOTIONAL DISORDERS ARE CHARACTERIZED BY AVERSIVE REACTIONS TO EMOTIONAL EXPERIENCES

Perceptions of emotions as uncontrollable and intolerable, which, in our definition, are included within the purview of the trait of neuroticism (see

Figure 3.3; Barlow et al., 2014a, 2014b), have also been demonstrated across a range of disorders, including depression, GAD, and social anxiety disorder (Boelen, Vrinssen, & van Tulder, 2010; Boswell, Thompson-Hollands, Farchione, & Barlow, 2013b; Lee, Orsillo, Roemer, & Allen, 2010). In fact, the ubiquitous nature of aversive reactions to emotional experiences across the emotional disorders has led to the identification of several overlapping constructs that, while referred to by different labels, all capture the tendency to view emotions negatively. As introduced in the previous chapter, these constructs include anxiety sensitivity, experiential avoidance, intolerance of uncertainty, and distress intolerance. Each of these constructs, along with other related constructs, and their role in our functional model of emotional disorders is described in detail below.

> The terms anxiety sensitivity, experiential avoidance, intolerance of uncertainty, *and* distress intolerance *all point to the tendency to view emotions negatively.*

In addition to being associated with anxiety, depressive, and related disorders, aversive reactions to emotions also have important implications for the intensity and duration of discrete affective experiences (Ostafin, Brooks, & Laitem, 2014). For example, Campbell-Sills and colleagues (2006) instructed 60 individuals with anxiety and depressive disorders to either suppress or accept emotions that arose from viewing a provoking film clip. They found that suppression, compared with acceptance, resulted in increased heart rate and subjective distress during the postfilm recovery period (Campbell-Sills, Barlow, Brown, & Hofmann, 2006). Others have used a similar laboratory paradigm to demonstrate the counterproductive effects of reacting negatively to emotions as they occur (Erisman & Roemer, 2012; Ford, Lam, John, & Mauss, 2018; Keng, Tan, Eisenlohr-Moul, & Smoski, 2017; Troy, Shallcross, Brunner, Friedman, & Jones, 2018). Experience sampling and daily diary studies have also been used to demonstrate the effects of aversive emotional reactivity. For example, Chapman, Rosenthal, and Leung (2009) instructed participants to respond to assessment prompts eight times over the course of 4 days; the 1st day was the baseline day, followed by instructions to simply observe emotions on the 2nd day, to suppress emotions on the 3rd day, and to observe emotions again on the 4th day. Negative emotions were paradoxically more frequent and intense on the days in which participants were instructed to suppress. These results have been replicated in similar studies (Catalino, Arenander, Epel, & Puterman, 2017; Chapman, Rosenthal, Dixon-Gordon, Turner, & Kuppens, 2017; Ford et al., 2018).

Treatment studies exploring the role of aversive reactivity to emotions in accounting for intervention effects also underscore the importance of this component of our emotional-disorders functional model. For example, following a course of cognitive-behavioral therapy for anxiety disorders at our Center, we found that reductions in negative reactivity toward emotions significantly predicted symptom improvements even after controlling for frequency of negative emotional experiences (Sauer-Zavala et al., 2012). In addition, several studies have shown that increased acceptance of emotions during treatment also uniquely predicts improvements in symptoms of anxiety and depressive disorders (e.g., Forman, Herbert, Moitra, Yeomans, & Geller, 2007; Hayes, Orsillo, & Roemer, 2010). How individuals relate to their emotional experiences seems to be just as important for psychological health as the frequency with which they occur. Chapter 6 discusses targeting aversive reactivity to emotions as a means to address emotional disorders, as well as neuroticism itself.

In summary, multiple lines of research converge to underscore the importance of aversive reactions to emotional experiences for maintaining both emotional disorders and neuroticism. Specifically, there is ample evidence linking the tendency to view emotions as negative experiences that should be avoided to the development of anxiety, depressive, and related disorders (see Abramowitz, Tolin, & Street, 2001; Purdon, 1999). Moreover, laboratory and experience-sampling data indicate the real-time emotional consequences of responding negatively to affective experiences. Indeed, efforts to avoid emotions, prompted by their negative evaluation, exacerbate the frequency and intensity of these experiences, possibly maintaining the neurotic temperament itself. The majority of this research has been in the context of specific psychological processes representing aversive reactivity to emotions (see Figure 3.3): anxiety sensitivity, experiential avoidance, distress intolerance, and intolerance of uncertainty.

Anxiety Sensitivity

Anxiety sensitivity has been defined as the belief that the physical symptoms associated with anxiety will have negative somatic, cognitive, and social consequences (Reiss, 1991). In the seminal articles that first describe this construct, the authors note that those exhibiting high levels of anxiety sensitivity are likely to misinterpret the physical sensations associated with emotions as danger signals, resulting in an exacerbation of affective experiences (McNally, 1996; Reiss et al., 1986). For example, elevated levels of anxiety sensitivity may lead an individual to view the increased heart rate that may accompany both anxiety and fear reactions as a sign of an impending heart attack, resulting in a further escalation of this emotional (and related physiological) experience. Or an individual may be distressed by sweating in emotion-eliciting situations due to the concern that others might notice, again increasing the intensity of that symptom.

Anxiety sensitivity was initially considered a one-dimensional construct, consisting of a single factor representing distress in response to physical sensations (McNally, 1996; Reiss et al., 1986). However, this construct is increasingly described as multidimensional, with three distinct factors that appear to be hierarchical in composition (e.g., Lilienfeld, 1996; Lilienfeld, Turner, & Jacob, 1993). Indeed, factor analytic work suggests that anxiety sensitivity is composed of a unifactorial structure at the higher order level and a multifactorial structure at the lower order level (Taylor, 1999). The three most replicable lower order dimensions of anxiety sensitivity include distress focused on physical symptoms, distress focused on publicly observable anxiety symptoms, and distress focused on cognitive dyscontrol.

Given that anxiety sensitivity refers to distress over physical sensations, it is not surprising that this construct has traditionally been studied in the context of panic disorder. Specifically, anxiety sensitivity predicts distress in response to panic-related symptoms (Rapee, Brown, Antony, & Barlow, 1992), which, as we describe in Chapter 3, represent surges of autonomic arousal associated with fear in the absence of danger. In addition to distress over the panic sensations themselves, anxiety sensitivity predicts anxious apprehension over the emergence of future attacks that, paradoxically, results in subsequent panic episodes (Schmidt, Lerew, & Jackson, 1997). Indeed, this aversive reactivity to the physical sensations associated with emotional experiences is significantly associated with panic attack frequency independent of the frequency/intensity of negative affect (Schmidt, Keogh, Timpano, & Richey, 2008). Moreover, anxiety sensitivity is such a robust risk factor for panic symptoms that this construct can prospectively predict the frequency and intensity of panic attacks 3 years following a baseline assessment (Maller & Reiss, 1992). More recent studies also support the utility of anxiety sensitivity in predicting the development of spontaneous panic attacks throughout extended follow-up periods (Schmidt, Zvolensky, & Maner, 2006). Similarly, compared with those with lower levels of this construct at baseline, individuals with elevated anxiety sensitivity were five times more likely to develop a future anxiety disorder.

Emerging literature now suggests that anxiety sensitivity may also be an important risk factor for the broad range of anxiety and related disorders (Maller & Reiss, 1992). For example, this construct has been theoretically linked to the development and maintenance of PTSD (e.g., Taylor, 2003), specific phobias (e.g., McNally & Steketee, 1985), and social phobia (e.g., Rapee & Heimberg, 1997). In one study, higher levels of anxiety sensitivity were found among women who developed PTSD in response to intimate partner violence compared with those experiencing such violence who did not develop this condition (Lang, Kennedy, & Stein, 2002). Similarly, Elwood and colleagues found that anxiety sensitivity specifically predicts the avoidance and numbing symptoms of PTSD among female adult sexual assault victims (Elwood, Mott, Williams, Lohr, & Schroeder, 2009). Elevated anxiety sensitivity has also been found in patients with GAD and OCD relative to individuals without anxiety disorders (Zinbarg, Barlow, & Brown, 1997).

There is some evidence suggesting that the three dimensions of anxiety sensitivity correspond to distinct anxiety disorder presentations. For example, anxiety focused on physical symptoms is, unsurprisingly, most strongly associated with panic-related phenomena (Zinbarg, Brown, Barlow, & Rapee, 2001; Zinbarg et al., 1997), whereas anxiety focused on publicly observable symptoms is most strongly related to a diagnosis of social anxiety disorder (McWilliams, Stewart, & MacPherson, 2000). In parallel, anxiety focused on the cognitive dyscontrol dimension appears to be most strongly related to GAD (Rodriguez, Bruce, Pagano, Spencer, & Keller, 2004). Concerns of cognitive dyscontrol are consistent with commonly occurring cognitive content in this condition (i.e., the belief that difficulty concentrating is a sign of "going crazy").

Of course, despite some specificity in dimensions of anxiety sensitivity predicting various anxiety disorders, there is also a great deal of overlap. For example, as in panic disorder, PTSD risk may be elevated by the anxiety sensitivity dimension reflecting anxiety focused on physical symptoms (e.g., Pole, 2007). Exposure to traumatic events often results in a wide range of physical sensations, and those with a preexisting sensitivity to these feelings may be more emotionally reactive during the trauma and/or learn to be emotionally reactive to reminders of the trauma. Additionally, anxiety sensitivity related to cognitive dyscontrol is also associated with posttraumatic stress-relevant avoidance symptoms among trauma-exposed adults, even after researchers control for negative affect and number of trauma exposures (Vujanovic, Zvolensky, & Bernstein, 2008). This finding suggests that, even within a given anxiety disorder, different anxiety sensitivity dimensions may serve different predictive functions.

Beyond anxiety disorders, individuals with major depressive disorder (MDD) also display high levels of anxiety sensitivity relative to controls (Taylor, Woody, Koch, McLean, & Anderson, 1996). Similar to the anxiety disorder literature described above, a multidimensional view has also implicated specific anxiety sensitivity dimensions in depression (Taylor et al., 1996). For example, anxiety focused on physical sensations at baseline predicted increases in depressive symptoms at a 1-year follow-up assessment (Grant, Beck, & Davila, 2007). Additionally, Schmidt, Lerew, and Joiner (1998) found that anxiety focused on cognitive dyscontrol also predicted future depressive symptoms. Moreover, Viana and Rabian (2009) recently found that anxiety focused on publicly observable symptoms and anxiety focused on cognitive dyscontrol significantly predicted depression symptoms even after controlling for worry and GAD symptoms. Simon and colleagues (2003) found that anxiety sensitivity is even more elevated among patients with bipolar disorder compared with those with unipolar depression and that heightened levels of this construct have been found during manic states even after researchers control for anxiety disorder comorbidity (Simon et al., 2005). Anxiety sensitivity is also elevated across the broader spectrum of emotional disorders, including for eating and somatic symptom disorders (Khalsa & Feinstein, 2018; Thompson-Brenner, Boswell, Espel-Huynh, Brooks, & Lowe, 2018a). Finally, there is emerging research that anxiety sensitivity is heightened in individuals with borderline personality and substance use disorders (see Barlow & Farchione, 2018; Sauer-Zavala & Barlow, 2014).

Experiential Avoidance

Another transdiagnostic construct that exemplifies aversive reactions to emotions and has received considerable empirical attention is experiential avoidance (Hayes, Wilson, Gifford, Follette, & Strosahl, 1996). Experiential avoidance is traditionally described as consisting of two related parts: (1) the unwillingness to remain in contact with aversive private experience (including bodily sensations, emotions, thoughts, memories, and behavioral predispositions), and (2) action taken to alter the aversive experiences or the events that elicit them (Hayes et al., 1996). Thus this construct relates to both the aversive-reactivity and avoidant-coping components of our emotional-disorders functional model. The term *experiential avoidance* is relatively new, adopted by Hayes and colleagues (1996) as a key mechanism in acceptance and commitment therapy (ACT); however, these authors indicate that this putative pathological process is recognized by a wide number of theoretical orientations and is thought to be critical to the development and maintenance of a range of psychopathology (Hayes, Strosahl, & Wilson, 1999). According to Hayes et al. (1996), experiential avoidance includes both avoidance and escape in all of their forms, as long as they are used as methods of altering the form and frequency of emotional experiences.

A number of studies have attempted to understand the role experiential avoidance plays in the generation of emotions in response to distressing stimuli. For example, in one study, Karekla, Forsyth, and Kelly (2004) evaluated this construct in relation to an acute state of stress induced by a carbon dioxide challenge; participants included two groups, individuals low in experiential avoidance and individuals who demonstrated elevated levels of this construct. Although there were no significant differences between the groups on physiological reactions to the stimulus, those high on experiential avoidance reported significantly greater subjective panic symptoms compared with less avoidant individuals. In a similar study using the carbon dioxide challenge, Feldner, Zvolensky, Eifert, and Spira (2003) assigned individuals high or low in experiential avoidance to either suppress or simply observe their bodily sensations. Participants high in experiential avoidance reported greater displeasure and higher levels of anxiety in response to the laboratory stressor compared with the low-experiential-avoidance group, and these findings were even more pronounced when participants were given specific instructions to suppress the experience. Interestingly, consistent with the findings of Karekla and colleagues (2004), no differences were found between high and low experiential avoiders on heart rate, suggesting that this construct may be related to how bodily arousal is perceived rather than how it actually occurs.

Using a different laboratory paradigm, Sloan (2004) explored reactions to pleasant, unpleasant, and neutral emotion-eliciting film clips as function of experiential-avoidance level. Specifically, participants viewed a series of brief films designed to provoke positive and negative (and neutral) emotions, and their responses were assessed using physiological and self-report measures. Individuals high in experiential avoidance demonstrated greater heart rate and electromyographic activity of smile and frown muscles in response to the neutral film clip compared with those with lower levels of this construct. Additionally, although the high experiential avoiders reported greater subjective responses to the emotional film clips for both negative and positive valence, this group showed decreased heart rate reactivity to the fear and disgust film clips relative to the low-experiential-avoidance group; the authors speculated that decreased heart rate reactivity may be a physiological marker of avoidance.

In addition to understanding the consequences of experiential avoidance on discrete emotional experiences, ample research has been conducted to relate this construct to various forms of psychopathology. Self-report studies suggest that high levels of this construct are present in anxiety disorders (Karekla et al., 2004). For example, Roemer, Salters, Raffa, and Orsillo (2005) conducted two early studies aimed at understanding the role of experiential avoidance in the development of GAD. In a large sample of female undergraduate students, experiential avoidance was a significant predictor of GAD severity. Next, in a study that included individuals who met DSM criteria for GAD, experiential-avoidance scores were found to be higher than in the nonclinical sample used in the previous study. Moreover, experiential avoidance predicts GAD symptoms even when the frequency of negative affect is partialed out (Lee et al., 2010). Similarly, cross-sectional studies in nonclinical samples indicate that experiential avoidance is also associated with symptoms of social anxiety (Glick & Orsillo, 2011; Mahaffey, Wheaton, Fabricant, Berman, & Abramowitz, 2013). Moreover, in a large sample of individuals diagnosed with social anxiety disorder, experiential avoidance predicted impairments in daily life, free time, and social contacts above and beyond dysfunctional attitudes and the tendency to experience negative emotions (Gloster et al., 2011). Further, in addition to the biological challenge experiments described previously (e.g., Feldner et al., 2003; Karekla et al., 2004), in which those higher in experiential avoidance displayed greater panic-like reactivity, individuals with panic disorder (or a history of panic attacks) displayed higher levels of experiential avoidance than healthy controls, even after controlling for level of depressive symptoms (Baker, Holloway, Thomas, Thomas, & Owens, 2004; Tull & Roemer, 2007).

Beyond anxiety disorders, there is also evidence to suggest that high levels of experiential avoidance are present among other emotional disorders. For example, individuals with depressive disorders demonstrate elevations on this construct (Berking, Neacsiu, Comtois, & Linehan, 2009; Cribb, Moulds, & Carter, 2006; Hayes, Luoma, Bond, Masuda, & Lillis, 2006; Shahar & Herr, 2011). Additionally, avoidant coping has been shown to mediate the relationship between experiential avoidance and depressive symptoms (Cheavens & Heiy, 2011). A number of studies have also investigated the role of experiential avoidance in the development of PTSD among individuals who have experienced various traumas (e.g., sexual assault survivors, combat veterans). Specifically, experiential avoidance has been shown to predict psychological distress and PTSD symptom severity (Boeschen, Koss, Figueredo, & Coan, 2001; Orcutt, Pickett, & Pope, 2005; Plumb, Orsillo, & Luterek, 2004; Tull, Gratz, Salters, & Roemer, 2004). Indeed, experiential avoidance has also been shown to mediate the relationship between negative affect and PTSD symptoms (Maack, Tull, & Gratz, 2012; Pickett, Lodis, Parkhill, & Orcutt, 2012).

It has also been suggested that substance use functions to escape negative emotions and that some substance-abusing individuals may display high levels of experiential avoidance (Hayes et al., 1996). In a study by Stewart, Zvolensky, and Eifert (2002), experiential avoidance was a significant predictor of drinking for reasons of either negative (coping) or positive (enhancement) reinforcement. However, in contrast, Forsyth, Parker, and Finlay (2003) did not find experiential avoidance to predict addiction severity or drug of choice in a sample of substance abusing veterans.

Distress Intolerance

Distress (in)tolerance is an additional construct that has been employed to describe aversive reactivity to emotions. The literature generally characterizes two broad forms of this construct (Leyro, Zvolensky, & Bernstein, 2010): (1) one's perceived capacity to endure aversive states (e.g., negative emotions, physical discomfort) and (2) the objective behavioral act of withstanding these distressing states when challenged by a stressor. Though the authors describe distress tolerance as related to, yet distinct from, other forms of aversive reactivity (e.g., anxiety sensitivity, experiential avoidance), by definition these constructs appear to have a great deal of conceptual overlap. Indeed, Leyro and colleagues (2010) point out that numerous conceptualizations and assessment models are subsumed under this term, including tolerance of ambiguity, intolerance of uncertainty, and discomfort intolerance, which specifically refers to the capacity to withstand uncomfortable physical sensations and therefore would be closely linked to anxiety sensitivity.

With regard to one's perceived capacity to withstand negative emotional and physical states (Simons & Gaher, 2005), this conceptualization of distress tolerance is typically measured via self-report indices. Specifically, the Distress Tolerance Scale (Simons & Gaher, 2005) is a popular questionnaire focused on the extent to which participants believe they can endure negative emotions (e.g., "I'll do anything to avoid feeling distressed or upset"), whereas the Discomfort Intolerance Scale (Schmidt et al., 2006) measures tolerance of uncomfortable physical states (e.g., "When I begin to feel physically uncomfortable, I quickly take steps to relieve the discomfort"). In contrast, behavioral indicators of distress tolerance typically measure the duration of time (i.e., latency to quit) that an individual can withstand exposure to a specific task, typically presented in a laboratory setting. For example, behavioral distress tolerance has been evaluated in the context of stressful or frustrating cognitive tasks, such as the Paced Auditory Serial Addition Test (PASAT), the Mirror-Tracing Persistence Test (MTPT), and the Anagram Persistence Task. Interestingly, the behavioral distress tolerance tasks that assess ability to withstand difficult physical sensations are the same as those used in laboratory tests of anxiety sensitivity procedures (e.g., voluntary hyperventilation or breath holding, carbon-dioxide-enriched air challenge [CO_2 challenge]), further underscoring the overlap of these constructs.

Despite lack of correspondence between self-reported perceptions of distress tolerance and one's actual ability to withstand aversive states (Ameral, Reed, Cameron, & Armstrong, 2014), both forms of this construct are associated with a wide variety of psychopathological symptoms and disorders (Leyro et al., 2010). For example, low levels of distress tolerance are associated with severity of depressive symptoms (Buckner, Keough, & Schmidt, 2007; Dennhardt & Murphy, 2011; Gorka, Ali, & Daughters, 2012), and predict poorer treatment outcomes in this population (Williams, Thompson, & Andrews, 2013). Distress tolerance is also consistently associated with anxiety disorder symptoms in both adults (Keough, Riccardi, Timpano, Mitchell, & Schmidt, 2010) and children (O'Neil Rodriguez & Kendall, 2014). In fact, this construct emerges as a transdiagnostic risk factor, with demonstrated relationships with the onset of PTSD, panic disorder, OCD, GAD, and social anxiety disorder symptoms (Marshall-Berenz, Vujanovic, Bonn-Miller, Bernstein, & Zvolensky, 2010; Norr et al., 2013). Moreover, intolerance of distress is also associated with substance dependence, the degree to which a former substance user can remain abstinent, and substance use treatment retention (Quinn, Brandon, & Copeland, 1996). This construct has also been linked to antisocial (Daughters, Sargeant, Bornovalova, Gratz, & Lejuez, 2008) and borderline personality (Bornovalova et al., 2008) disorders, as well as eating disorders (Anestis, Selby, Fink, & Joiner, 2007) and emotion-related risk taking (MacPherson, Magidson, Reynolds, Kahler, & Lejuez, 2010). Thus, like experiential avoidance and anxiety sensitivity, distress tolerance has transdiagnostic relevance to various emotional disorders and other psychopathological conditions involving emotional disturbance.

Intolerance of Uncertainty

Intolerance of uncertainty has been described as difficulty enduring the experience of not knowing and has been shown to predict a range of cognitive, emotional, and behavioral responses aimed at avoiding or resolving the aversive experience (Carleton, 2016). Although intolerance of uncertainty has been considered as a symptom, particularly for GAD, researchers have also described this construct as a core maintaining mechanism for a range of emotional disorders that can explain a wide swath of avoidant coping behaviors (e.g., Carleton, 2012, 2016; Einstein, 2014). Specifically, this construct has demonstrated relationships with GAD (Ladouceur et al., 1999), social anxiety disorder (Boelen & Reijntjes, 2009), panic disorder (Smith, Albanese, Schmidt, & Capron, 2019), and OCD (Hezel, Stewart, Riemann, & McNally, 2019; Holaway, Heimberg, & Coles, 2006; Tolin, Abramowitz, Brigidi, & Foa, 2003). Indeed, meta-analytic findings suggest a strong positive correlation between intolerance of uncertainty and anxiety-related difficulties, as well as higher levels of this construct in clinical populations compared with healthy controls (Gentes & Ruscio, 2011).

There is also empirical support for relevance of intolerance of uncertainty to additional conditions beyond anxiety disorders. Indeed, correlational data suggest that this construct is strongly associated with depression (Gentes & Ruscio, 2011). Further underscoring its transdiagnostic relevance, not only is intolerance of uncertainty higher in clinical samples of individuals with depression compared with healthy controls, but the distribution of levels of this construct also appears comparable across depression and anxiety-related conditions (Carleton, 2012). Moreover, meta-analytic results have also demonstrated elevated levels of intolerance of uncertainty in individuals with eating disorders compared with healthy individuals (Brown et al., 2017).

In addition to correlational studies, experimental manipulations that induce intolerance of uncertainty shed light on its consequences. For example, using a previously validated procedure, Mosca, Lauriola, and Carleton (2016) asked participants to progressively consider potential outcomes of a possible negative future life event, followed by reading statements designed to induce high or low intolerance of uncertainty. The authors reported significantly higher levels of worry (after controlling for baseline worry levels) in the high intolerance of uncertainty manipulation condition, compared with the low intolerance of uncertainty and control conditions. Moreover, in a recent prospective study, general intolerance of uncertainty and intolerance of uncertainty relevant to specific DSM disorders (i.e., social anxiety, GAD, and OCD) both predicted symptoms of these conditions (Shihata, McEvoy, & Mullan, 2017). This research may suggest that, although this construct may present as a general transdiagnostic process implicated in multiple difficulties, consideration of condition-specific areas in which uncertainty is a particularly difficulty (e.g., places that may produce physical sensations for panic disorder) may help clarify why one disorder emerges instead of another. This notion is consistent with the theory of divergent trajectories proposed by Nolen-Hoeksema and Watkins (2011), as well as specific psychological vulnerabilities (e.g., Barlow, 2002) described later in this chapter.

Aversive Reactivity and Neuroticism

We consider aversive reactivity to be an important component of neuroticism (see Figure 3.3). Originally, as noted throughout this book, we define this dimension of temperament as the propensity to experience negative emotions, coupled with the perception that the world is threatening and the belief that one is ill equipped to cope. Aversive reactivity represents a specific instance of an individual's sense of uncontrollability/limited self-efficacy—the belief that *emotional experiences* are dangerous, long-lasting, and intolerable and should be avoided. Indeed, we consider aversive reactivity to be a particularly important example of uncontrollability given that this construct is associated with the maintenance of frequently occurring negative affect (Campbell-Sills et al., 2006; see the next section, concerning clinical examples of the effects of aversive reactivity). In sum, the general tendency to experience negative emotions and aversive reactivity to these emotional experiences are separate constructs, though we consider both within the broader purview of the neurotic temperament.

> *Aversive reactivity is the belief that emotional experiences are dangerous and should be avoided.*

Thus how neuroticism is measured may explain the mixed literature about aversive reactivity and its utility for predicting emotional disorders. For example, when controlling for negative affect (i.e., the general tendency to experience negative emotions), anxiety sensitivity remains a significant predictor of the onset and course of most mood and anxiety disorders (Collimore, McCabe, Carleton, & Asmundson, 2008; Cox, Enns, Walker, Kjernisted, & Pidlubny, 2001; Kotov, Watson, Robles, & Schmidt, 2007; Norton, Cox, Hewitt, & McLeod, 1997; Reardon & Williams, 2007). Similarly, laboratory studies have shown that anxiety sensitivity is a significant predictor of fear in response to inhalation of carbon dioxide–enriched air independent of trait anxiety in both adults (Zinbarg et al., 2001; Zvolensky,

Feldner, Eifert, & Stewart, 2001) and youth (Leen-Feldner, Feldner, Bernstein, McCormick, & Zvolensky, 2005).

Similarly, experiential avoidance predicts anxiety disorder symptoms above the contributions of negative affect (Lee et al., 2010), as well as mediating the relationship between the frequency of negative emotions and anxiety symptoms (Maack et al., 2012; Pickett et al., 2012). Although limited empirical work has been conducted to explore the relationship between negative affect and distress tolerance, one study demonstrated that the tendency to experience negative emotions was positively associated with the self-reported perception of one's inability to tolerate emotional distress (i.e., the Distress Tolerance Scale; Simon & Gaher, 2005), but not with self-report measures of physical discomfort tolerance or behavioral measures of distress tolerance.

Finally, several interesting studies have been conducted to explore the relationships between negative affect, intolerance of uncertainty, and the emergence of clinical disorders. For example, Lommen, Engelhard, and van den Hout (2010) recruited participants who were high and low in the general tendency to experience negative emotions and asked them to complete a conditioning task in which one stimulus (CS+: a colored circle) was followed by an electric shock and another stimulus (CS–: a different colored circle) was not. After the acquisition phase, degraded colored circles on a continuum between CS+ and CS– were presented and could be avoided by the participants. Individuals in the high-negative-affect group were more likely to avoid degraded stimuli. Thus, by engaging in avoidance that prevents disconfirmation of irrational fears, individuals with higher levels of negative affect may be at risk of developing emotional disorders. Indeed, McEvoy and Mahoney (2012) demonstrated that intolerance of uncertainty mediates the relationship between negative affect and symptoms of social anxiety disorder, GAD, panic disorder, agoraphobia, and OCD. Taken together, these findings suggest that emotional-disorder symptoms are not simply a product of high levels of negative affect; instead, the combination of strong negative emotions *and* how one relates to them when they occur (both considered important components of neuroticism in our model) is necessary for the development of these disorders.

Other research, however, has found these aversive-reactivity constructs to be largely indistinguishable from more broadly defined neuroticism, consistent with our view that this trait encompasses both negative affect and reactions to it. Specifically, several studies have included these constructs (i.e., anxiety sensitivity, intolerance of uncertainty, experiential avoidance) in factor analyses and concluded that they are isomorphic with neuroticism (Naragon-Gainey & Watson, 2018; Spinhoven, Drost, de Rooij, van Hemert, & Penninx, 2016). However, the unique forms of aversive reactivity are described by these authors as "proximal individual differences that can better describe who is likely to develop *which* specific symptoms beyond the broad risk conferred by affective traits" (Naragon-Gainey et al., 2018, p. 1177). Thus, in addition to understanding the relationship between aversive reactivity and neuroticism, it is also important to consider the extent to which each of these discrete constructs (anxiety sensitivity, experiential avoidance, distress intolerance) is distinct from the others—a topic to which we return below in describing the specific psychological vulnerability component of the triple vulnerability model of etiology introduced in Chapter 2.

The Effect of Aversive Reactions to Strong Emotions in the Context of Clinical Disorders

The consequences of aversive reactions to emotions can be clearly seen across the emotional disorders. In Figure 4.1, we see that precipitating events prompt negative emotional reactions, though the likelihood and strength of this response depends on an individual's general propensity to experience negative emotions, along with specific learning histories that may make a given stimulus emotionally salient (see the section "Specific Psychological Vulnerability" later in the chapter). Once negative affect is activated, how

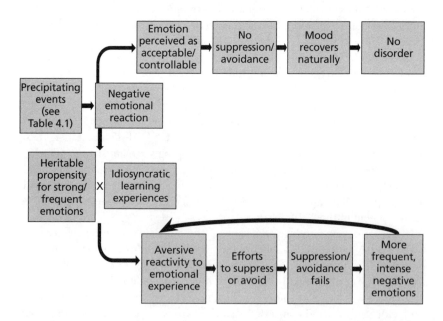

FIGURE 4.1. Model of mechanisms leading to the persistence of emotional distress and emotional disorders vs. normal emotional experience. Based on Bullis et al. (2019).

an individual reacts to these emotions has important implications for the trajectory of the experience. Specifically, aversive reactions to emotional experiences are likely to prompt efforts to control, suppress, or otherwise escape negative emotions; although this avoidant coping may provide temporary relief, it has been shown to exacerbate negative emotions in the long run (Campbell-Sills & Barlow, 2007), thereby maintaining the neurotic temperament. The more intense emotional experiences become, the more aversive they will seem, leading to a stronger pull to avoid them; and, when this avoidance is frequent/chronic and takes the form of DSM criteria, it may serve to push an individual across the diagnostic threshold for an emotional disorder (e.g., worry in GAD, situational avoidance in agoraphobia; see the section "Avoidant Emotional Coping" later in the chapter; Abramowitz et al., 2001).

To understand the crucial role that aversive reactivity plays in the development of emotional disorders, it is worth considering how common the precipitating or "setting" events (see Table 4.1) for these conditions are in the general population. Studies have indicated that up to one-third of the population experiences nonclinical panic attacks (i.e., attacks that do not occur in the context of any disorder), whereas the prevalence for panic disorder is only 2–3% (see Norton, Cox, & Malan, 1992). That is, these nonclinical attacks, while intense and perhaps triggered by stress, are not accompanied by anxiety. Neuroticism, however, may potentiate the reoccurrence of the initial attack in those who go on to develop panic disorder via the susceptibility of the individual to aversive conditioning. Thus, when physical symptoms associated with initial panic attacks (e.g., increased heart rate, shortness of breath) occur in the context of neuroticism, these symptoms are

TABLE 4.1. Precipitating "Setting Events" for Emotional Disorders

Precipitating "setting event"	Disorder
Nonclinical panic attack	Panic disorder
Ego-dystonic intrusive thoughts	Obsessive–compulsive disorder
Uncomfortable somatic sensations	Illness anxiety disorder/panic disorder
Weight and shape concerns	Eating disorders
Interpersonal conflict	Borderline personality disorder
Trauma	Posttraumatic stress disorder
Insufficient sexual arousal/erectile failure	Sexual dysfunction
Restless, unsatisfying sleep	Insomnia disorder
Bullying, unsatisfying social interactions	Social anxiety disorder
Loss	Persistent complex bereavement, depression

viewed as dangerous and are likely associated with future negative outcomes (e.g., heart attack). Here, aversive reactivity serves to intensify anxiety and its related physical symptoms, possibly triggering additional attacks (Barlow, 1988; Clark, 1986). In this model of panic disorder, it is neuroticism (i.e., the propensity for intense negative affect and aversive reactivity) that drives the development of panic disorder, not just the panic attack itself (Bouton et al., 2001).

Similarly, most people in the general population experience the ego-dystonic intrusive thoughts that characterize OCD while under stress, such as thoughts of harming family members, that are quickly dismissed (Rachman & de Silva, 1978), but for individuals who go on to develop OCD, these thoughts produce intense anxiety or associated negative emotions and are believed to be indicative of impending catastrophic consequences (i.e., Shafran, Thordarson, & Rachman, 1996) or morally reprehensible (Nelson, Abramowitz, Whiteside, & Deacon, 2006). These aversive reactions prompt the avoidance of the thoughts and associated strong negative emotions, which reinforces the view of this internal experience as dangerous. More-over, individuals with GAD may find unexpected, uncontrolled emotional reactions to surprising or mildly threatening situations (such as a family member being late arriving home) particularly aversive, resulting in worry or checking behavior to regulate this emotional experience (repeated phone calls to check on family members; Newman & Llera, 2011). More examples of the precipitating events that prompt aversive reactions, along with associated avoidant coping strategies employed (described in detail in the following section), can be seen in Table 4.1. In sum, the typical triggers for an emotional response associated with many DSM diagnoses (e.g., panic attacks, intrusive thoughts, social evaluation) are relatively normal and occur frequently in the population; however, the intensity of the negative emotional reaction to the triggers and one's attempts to cope with or down-regulate this reaction are at the shared core of emotional disorders.

AVOIDANT EMOTIONAL COPING

Given these aversive reactions to negative emotional experiences, it is not surprising that individuals with emotional disorders also display a range of behavioral and cognitive strategies aimed at escaping or avoiding them (Aldao, Nolen-Hoeksema, & Schweizer, 2010; Baker et al., 2004; Moore, Zoellner, & Mollenholt, 2008; Tull & Roemer, 2007; Turk, Heimberg, Luterek, Mennin, & Fresco, 2005). Indeed, extensive evidence has been building for decades supporting the functional relationship of negative reactivity to emotional experiences and the subsequent use of avoidant strategies. Avoidant coping includes information-processing biases minimizing emotion-eliciting stimuli, overt avoidance of situations that may provoke strong emotions, more subtle behaviors designed to dampen emotional experiences, forms of repetitive thought (i.e., worry, rumination) that serve to shift focus away from affective components of the stressor, and other cognitive suppression techniques (e.g., thought suppression, dissociation, distraction); these forms of emotional avoidance are described in detail below.

Avoidant coping, regardless of form, is negatively reinforced, as it has been shown to lead to immediate short-term reductions in negative affect (e.g., Hayes et al., 1996). Unfortunately, this avoidance of emotional experiences paradoxically produces rebound effects in which the suppressed emotions return with greater frequency and intensity (Rassin, Muris, Schmidt, & Merckelbach, 2000b; Wegner, Schneider, Carter, & White, 1987), essentially maintaining the frequent negative affect that is a part of the neurotic temperament. For example, the behavioral avoidance associated with each anxiety disorder serves to reinforce the dangerousness of the avoided stimuli (e.g., parties, public transportation; Craske, Treanor, Conway, Zbozinek, & Vervliet, 2014), as well as the experience of emotions themselves. Similarly, withdrawal and hypersomnia in depression may produce short-term relief from daily stressors and negative emotional experiences but increase depressive symptoms in the long term (Franzen & Buysse, 2008). Additionally, emotional suppression has been shown to predict increased physiological arousal, paradoxically (Hofmann, Heering, Sawyer, & Asnaani, 2009), as has rumination, which is implicated in a cycle of intensifying negative affect that continues until a behavioral form of avoidance (reassurance seeking, substance use, binge eating, and the like) interrupts the cycle (Selby, Anestis, Bender, & Joiner, 2009).

In the following subsections, we review various forms of avoidance relevant for emotional disorders. Some of these strategies have been studied transdiagnostically, whereas others have been traditionally associated with a particular DSM disorder, despite occurring across a range of conditions. In each case, avoidant coping serves as an escape from negative emotional experiences that are viewed as uncomfortable and/or intolerable.

Overt Situational Avoidance

Overt situational avoidance has always been recognized as a hallmark of anxiety disorders, particularly social anxiety disorder, specific phobia, panic disorder, and agoraphobia, as well as other emotional disorders, including PTSD and depression (American Psychiatric Association, 2013). For example, clinicians and researchers alike are familiar with the reluctance of patients with social anxiety to enter or remain in situations in which they might be observed or evaluated by others (e.g., classes with a public speaking component, parties). Similarly, in the context of specific phobias, patients go to great lengths to avoid coming in contact with feared stimuli (e.g., spiders, injections). In panic disorder and agoraphobia, patients may avoid situations/ places in which they previously experienced panic attacks or in which they believe they might have one in the future and from which escape would be difficult. These situations can include transportation (e.g., driving long distances, air travel, open spaces—e.g., bridges, parking lots, arenas), enclosed places (e.g., grocery stores, malls, theaters, elevators, restaurants), crowds, and, in extreme cases, leaving the house. Beyond anxiety disorders, evidence for overt situational avoidance is also present. For example, patients with traumatic stress disorders may seek to avoid locations that are reminiscent of their trauma, whereas patients with depression may eschew activities that were previously pleasurable. By focusing on the different specific forms of overt avoidance, it is possible to lose sight of the fact that, across diagnoses, these behaviors function to reduce or prevent intense emotions.

Subtle Forms of Behavioral Avoidance and Safety Behaviors

More subtle forms of avoidance are also typical across most emotional disorders. For instance, in GAD, excessive planning and researching, reassurance seeking, or checking in on the safety of loved ones can be conceptualized as attempts to gain control over and reduce aversive emotional experiences (Santanello & Gardner, 2007). These behaviors resemble compulsions in OCD (Newman & Llera, 2011; Zinbarg, Craske, & Barlow, 2006), although they are usually experienced as ego-syntonic (reasonable) by patients rather than ego-dystonic (bizarre), as in OCD. Of course, compulsions in OCD, which at times can be subtle, have long been recognized for their avoidant function (Barlow, 2002). Common compulsions include washing, cleaning, checking, repeating, ordering, and thought sequences that are carried out in a patient's mind in order to "undo" an emotion-eliciting obsession. In social anxiety, subtle avoidance can include behaviors such as decreased eye contact or standing farther away from people during conversations, as well as refraining from asking for help in stores or participating during work meetings or classes. In panic disorder, this phenomenon may manifest as avoiding activities that produce anxiety-like somatic sensations, such as exercise, drinking coffee, or even having heated conversations with loved ones (i.e., interoceptive avoidance; Barlow, 1988). In PTSD, subtle behavioral avoidance may include positioning oneself in proximity to a doorway or planning an exit strategy. Although the preceding strategies are often relegated to particular discrete diagnoses, it is worth noting that they may appear across the range of emotional disorders. In addition, there are various transdiagnostic forms of subtle behavioral avoidance that frequently manifest across diagnostic boundaries. For example, drugs and alcohol are often used to prevent or reduce the full impact of emotional experiences.

Perfectionism

The accepted definition of what has been called "clinical perfectionism" is the "pursuit of high standards despite negative consequences, along with basing self-worth on achievement" (Fairburn, Cooper, & Shafran, 2003). This construct's relationship to emotional disorders has been studied for decades (e.g., Antony, Purdon, Huta, & Swinson, 1998). Although it has previously been most closely associated with OCD and eating disorders, a recent meta-analysis demonstrated that perfectionism is indeed associated with the wide range of disorders characterized by negative affect (Limburg, Watson, Hagger, & Egan, 2017). Although many patients describe their perfectionistic approach to activities as likely to increase their anxiety, much as with many compulsions (Cross & Cross, 2015), it still constitutes emotional avoidance given that perfectionism can serve as a way to escape uncertainty about one's eventual performance or guilt if outcomes do not meet personal standards (van der Kaap-Deeder et al., 2016). In a clinical context, many patients have described uncertainty or guilt over poor performance as worse than the anxiety that results from painstaking attention to detail or overworking. It is also worth noting that individuals can be both low achieving and perfectionistic; for instance, procrastination (another form of subtle behavioral avoidance) has been associated with perfectionism, with some individuals reporting being unable to begin activities they feel they will not be able to complete perfectly (Sirois, Molnar, & Hirsch, 2017).

Safety Behaviors

Carrying a talisman or security item represents an additional form of subtle avoidance that occurs widely across emotional disorders. Safety behaviors may include carrying around medications or even empty medication bottles, making sure to always have a cell phone or water on hand, or only doing certain activities with a "safe" person. Using a clinical example to indicate how safety behaviors can undermine one's perception of their ability to cope with emotions (and thus contribute to one's overall aversive reactivity to emotional experiences), we describe conducting a flight exposure with a patient diagnosed with panic disorder. Here, our patient successfully completed a round-trip flight with his therapist and did not experience a panic attack. When queried about his perception of this experience, he noted that "the only reason [he] didn't panic, was because [he] knew he could have taken the Xanax [he] had packed if [he] needed it." As a result of engaging in the safety behavior of carrying his medication, this patient undermined the goal of the exposure, which was to provide evidence that he could experience/tolerate the emotions that arose as a function of flying.

Summary

Behavioral avoidance in all forms, whether overt or subtle, is a consequence of negative affect, representing attempts to down-regulate the emotional experience. Assessing and addressing such behavioral avoidance, even very subtle avoidance, is an important transdiagnostic element of most cognitive-behavioral treatments for emotional disorders, including the use of fear and avoidance hierarchies in anxiety disorder protocols or activity scheduling in depression treatments. Some treatment protocols posit behavioral avoidance as constituting the core of the dysfunction, as in the example of behavioral activation, a well-supported treatment for depression, which is based on the notion that depressive symptoms are maintained by chronic avoidance of engagement or activity (Manos, Kanter, & Busch, 2010). These approaches to countering emotional avoidance are described in more detail in Chapter 6.

Cognitive Avoidance Techniques

In addition to engaging in problematic avoidant behaviors, individuals with emotional disorders also engage in cognitive coping motivated by avoidance. At an information-processing level, patients with anxiety and depressive disorders exhibit strong biases toward negative information, but then tend to quickly turn their attention away from such negative information—the so-called "seek to avoid" pattern (MacLeod & Mathews, 2012; Mathews & MacLeod, 2005). Thus it is not surprising that these individuals display deficits in emotional clarity (Baker et al., 2004; Campbell-Sills et al., 2006; McLaughlin, Mennin, & Farach, 2007; Tull & Roemer, 2007). For example, Thompson et al. (2015) demonstrated in a series of studies, one of which included patients with MDD, that after controlling for current levels of both negative and positive emotion, neuroticism was related to lower clarity of negative (but not positive) emotion. Indeed, low emotional clarity has been conceptualized as an unwillingness to engage with emotions in order to accurately label them (Gratz & Roemer, 2004). Clinically, this may manifest as patients labeling all negative emotional experiences as feeling "bad," rather than being able to differentiate into more nuanced categories such as "annoyed," "frustrated," or "angry." Similarly, when asked how they are feeling or what triggered an emotional response, patients may simply respond "I don't know" as a way to refrain from any in-depth engagement with emotion-eliciting content.

Emotion Suppression

Additionally, emotion suppression is a strategy in which individuals deliberately attempt to push unpleasant emotions (including emotion-inducing cognitions) out of awareness (Gross & Levenson, 1993). High levels of emotion suppression have been demonstrated across emotional disorders, including depression, GAD, OCD, and PTSD (Purdon, 1999) and have also been shown to exacerbate symptoms across these disorders (Abramowitz et al., 2001). Paradoxically, this strategy has long been shown to produce rebound effects in which the suppressed emotionally salient thoughts return with greater frequency and intensity (Rassin, Merckelbach, & Muris, 2000a; Wegner, 1987). As noted previously, emotional suppression is also associated with increased physiological arousal (Hofmann et al., 2009). As with many of the avoidant strategies described in this chapter, it is thought that emotion suppression is a negatively reinforced behavior given that it produces short-term reductions in negative affect. Moreover, the repeated practice of pushing away emotions reinforces the notion that emotions are dangerous, long-lasting, and uncontrollable, thereby solidifying the aversive-reactivity piece of the emotional-disorders functional model.

Repetitive Negative Cognitive Activity

Rumination and worry can also be considered as forms of cognitive avoidance. Both cognitive processes refer to repetitively and passively focusing on negative mood and its possible causes, meanings, and consequences, with rumination chiefly concerned with past events and worry more future-oriented (Nolen-Hoeksema, 1991; Segerstrom, Tsao, Alden, & Craske, 2000). Rumination and worry can both be considered avoidant strategies, as a passive focus on surface matters may serve to protect individuals from more distressing affect-laden concerns (Lyubomirsky, Tucker, Caldwell, & Berg, 1999; Lyubomirsky & Nolen-Hoeksema, 1995). Thus these different forms of repetitive negative thinking, despite some small definitional differences, seem to serve a similar function (Ruscio et al., 2015) and have been described as "two sides of the same coin" (Topper, Molenaar, Emmelkamp, & Ehring, 2014).

Worry, specifically, refers to repetitive thinking about worst-case scenarios involving potential future events. Worry is most commonly associated with GAD; however, there is evidence that it occurs across the emotional disorders, albeit with a more specific focus (e.g., worry about gaining weight in eating disorders, worry about being evaluated in social anxiety disorder). The emergence of worry as an important clinical feature can be traced to DSM-III-R (American Psychiatric Association, 1987), wherein GAD was elevated from its previous status in DSM-III as a residual disorder (i.e., only to be diagnosed in those individuals who were impaired by anxiety but did not meet criteria for another anxiety disorder). Indeed, this change marked the recognition that pathological worry, along with associated physiological states (i.e., muscle tension), represented an important clinical phenomenon in its own right (Barlow et al., 1986). Then, in DSM-IV (American Psychiatric Association, 1994), the uncontrollability of the worry process became the prominent modifier of worry, and the "unrealistic" modifier was dropped (Brown et al., 1994a).

As noted above, the worry process often cycles across a number of relatively minor matters and seems to serve an avoidant function in that it presents the illusion of decreasing the likelihood of already low-base-rate negative events, as well as distracting oneself from negative affect and its associated arousal (Borkovec & Roemer, 1995; Llera & Newman, 2010). In a sophisticated study focusing on patients with GAD, Llera and Newman (2014) established a nuanced avoidant function of worry with their observation that, although worry increases and sustains negative emotionality, the worry process avoids the sharp upward shifts in negative affect that typically accompany negative events. Since the 1980s, psychological treatments have focused largely on this uncontrollable worry process, along with associated muscle tension (e.g., Barlow, Rapee, & Brown, 1992; Eustis, Hayes-Skelton, Roemer, & Orsillo, 2016).

Rumination refers to repetitively and passively focusing on negative mood and its possible causes, meanings, and consequences. Rumination can also be conceptualized as an avoidant strategy, as passive focus on surface matters may serve to protect individuals from more distressing concerns (Lyubomirsky et al., 1999; Lyubomirsky & Nolen-Hoeksema, 1995). As with worry, the avoidant function of rumination is not often successful, as it has been shown to intensify negative affect (Nolen-Hoeksema, Wisco, & Lyubomirsky, 2008; Ruscio et al., 2015), leading to more rumination, in what Selby, Anestis, and Joiner (2008) describe as an emotional cascade. This continues until a maladaptive avoidant behavior (reassurance seeking, substance use, binge eating, and the like) interrupts the cycle. As noted, rumination appears to be prominent across emotional disorders (see Aldao et al., 2010) and prospectively predicts increases in anxiety and depressive symptoms.

Summary

Overall, aversive reactions to frequently occurring negative emotions appear to lead to the use of avoidant coping that is common to all emotional disorders. Although the typical avoidant coping strategies employed may differ across the anxiety and depressive disorders, these behavioral and cognitive approaches function to reduce the frequency and intensity of emotional experiences in the short term; unfortunately, there is ample

Avoidant coping strategies reduce the frequency and intensity of emotional experiences in the short term but increase them over time.

evidence to suggest that this approach to emotions paradoxically increases their occurrence over time. This functional relationship, driven at its core by the neurotic temperament, accounts for the development of emotional disorders, as well as the maintenance of this trait itself.

SPECIFIC PSYCHOLOGICAL VULNERABILITY: THE DEVELOPMENT OF EMOTIONAL DISORDERS

Despite clear overlap in the functional relationships that maintain emotional disorders (i.e., aversive reactions to emotions that prompt avoidant coping), there are still obvious phenotypic differences that constitute discrete DSM disorders. Given that a host of behaviors can serve to distract from emotional experiences, why does a particular constellation of avoidant behaviors coalesce within a given disorder, forming the basis for a DSM diagnosis? The third component of Barlow's triple vulnerability theory (Barlow, 2002) refers to specific psychological factors that may explain why a particular emotional disorder may emerge from the high level of neuroticism conferred from generalized biological and psychological vulnerabilities described in Chapter 2. In summary, the generalized biological vulnerability refers to genetic and neurobiological risk factors that interact with the generalized psychological vulnerability—early life experiences that result in a sense of unpredictability and uncontrollability of salient life events.

The co-occurrence of generalized biological and psychological vulnerabilities may be sufficient to result in the development of some disorders, particularly GAD, which has been described as the phenotypic expression of high levels of neuroticism (Brown et al., 1994a). Depression also represents the expression of high levels of this trait, perhaps with increased hopelessness and low positive affectivity (Abramson et al., 1989; Alloy et al., 2012). Beyond GAD and depression, the pathway to other emotional disorders likely depends upon the development of specific foci for anxiety or distress. In other words, the neurotic temperament evolves into these disorders via learning experiences that create conditions for a specific focus of anxious reactions. These learning experiences may be the result of an individual's own experiences with the environment, in which direct aversive contact with an object, situation, or context results in classically conditioned fear and anxiety responses. Alternatively, there is evidence to suggest that some specific emotion-related behaviors might also be the result of observational learning and behavioral modeling by primary caregivers or other close associates. Early evidence for this notion was reported in a large study investigating pathways to fear acquisition in American and Australian children and adolescents; the majority of respondents attributed the onset of their fear to vicarious and instructional factors, although those who endorsed the highest level of fear also acknowledged direct conditioning experience in combination with these sources (Ollendick & King, 1991).

Evidence for the observational learning of fear comes from both animal models and human studies. For example, early studies showed that laboratory-reared rhesus monkeys who were not initially afraid of snakes acquired intense fear responses after spending several sessions observing wild-reared monkeys exhibit fear in the presence of snakes (Cook, Mineka, Wolkenstein, & Laitsch, 1985; Mineka, Davidson, Cook, & Keir, 1984). Similar effects have been observed in humans. In a study conducted by Gerull and Rapee (2002), mothers were instructed to display negative reactions to either a toy snake or a toy spider, with their toddlers observing their mother's reactions. Toddlers displayed significantly greater avoidance behavior in the presence of objects to which their mothers displayed fear or disgust expressions than to neutral-reaction objects, suggesting the toddlers acquired a conditioned association through observational learning. However, due in large part to the ethical concerns surrounding the promotion of acquired fear in children in the context of a laboratory setting, few additional experimental studies of the transmission of anxiety or fear directly related to psychological disorders have been conducted.

Despite limited experimental data, studies using retrospective reports provide evidence for the notion that pathological fear and anxiety may develop out of observational learning experiences. To date, the most support for the relationship between these types of experiences and the development of emotional disorders has been amassed in the context of panic disorder. For example, patients with panic disorder recalled more parental encouragement of sick-role behavior in response to somatic symptoms associated with panic attacks (e.g., racing heart, dizziness, shortness of breath, or strong nausea) during childhood relative to healthy control participants, whereas no differences between groups were found in parental encouragement of sick-role behavior in response to cold symptoms (Ehlers, 1993). Another study replicated these results, finding that level of anxiety sensitivity in adults was positively related to the degree of parental encouragement of sick-role behavior in response to somatic symptoms (Watt, Stewart, & Cox, 1998). In an attempt to more directly relate these early learning experiences to current anxiety reactivity in provoking situations, another study examined the relationship between self-reported experiences of early modeling related to panic symptoms and the results of a panic-relevant biological challenge. The authors found that individuals who endorsed parenting-related messages communicating the threat value of somatic symptoms were more likely to display increased reactivity to the biological challenge (Leen-Feldner, Blumenthal, Babson, Bunaciu, & Feldner, 2008).

In addition to parental influences facilitating a preoccupation with physical symptoms, there is also evidence that childhood experiences with illness differentially predict the emergence of panic disorder versus other emotional disorders. For example, women diagnosed with panic disorder were more likely to have had a history of physical diseases than women with social anxiety disorder; indeed, patients with panic disorder may have learned in childhood that unexpected bodily sensations are dangerous—creating a specific vulnerability for panic disorder (Rudaz, Craske, Becker, Ledermann, & Margraf, 2010). These patterns also extend to individuals with relatives who had physical illnesses while they were growing up. Patients with a family member who had chronic obstructive pulmonary disease were more likely to have a specific sensitivity to interpreting their own respiratory symptoms as potentially hazardous than those without such family history (Craske, Poulton, Tsao, & Plotkin, 2001).

With regard to direct learning experiences, there is evidence to suggest that one's first panic attack can itself serve as a conditioning trial in which internal bodily sensations that accompany the early onset of the attack become associated with the rest of the attack. In other words, modest increases in heart rate and/or respiration serve as conditioned signals that can elicit a full-blown attack (Bouton et al., 2001). Indeed, animal research clearly demonstrates that interoceptive experiences can serve as conditioned stimuli; for example, in dogs, when distention of the intestine was paired with carbon dioxide administered directly to the trachea (i.e., the unconditioned stimulus), intestinal distention quickly began to elicit respiratory changes (i.e., the conditioned response) that mirrored the unconditioned response (see Razran, 1961). Similarly, when a small injection of ethanol repeatedly preceded the administration of a larger dose, rats began to mount a compensatory response to the initial dose that was associated with greater tolerance of the larger one (Greeley, Lê, Poulos, & Campbell, 1984). These results indicate that animals demonstrate the ability to link a weak interoceptive event with a subsequent, more intense experience.

In individuals who develop panic disorder, early warning signs of an impending attack (e.g., changes in heart rate, sweating) can be associated with full-blown panic, and, because these early-onset cues are presumably similarly to the unconditioned stimulus's later effects, they may be especially easy to condition (see Rescorla & Furrow, 1977; Rescorla & Gillan, 1980). Indeed, there is evidence to suggest that patients with panic disorder report increased anxiety prior to panic attacks (Başoglu et al., 1994; Kenardy, Fried, Kraemer, & Taylor, 1992; Kenardy & Taylor, 1999), and the single best predictor of panic in response to laboratory provocation is baseline level of anxiety (see Barlow, 1988). Additionally, the majority of individuals with panic disorder clearly recall their first attack and report that anxious apprehension regarding the onset of subsequent attacks developed shortly thereafter (Craske, Miller, Rotunda, & Barlow, 1990; Öst & Hugdahl, 1983). Of course, as noted previously, panic attacks are ubiquitous in the general population, suggesting that several factors potentiate the development of panic disorder; these factors include the tendency to experience negative emotions, coupled with the perception that negative events (in this case, panic attacks) are unpredictable and uncontrollable (e.g., Mineka, Cook, & Miller, 1984; Sanderson, Rapee, & Barlow, 1989)—both included within our definition of neuroticism. Thus initial panic attacks, probably triggered by stress and occurring against the backdrop of the neurotic temperament, evidence enhanced interoceptive conditioning and aversive reactions to this intense emotional event. Nonclinical panic attacks are less subject to these aversive reactions.

Similar to panic disorder, in which the importance of physical sensations is emphasized via parenting messages and early learning experiences, individuals with social anxiety disorder also relate characteristic early experiences that suggest that social evaluation is dangerous. For example, parents of patients with social anxiety disorder are significantly more socially fearful and concerned about what others think of them than parents of patients with panic disorder (Bruch & Heimberg, 1994; Rapee & Melville, 1997), and these views are passed along to children (Lieb et al., 2000). Indeed, these messages from parents, along with socially related negative events (e.g., being laughed at by peers), may contribute to negative beliefs about one's social abilities ("I'm boring) and rigid standards ("I must be seen as completely competent") that can portend the development of social anxiety (Wells et al., 1995). Direct learning experiences are also relevant for the development of social anxiety disorder; however, although negative social experiences (i.e., bullying) are associated with social anxiety (Pabian & Vandebosch, 2016), many individuals who undergo such events do not develop emotional disorders. Here again, neuroticism sets the stage for these events to detrimentally affect the mental health of those who experience them.

In fact, this model can be applied to nearly every emotional-disorder diagnosis. With regard to OCD, a key specific vulnerability is the belief that certain thoughts are dangerous and unacceptable (Barlow, 2002). *Thought–action fusion* is a term that refers to a cognitive error common in OCD, in which patients believe that having a thought about an event makes it more likely to occur ("I had a thought about my mom having cancer, so now she's more likely to be diagnosed") and that thinking about an action is morally equivalent to performing that behavior ("thinking about hitting my child is as wrong as actually hitting her"). The specific vulnerability for increased thought–action fusion may be the result of childhood incidents in which excessive feelings of responsibility and guilt develop and unpleasant thoughts are associated with evil intent (Salkovskis, Shafran, Rachman, & Freeston, 1999). Indeed, several studies have demonstrated that the strength of fundamental religious beliefs emphasizing that thoughts themselves can be evil or sinful are associated with thought–action fusion and OCD severity (Rassin &

Koster, 2003; Steketee, Quay, & White, 1991). This is not to say that religious beliefs cause OCD, but rather that believing that certain thoughts are unacceptable and must be suppressed may put one at greater risk of developing OCD (Amir, Cashman, & Foa, 1997; Parkinson & Rachman, 1981; Salkovskis & Campbell, 1994).

The Influence of Neuroticism on Specific Psychological Vulnerability

The interaction of early specific learning experiences and neuroticism is only beginning to be understood; however, there is evidence that higher levels of neuroticism may increase the impact of these life events on subsequent mental health. For example, in one study (i.e., Hooker, Verosky, Miyakawa, Knight, & D'Esposito, 2008), participants learned object–emotion associations by observing specific facial expressions (portraying fear, happiness, or a neutral expression) paired with specific objects. Fear association learning relative to neutral or reward association learning resulted in greater amygdala–hippocampus activation, and this effect was modulated by temperament. Specifically, neuroticism was positively related to the degree of amygdala and hippocampus activation during fear learning, and, in turn, greater amygdala–hippocampal activation during fear learning was associated with better long-term memory of learned associations. Greater neuroticism also predicted faster behavioral response times when both predicting and recognizing fear expressions. These findings support assertions that neuroticism is associated with both heightened sensitivity to fear associations and enhanced fear conditioning during observational learning.

Taken together, the evidence suggests that both classical conditioning through direct experiences and observational or instructional learning play an important role in the acquisition of specific pathological expressions of fear and anxiety, and neuroticism may potentiate these learned associations. Hence, if an individual high in neuroticism is confronted with learning experiences that solidify fear associations, these associations may develop into the foci of an anxiety disorder. For example, if an individual learns that physical illness is dangerous, either through witnessing their family's reaction whenever anyone becomes ill or parental reinforcement of sick-role behaviors, the individual may focus anxiety on physical sensations, leading to the development of panic disorder or hypochondriasis. These negative beliefs about physical sensations (aversive reactivity), coupled with the general tendency to experience negative emotions, increase the likelihood that an initial panic will result in strong associations (conditioning) with similar somatic sensations and, hence, panic disorder. Similarly, if the individual learns that disapproval from others has negative, even dangerous consequences (or experiences negative social consequences firsthand), social evaluation may become the focus of anxiety, leading to the development of social anxiety disorder. If the individual learns that having an aggressive thought is as reprehensible as acting on the thought (thought–action fusion) and attempts to suppress or avoid that thought, then intrusive, ego-dystonic thoughts may become the focus of anxiety, leading to the development of OCD. Hence, generalized biological and psychological factors that compose neuroticism, when lined up with specific forms of learning experiences, may provide the optimum conditions for the development of specific discrete emotional disorders.

CONCLUSIONS

We have proposed a functional model whereby the neurotic temperament may be causally related to the distress and impairment associated with DSM disorders. Specifically, emotional disorders are characterized by the frequent experience of negative emotions, coupled with aversive reactions to these experiences that, in turn, lead to attempts to escape or avoid them. Aversive reactivity to emotional experiences is so ubiquitous among common mental health conditions that several constructs have emerged to describe this phenomenon; these include anxiety sensitivity, experiential avoidance, distress intolerance, negative urgency, and intolerance of uncertainty. Although these constructs are largely overlapping, there may be some differences in emphasis (e.g., anxiety sensitivity focusing on physical symptoms) that differentially predict particular DSM disorder constructs (e.g., panic disorder). These differences may be accounted for by Barlow's (1991) specific psychological vulnerability, in which a specific focus of one's anxiety/distress emerges as a function of early learning experiences (i.e., negative life events, parental modeling).

Despite the phenotypic differences between disorders that can be accounted for by a specific psychological vulnerability, it is clear that shared functional mechanisms apply to the broader groups of emotional disorders and may inform more efficient strategies designed to explicitly target the processes that maintain symptoms across diagnostic boundaries. The incorporation of these processes into more dimensional models of classification for psychopathology are described in Chapter 5, and treatment approaches for addressing neuroticism (i.e., negative affect and aversive reactivity) and related emotional disorders are described in Chapter 6.

5

Nosology and Assessment

As we have noted, neuroticism is strongly associated with psychopathology (see Barlow et al., 2014b), underscoring the question of how this trait can be incorporated into nosological schemes. In early versions of the *Diagnostic and Statistical Manual of Mental Disorders* (DSM; American Psychiatric Association, 1952, 1968), neuroticism itself was not discussed; however, the broad diagnostic category of neuroses reflected the propensity to experience and react negatively to strong emotions in its general description of the conditions falling within its purview. Dictated by the zeitgeist in the field of psychiatry, the term *neuroses* fell out of favor due to its association with a psychodynamic etiology (Barlow, 1982). Indeed, this diagnostic label was removed from DSM-III and its successors, replaced by objective symptom criteria without references to etiological underpinnings. As noted in Chapter 3, these changes, while increasing diagnostic reliability and prompting a surge of meaningful treatment development and outcome work, prioritized the identification of differences between diagnostic categories rather than recognizing what they share. More recently, the tide has turned again, with researchers and clinicians criticizing the validity of the DSM categories and advocating for a more dimensional system that includes temperamental elements. In this chapter, we review how what we call neuroticism has been considered within the field's official nosological systems (i.e., DSM and the International Statistical Classification of Diseases and Related Health Problems [ICD]), as well as within four prominent proposals for dimensional classification schemes. Finally, we describe the challenges that limit the clinical utility each of these approaches and advocate for the inclusion of a functional assessment that describes intermediate, mechanistic constructs to connect psychopathology to temperamental vulnerabilities.

NEUROTICISM AND THE DSM AND ICD SYSTEMS

Over the past century, the influence of neuroticism on the official nomenclature for mental disorders has varied significantly. In the following section, we review the impact of temperament on the understanding of mental health classification in the DSM and ICD systems.

Neuroticism, Neuroses, and Early Editions of the DSM

In 1918, the Bureau of the Census and the American Medico-Psychological Association (the precursor to the American Psychiatric Association) released the *Statistical Manual for the Use of Institutions for the Insane*, a first attempt at a standardized nomenclature for psychopathology that can be considered the precursor to the DSM series. The *Statistical Manual* included 22 diagnoses, most of which were psychotic conditions that were assumed to have biologically based etiological factors (Grob, 1991). This early approach was heavily influenced by the Kraepelinian tradition, named for German psychiatrist Emil Kraepelin, who believed that a taxonomy of mental illness could be derived through careful observation of the signs, symptoms, and course of the diseases exhibited by hospitalized psychiatric patients (Compton & Guze, 1995). Nine updates to the *Statistical Manual* followed before the first edition of the DSM was published in 1952. Psychodynamic theory had little influence on diagnostic schemes in the *Statistical Manual*; however, following the perceived success based on anecdotal case studies of psychoanalysis in treating veterans who had experienced trauma during the world wars, this orientation to understanding psychopathology began to exert a more dominant effect and was carried forward into early editions of the DSM.

Indeed, when the *Diagnostic and Statistical Manual of Mental Disorders* was officially released, it included 102 broadly construed categories that were based upon psychodynamic etiological explanations. Two major classes of disorders were described: (1) conditions assumed to be caused by organic brain dysfunction (e.g., substance intoxication) and (2) conditions presumed to result from the effects of socioenvironmental stressors on an individual's biological constitution, along with the patient's inability to adapt to these stressors (American Psychiatric Association, 1952). The latter class was further subdivided into psychoses, which contained severe conditions such as manic-depressive disorder and schizophrenia, and neuroses, which included anxiety, depressive, and personality disorders.

As noted in Chapter 1, the term *neurosis* was originally used by Scottish physician William Cullen to describe physical symptoms without an obvious medical cause (see Bailey, 1927). Freud adopted the term to describe symptoms that, in his estimation, arose from the failure of the ego to contain the increased insistence of the id. He viewed the symptoms of what we now consider anxiety, depressive, and related disorders as substitutes for the id's instinctual impulses, which had been reduced, displaced, and distorted to odd compulsions, rather than the gratification of the id's desire. In the early DSM system, *neuroses* referred to chronic, interfering distress (in the absence of delusions or hallucinations), which obstensibly associates the experience and reaction to negative emotions (i.e., neuroticism) with this class of conditions. Of course, the etiology of this distress, assumed to result from unconscious conflicts, differs from Eysenck's (1947) biologically based neuroticism.

There were, even as the first edition of the DSM was being developed (and in the years shortly after its release), signs that the predominant psychodynamic approach to psychiatry might not go unchallenged for much longer. First, Eysenck was active, and his work on temperament was beginning to exert influence during the same time period in which the early editions of the DSM were being published. As described in Chapter 1, although Eysenck drew inspiration from the Freudian label of neurosis when he coined the term *neuroticism* in 1947 (5 years prior to the DSM's publication), he was not keen to use a label that might suggest that unobservable psychic conflicts were responsible for negative emotionality. He did, however, wish to highlight the connection between his trait and psychopathology, noting that individuals with neuroses would likely exhibit the tendency to experience negative emotions. Eysenck, of course, favored a biological approach in which genetically mediated brain mechanisms were thought to influence the extent to which individuals respond to environmental stressors with distress. Additionally, the release of psychiatric drugs (e.g., lithium, chlorpromazine, monoamine oxidase inhibitors, tricyclic antidepressants, diazepam) in the 1940s and 1950s may have also been responsible for increasing skepticism toward analytic approaches, as their effect on symptoms was thought to underscore a biological etiology of mental disorders.

Despite these rumblings of sea change, the second edition of the DSM, published in 1968, remained largely influenced by psychodynamic traditions, though minor amendments foreshadowed the paradigm-shifting changes included in subsequent editions. For example, the psychodynamic term *reaction*, referring to the maladaptive responses of an individual to environmental stimuli, was removed in an attempt to make clear that the etiology of many disorders falling under the umbrella of neuroses was unknown. Perhaps in an attempt to stave off a firestorm of criticism from analysts, the following disclaimer was released to explain this change:

> Some individuals may interpret this change as a return to a Kraepelinian way of thinking, which views mental disorders as fixed disease entities. Actually, this was not the intent of the APA committee on Nomenclature and Statistics. [The Committee] tried to avoid terms which carry with them implications

regarding either the nature of a disorder or its causes. In the case of diagnostic categories about which there is current controversy concerning the disorder's nature or cause, the Committee has attempted to select terms which it thought would least bind the judgment of the user. (Spitzer & Wilson, 1968, p. 490)

DSM-III and the Death of Neuroses

During the 1960s and 1970s, psychiatry endured a great deal of criticism. Indeed, the emphasis on psychodynamically based etiology in the DSM classification system, in lieu of clear, descriptive diagnostic criteria, resulted in uncertain demarcations between mental health and illness, as well as relatively low diagnostic reliability (Millon & Klerman, 1986). These critiques led to financial constraints when, in the early 1970s, the National Institute of Mental Health (NIMH) reduced research support to conduct treatment trials for psychodynamic approaches; such studies were considered nonrigorous given lack of uniformity in classification (Wilson, 1993). Moreover, insurance companies were increasingly less likely to reimburse psychiatrists for their services, as nonmedical licensed professionals (i.e., psychologists, social workers) offered similar services at less expensive rates, forcing the field of psychiatry to defend its practice as the treatment of legitimate medical *diseases* (Mayes & Horwitz, 2005). At the same time, psychotropic medications were being prescribed more and more frequently to treat common mental health conditions (Redlich & Kellert, 1978), further underscoring the loosening grip of psychoanalysis on psychiatry.

The mounting critiques of a psychodynamically oriented psychiatry opened the door for more biologically inclined researchers and clinicians to gain a foothold. These individuals, sometimes referred to as neo-Kraepelinians due to their emphasis on observable disorder features (rather than unobservable, theoretically based notions of etiology), were responsible for several important developments in the field (Kawa & Giordano, 2012). For example, in the early 1970s, a group of psychiatrists at Washington University, one of the few psychiatry departments in the nation at that time without an ardent psychoanalyst as chair, published operational diagnostic criteria for several common mental disorders, known as the Feighner Criteria for the first author of the resultant manuscript (Feighner et al., 1972). Subsequently, the Research Diagnostic Criteria (Spitzer, Endicott, & Robins, 1978) were developed with a similar goal to enable investigators to apply a consistent set of criteria in order to select samples of patients with similar psychiatric conditions in a reliable fashion. These efforts heavily influenced the approach to diagnosis included in the third edition of the DSM (American Psychiatric Association, 1980).

Indeed, DSM-III introduced 61 new mental disorders (increasing the number of discrete diagnoses from 163 to 224), each with clear criteria to indicate whether a particular presentation warranted the use of a diagnostic label. This approach was in contrast to previous editions of the DSM that relied on narrative descriptions of each disorder and resulted in poor interrater reliability (Blashfield, Keeley, Flanagan, & Miles, 2014). Perhaps the most controversial change in DSM-III was the removal of the psychodynamic term *neurosis* (Barlow, 1982). Of course, the real debate was over the role of psychodynamic formulations in psychiatry's official classification system—but the inclusion of neurosis in the nomenclature became the symbolic focal point (Bayer & Spitzer, 1985). On one side of this division were those who believed that, in order for the field to advance, an atheoretical nosological system was necessary. Led by Robert Spitzer, who had been involved in the development of DSM-II and was engaged in diagnostic research, a task force on nomenclature for DSM-III was formed. The task force asserted that the field could not determine, with certainty, the causes of many psychiatric conditions and indicated that, when etiology was unknown, "classification should be based on shared phenomenological characteristics" (Bayer & Spitzer, 1985, p. 188); this approach would allow clinicians and researchers with different theoretical orientations to use the same diagnostic system. Given that the term *neurosis* asserted etiological constructs instead of descriptive features—as noted in DSM-II, intrapsychic conflict was responsible for symptom expression of neuroses (American Psychiatric Association, 1968)—it was removed from subsequent versions of the manual.

Although the task force was ostensibly atheoretical, many viewed the new nomenclature as anti-analytic. Some critics noted that decades of clinical experience had established the validity of an etiology based on psychodynamic theory. They decried the objective symptom criteria of DSM-III as "a generous measure of linguistic and conceptual sterility [that would] paralyze the creative and intuitive activity of that large part of psychiatry that lies outside the conceptual pale of the task force" (see Bayer & Spitzer, 1985, p. 189). Others believed that, despite its historical ties to psychoanalytic theory, the term *neurosis* did not require the assumption of intrapsychic conflict and that this diagnostic label could be descriptively defined such that it would align with the goals of the task force without an unnecessary rupture with the past. In response to these criticisms, Spitzer and the nomenclature task force included the term parenthetically to be used following the official disorder names (i.e., *anxiety disorder [anxiety neurosis]*). By the publication of DSM-IV in 1994, the term was entirely omitted (American Psychiatric Association, 1994).

Despite challenges to its development, the advent of DSM-III's empirically based system of classification represented a substantial advance over previous methods and sparked meaningful treatment outcome research (e.g., Mayes & Horwitz, 2005); see Chapter 3 in this volume for a summary of DSM-III's influence. Indeed, for the first time, researchers could objectively track diagnostic status in a reliable manner over time and in response to treatment. In tandem, psychotherapeutic (and pharmacological) treatments were increasingly tailored to address each specific form of psychopathology articulated in DSM, resulting in numerous interventions with demonstrated efficacy in a variety of formats, uses, and settings (Barlow, 1996, 2004; Barlow, Gorman, Shear, & Woods, 2000; Heimberg et al., 1998).

Beyond objective descriptive symptom sets for each diagnosis, another (arguably less controversial) new feature of DSM-III was the inclusion of a multiaxial system to facilitate a more comprehensive depiction of the patient's condition (American Psychiatric Association, 1980). The five axes described: (I) the presence of mental disorder categories, (II) personality dysfunction and intellectual disability, (III) medical disorders that may affect the patient's psychiatric function, (IV) stressors in the social environment, and (V) an assessment of overall adaptive functioning. Despite the intent to capture temperamental features and other long-standing difficulties (i.e., intellectual disability) on Axis II, this section of DSM-III included categorical personality disorder diagnoses that were, like Axis I disorders, based on symptom criteria. Thus Axis II did not provide clinicians with information on levels of more traditionally relevant personality characteristics (e.g., neuroticism, extraversion) that might influence symptom expression and responsiveness to treatment.

Neuroticism in the ICD System

The ICD, maintained by the World Health Organization (WHO), represents the international standard for diagnosis, epidemiology, and clinical management of disease. The sixth edition of the ICD, released in 1949 (just 3 years prior to the publication of the DSM), was the first to include a section on mental disorders. Some have argued that, in general, the current ICD system is less attached to clear diagnostic criteria unless they are independently validated, allowing clinicians to make more judgments in the classification of disorder than they would under the DSM model (Tyrer, 2014).

ICD-9, ICD-10, and ICD-11(World Health Organization, 1979, 1999, 2019) run parallel to DSM-III, DSM-IV, and DSM-5, respectively (American Psychiatric Association, 1980, 1994, 2013) and, in contrast to the DSM approach, maintain references to neuroses/neuroticism. Specifically, "Neurotic, Stress-Related, and Somatoform Disorders" is a discrete class of psychopathology in the ICD system that includes phobic anxiety disorders (i.e., agoraphobia, social phobia, specific phobia), other anxiety disorders (i.e., GAD, panic disorder, mixed anxiety and depressive disorder), obsessive–compulsive disorders, adjustment and stress-related disorders (i.e., acute stress reaction, PTSD, adjustment disorder), dissociative disorders, somatoform disorders, and other neurotic disorders. Although neuroticism is not formally assessed within the ICD system, the inclusion of the word *neurotic* in the chapter title portends the importance of negative emotionality within this class of conditions. Within the other neurotic disorders subgrouping, the ICD includes the diagnosis of "neurasthenia," which refers to extreme fatigue or weakness following disproportionate effort in occupational and social settings; this fatigue may be accompanied by distracting recollections, difficulty concentrating, and "inefficient thinking." The term *neurasthenia* emerged in the mid-1800s, coined by two American physicians, Van Deusen (1869) and George Beard (1869), to describe isolated farm wives and bored society women, respectively.

Assessment of Symptoms in a Categorical Approach to Nosology

Given the limited role for personality in the DSM system, it is not surprising that the study of mental health conditions and personality/temperament have proceeded independently, with a few exceptions (described in detail in Chapter 3). These divergent paths have implications for assessment. For example, a number of semistructured interviews that assess the diagnostic criteria for each disorder have emerged. The first was the Schedule for Affective Disorders and Schizophrenia (SADS; Endicott & Spitzer, 1978), which predated DSM-III and provided in-depth information on schizophrenia and affective disorders. Following publication of DSM-III, the Anxiety Disorders Interview Schedule (ADIS), which provided in-depth information on anxiety, depression, and related disorders, appeared. First written in 1981 to correspond with DSM-III (Barlow, 1987; Di Nardo, O'Brien, Barlow, Waddell, & Blanchard, 1983), the ADIS was later updated to correspond to DSM-III-R (Barlow, 1988; Di Nardo, Moras, Barlow, Rapee, & Brown, 1993), DSM-IV (Brown, Barlow, & Di Nardo, 1994a; Di Nardo, Brown, & Barlow, 1994), and DSM-5 (Brown & Barlow, 2014). The Structured Clinical Interview for DSM Disorders (SCID; Williams et al., 1992), published by the American Psychiatric Association to specifically correspond with DSM disorder criteria, covers more disorders than the SADS or the ADIS but provides less in-depth information on each disorder.

These semistructured diagnostic interviews, based on a categorical or prototypical classification, have influenced the field in several ways. First, they have contributed to the meaningful conduct of clinical trials, allowing researchers to define their sample adequately and to determine whether patients no longer meet criteria for targeted disorders following research treatment. Second, in clinical settings, semistructured interviews assist clinicians faced with challenging

> *The study of mental health conditions and temperament have proceeded independently.*

differential diagnosis decisions and facilitate communication across professionals. Finally, as training programs frequently use structured diagnostic interviews to familiarize trainees with diagnostic criteria, symptom-focused categorical conceptualizations of psychopathology have become ingrained in our mental health system.

Beyond comprehensive interview tools, more narrowly focused clinician-rated and self-report measures of individual diagnoses have also proliferated in the post-DSM-III era. For anxiety, depressive, and related disorders, examples of interview-based measures include the Panic Disorder Severity Scale (Shear et al., 1997), the Liebowitz Social Anxiety Scale (LSAS; Liebowitz, 1987), the Yale–Brown Obsessive–Compulsive Scale (YBOCS; Goodman et al., 1989), the Generalized Anxiety Disorder Severity Scale (GADSS; Shear, Belnap, Mazumdar, Houck, & Rollman, 2006) and the Hamilton Depressive Rating Scale (HDRS; Williams, 1988). Additionally, numerous self-report measures of severity for discrete DSM disorders have also been developed.

Assessment of Personality in a Categorical Approach to Nosology

In general, personality assessment remained largely separate from symptom assessment. In contrast to determining the presence and severity of psychopathology that, guided by a shared nomenclature (i.e., the DSM categories), was relatively uniform in approach across tools, the characterizing of personality varied widely, based on the theoretical perspective of the assessor. In a groundbreaking and influential text, Wiggins (2003) described five paradigms for personality assessment: personological, psychodynamic, interpersonal, multivariate, and empirical. Indeed, without a uniform system for determining how to approach this phenomenon, different paradigms of personality assessment produced fundamentally different answers to the question "What is personality and how do we measure it?" (Wiggins, 2003, p. 1). For example, the personological tradition highlights an individual's life story, which is assessed by gleaning themes from personal narratives. Personality assessment according to the psychodynamic paradigm emphasizes implicit and unconscious dynamics using more indirect methods such as interpretations of inkblots (i.e., the Rorschach inkblot task; Rorschach, 1942) and storytelling tasks (i.e., the Thematic Apperception Test [Murray, 1943]; the Object Relations Inventory [Blatt, Wein, Chevron, & Quinlan, 1979]; and the Washington University Sentence Completion Task [Hy & Loevinger, 1996]). The interpersonal paradigm is aimed at understanding how people relate to others, including themes of agency and communion; a number of assessment tools grounded in an 8-point interpersonal circumplex with two orthogonal axes (i.e., agency and communication) have been developed (e.g., the Interpersonal Adjectives Scale [Wiggins, 1995]; the Inventory of Interpersonal Problems—Circumplex [Alden, Wiggins, & Pincus, 1990]; the International Personality Item Pool—Interpersonal Circumplex [Markey & Markey, 2009]). In the multivariate approach, important differences in personality emerge by factor analyzing the ways in which people describe one another, and, as described in Chapter 1, five broad domains of personality have consistently been extracted. The gold-standard assessment tool for the multivariate paradigm is the Revised NEO Personality Inventory (NEO-PI-R; Costa & McCrae, 1992), though Wiggins (2003) also places Eysenck's Personality Questionnaire (Eysenck & Eysenck, 1975) within this approach to understanding individual differences. Finally, the empirical paradigm determines important dimensions of personality based on correlations with relevant criterion variables. Instead of the theoretical approach driving the development of the assessment tool, important items of the Minnesota Multiphasic Personality Inventory (MMPI), for example, were identified on the basis of their ability to predict outcomes (regardless of their face validity). Perhaps the lack of integration between diagnostic and personality assessment is, at least in part, due to the lack of a uniform approach to understanding an individual's character.

MODERN ATTEMPTS TO RECONCILE TEMPERAMENT AND PSYCHOPATHOLOGY

The categorical-prototypical approach to grouping mental health disorders, exemplified by DSM-III (American Psychiatric Association, 1980) and its successors, is not without shortcomings, prompting some to advocate for a return to a more dimensional understanding of psychopathology (Blashfield et al., 2014). For example, many diagnoses share similar criteria and often co-occur, raising suspicion that enhanced diagnostic reliability may have come at the expense of validity. In other words, as a field, we may be overemphasizing categories that are, in fact, minor variations of broader underlying syndromes (Andrews, 1990, 1996; Blashfield et al., 2014; Lilienfeld, 2014). As articulated throughout this book, it is now well known that many disorders share similar biological and psychological mechanisms that contribute to their development and maintenance (e.g., Brown et al., 1998; Brown & Barlow, 2009; Cisler, Olatunji, Feldner, & Forsyth, 2010; Deacon & Abramowitz, 2006; Duval, Javanbakht, & Liberzon, 2015; Fledderus, Bohlmeijer, & Pieterse, 2010; McEvoy & Mahoney, 2012), underscoring the possibility that current DSM categories may have limited validity.

Additionally, as treatment development and testing have largely corresponded to the discrete disorders included in the DSM system, the field has witnessed a proliferation of manuals in an attempt to provide coverage for the full range of psychopathology. This is problematic for several reasons. First, given the high degree of diagnostic comorbidity among DSM disorders (e.g., Brown et al., 2001a; Kessler et al., 1998), it is troubling that protocols geared toward single diagnoses provide little guidance on how to address commonly co-occurring conditions. Indeed, in addition to limited improvement for co-occurring conditions, some studies have shown that, when comorbid disorders are present, single-diagnosis protocols demonstrate poorer outcomes for the primary targeted disorder (e.g., Craske et al., 2007; Gibbons & DeRubeis, 2008; Steketee, Chambless, & Tran, 2001). Moreover, having numerous treatment protocols, each targeting a single disorder, substantially increases therapist burden. In order to provide care consistent with many empirically supported approaches, therapists may need to complete costly training for multiple interventions (McHugh, Murray, & Barlow, 2009), perhaps dampening their enthusiasm for using them.

In an effort to address the limits of categorical classification, some have suggested moving toward a system that includes dimensional elements (e.g., Maser et al., 2009). The most notable example is the alternative model for classifying personality disorders in DSM-5 (American Psychiatric Association, 2013), described in detail below. Briefly, this model was created in response to overlapping symptoms and high rates of comorbidity across DSM personality disorders, low reliability and great heterogeneity within specific diagnoses, and overreliance on the unspecified personality disorder category (Krueger, Hopwood, Wright, & Markon, 2014; Widiger & Trull, 2007). Thus a categorical approach to this group of disorders was seen as particularly weak and in need of replacement. The DSM-5 alternative model asks clinicians to make severity ratings on a range of traits, allowing for greater specificity in communicating the deficits that drive symptoms (Hopwood, Thomas, Markon, Wright, & Krueger, 2012). A similar model has been proposed for common Axis I disorders (Brown & Barlow, 2005, 2009), and an ambitious attempt to create a comprehensive dimensional taxonomy of all psychopathology is also under way (Kotov et al., 2017). Across these proposals, dimensional models communicate important features (e.g., hostility, grandiosity, intimacy avoidance) that may then become idiographic treatment targets, rather than relying on a categorical diagnosis and applying a one-size-fits-all treatment.

DSM-5 Alternative Model of Personality Disorders

Although calls for a dimensional approach to personality disorder diagnosis began shortly after the publication of DSM-III (see Zachar & First, 2015), the inclusion of such elements was seriously considered for the fifth edition of the manual (American Psychiatric Association, 2013). The Personality and Personality Disorder Work Group was tasked with examining competing proposals that mirrored some of the same arguments put forth during the development of DSM-III—reliance on clinical experience supporting, in this case, the existence of discrete personality diagnoses versus emerging empirical data suggesting that personality pathology could be better captured via dimensional ratings. In order to satisfy both sides of the debate, the Work Group concluded that a hybrid approach to diagnosis would strike a balance between introducing dimensional elements while still preserving extant DSM categories with demonstrated clinical support (Krueger, Skodol, Livesley, Shrout, & Huang, 2007b). Thus the alternative model of personality disorders (AMPD) is described as an empirical, pantheoretical approach to understanding personality pathology and ultimately making a personality disorder diagnosis (American Psychiatric Association, 2013). Although the AMPD was approved by the DSM-5 Task Force, the Board of Trustees of the American Psychiatric Association decided to retain the traditional categorical approach in the newest edition of the manual, essentially replicating DSM-IV's Personality Disorders section. The AMPD was relegated as an "alternative model" subject to future study.

In DSM-5, personality disorders can be coded with the AMPD by using the "Other Specified Personality Disorder" (301.89) diagnosis. Utilizing the AMPD then requires fulfillment of seven general criteria. First, Criterion A (level of personality function) involves an assessment of self- (e.g., identity and self-direction) and interpersonal (e.g., empathy and intimacy) functioning, as difficulties in these areas are thought to define what personality disorders have in common that distinguishes them from healthy personality and other forms of psychopathology (Pincus, 2011). Criterion A represents Wiggins's psychodynamic, interpersonal, and personological approaches to personality assessment (see the discussion earlier in this chapter), given its focus on self–other boundaries, dynamics of self-esteem regulation, and interpersonal relatedness (Hopwood, Schade, Krueger, Wright, & Markon, 2013a). Next, Criterion B involves the assessment of dimensional personality traits, organized into five broad domains, each with 25 specific facets; levels on these facets determine the presence of a specific personality disorder. Wiggins's empirical, multivariate approach to personality assessment is reflected in Criterion B, as the five broad traits (i.e., negative affectivity, detachment, antagonism, disinhibition, and psychoticism) included here are isomorphic with the five-factor model (FFM), albeit with different labels. The developers of the AMPD view this nosological scheme as "benefiting from the cumulative wisdom of [several] great paradigms of personality assessment, . . . at once both traditional and innovative" (Waugh et al., 2017, p. 4). Finally, Criteria C through G represent additional considerations when making a mental health diagnosis, including pervasiveness, stability, age of onset, discrimination from other mental disorders, and differentiation from the effect of substances, developmental state, or sociocultural environment.

With regard to its hybrid categorical/dimensional approach, the AMPD allows for the diagnosis of six specific personality disorder categories by utilizing algorithms that combine trait ratings; these include antisocial, avoidant, borderline, narcissistic, obsessive–compulsive, and schizotypal personality disorders (American Psychiatric Association, 2013). For example, after establishing the presence of Criterion A, antisocial personality disorder can be represented as a combination of the following trait facet dimensions: manipulativeness, callousness, deceitfulness, hostility, risk taking, impulsivity, and irresponsibility (see Waugh et al., 2017). Of course, maladaptive personality functioning can exist outside of these six algorithms and can be coded in the AMPD as "personality disorder—trait specified"; here, clinically significant traits are described, rather than using a shorthand category that represents a set constellation of traits.

Negative affectivity with the AMPD is meant to represent pathologically high levels of neuroticism; indeed, within DSM-5, this construct is defined as "frequent and intense experiences of high levels of a wide range of negative emotions (e.g., anxiety, depression, guilt/shame, worry, anger)" (American Psychiatric Association, 2013, p. 779). The negative affectivity domain is further broken down to the following facets: emotional lability, anxiousness, depressiveness, perseveration, submissiveness, and separation insecurity. With regard to the six personality disorder categories retained in DSM-5, facets of negative affectivity are involved in the identification of avoidant personality disorder (anxiousness), borderline personality disorder (anxiousness, depressivity, emotional lability, and separation insecurity), and obsessive–compulsive personality disorder (perseveration). Given that the AMPD is a classification system specifically for personality disorders, the majority of the empirical work related to its facets has focused on their association with traditional personality disorder categories. In a recent meta-analysis, for example, Watters, Bagby, and Sellbom (2019) examined 25 independent samples that included measurement of the AMPD traits and at least one traditional personality disorder diagnosis. Their findings suggest that there is general support for the facets proposed for each personality disorder, though discriminant validity was weak for several diagnoses (i.e., categorical diagnoses were associated with additional facets beyond the ones proposed by the AMPD).

Assessment

DSM-5 uses the Levels of Personality Functioning Scale (LPFS; Bender, Morey, & Skodol, 2011) to operationalize and measure the self and interpersonal dysfunction that characterizes Criterion A. This tool consists of four constructs (identity, self-directedness, empathy, and intimacy) and requires raters to match patient behavior to prototypical manifestations of each construct; these manifestations are ordered in terms of severity, allowing raters to determine the overall personality disorder severity for a given patient. Empirical research on the validity of Criterion A and its assessment suggests that LPFS scores of moderate or greater demonstrated 84.6% sensitivity and 72.7% specificity when classifying patients who met criteria for at least traditional personality disorder diagnosis (Morey, Skodol, & Oldham, 2014). Moreover, Criterion A provided significant incremental validity when predicting functional impairment and prognosis, beyond the combined contribution of 10 traditional personality disorder categories (Morey et al., 2014).

Of course, assessment of the personality traits included in the AMPD's Criterion B is most germane to our consideration of neuroticism within mental health classification systems. These traits can be systematically assessed with the Personality Inventory for DSM-5 (PID-5; Krueger, Derringer, Markon, Watson, & Skodol, 2012), which has versions for self-, other-, and clinician reports, as well as a short form. Overall, given that the traits included in the AMPD were gleaned from factor analytic work using the PID-5 in large representative population samples, it is not surprising that its factor structure was replicated in other samples (e.g., undergraduates, community samples, informant reports; Creswell, Bachrach, Wright, Pinto, & Ansell, 2016; Markon, Quilty, Bagby, & Krueger, 2013; Wright et al., 2012). Moreover, the PID-5 has received empirical support for its content validity (e.g., Anderson et al., 2013; Hopwood, Wright, Ansell, & Pincus, 2013b), as well as its stability (Wright et al., 2015). Additionally, with regard to criterion validity, the PID-5 traits significantly predicted future dysfunction, and individual changes in the traits over time were associated with changes in functioning (Wright et al., 2015). In contrast to the previous paradigm of assessing personality and mental disorders separately, the PID-5 represents an innovative step forward given its ability to characterize these related constructs simultaneously.

Personality Disorders in ICD-11

The WHO has recently (i.e., May 2019) released the 11th version of the ICD, which will go into effect in 2022. With regard to personality disorder diagnoses, the ICD-11 will formally adopt a five-domain dimensional trait model similar to the DSM-5 AMPD. ICD-11 domains include negative affectivity, detachment, disinhibition, dissociality, and anankastia (i.e., compulsivity). The first four traits are isomorphic with DSM-5 negative affectivity, detachment, antagonism, and disinhibition, respectively. The omission of DSM-5 psychoticism in ICD-11 makes sense given that this domain is more associated with schizotypal features, which the WHO has historically not considered within the personality disorder purview. The DSM-5 AMPD proposal did, at one point in its development, include a domain of compulsivity that was eventually dropped to promote brevity; of note, some have argued that two facets of the PID-5, perseveration and rigid perfectionism, can be used to assess for ICD-11 anankastia (Bach et al., 2017).

An additional, perhaps more radical, difference between the ICD-11 and the DSM-5 conceptions of personality disorders is the replacement of all categorical diagnoses with trait descriptors (Tyrer, Mulder, & Crawford, 2019; Tyrer, Reed, & Crawford, 2015). This shift, supported by field trials for ICD-11 (i.e., Kim, Blashfield, Tyrer, Hwang, & Lee, 2014; Kim et al., 2015; Mulder, Horwood, Tyrer, Carter, & Joyce, 2016; Tyrer, 2014; Tyrer, Tyrer, Yang, & Guo, 2016), represents a huge step forward for dimensional classification, as the ICD is the authoritative classification system of mental disorders for the WHO's 194 member states (including the United States). In response to recent criticism (see Herpertz et al., 2017), however, the ICD-11 proposal has added ratings of self- and interpersonal dysfunction to better align with DSM-5 Criterion A. Additionally, a specific borderline personality disorder pattern qualifier is now included, along with the dimensional ratings, despite the fact that this condition is naturally embedded within the trait model (i.e., composed of negative affectivity, dissociality, and disinhibition).

Assessment

Three assessment tools have been developed to capture personality dysfunction as conceptualized by the ICD-11 system. Specifically, the Personality Inventory for ICD-11 (PiCD; Oltmanns & Widiger, 2019) can be used to measure dimensional traits generally, whereas the Borderline Pattern Specifier (BPS; Oltmanns & Widiger, 2019) specifically determines whether borderline personality disorder is present. Additionally, the Standardized Assessment of Severity of Personality Disorder (SASPD; Olajide et al., 2018) is used to determine the severity level of personality dysfunction. Given that, at the time of this writing, the ICD-11 proposal is still quite new, limited psychometric studies of its personality disorder assessment tools have been conducted. However, in one study, the ICD-11 personality disorder diagnostic system aligns well with the DSM-5 AMPD, perhaps with better discriminant validity between conditions obtained with the PiCD compared with the PID-5 (McCabe & Widiger, 2020).

Dimensional Proposals for Emotional Disorders

Beyond personality disorders, mental health classification systems that include dimensional elements have also been described for emotional disorders (e.g., anxiety, depressive, and related disorders; Brown & Barlow, 2005, 2009). For example, in 2005, Brown and Barlow proposed incorporating dimensional severity ratings into extant diagnostic categories (an approach utilized in their structured diagnostic interview, the ADIS; Brown et al., 1994a). They argued that this method could be readily employed given that the categorical system would remain in place and the dimensional ratings could be dropped for settings wherein they would not be feasible to collect. Brown and Barlow (2005) argued that adding a dimensional severity rating for each diagnosis would provide important additional information. For example, categories that delineate whether a person does or does not have a disorder fail to indicate the severity of the condition, nor do they allow clinicians to characterize dysfunction that may fall just short of conventional diagnostic thresholds (i.e., subclinical presentations). However, given that this proposal builds on the existing DSM system, issues reviewed above that continue to plague this approach to classification remain.

Thus, in 2009, Brown and Barlow updated their proposal to reflect the existence of higher order dimensions of temperament that confer risk for the range of emotional-disorder presentations. As described in Chapter 3, there is strong evidence that neuroticism and, to a lesser degree, extraversion are important for the development and maintenance of anxiety, depressive, and related disorders (e.g., Brown et al., 1998; Brown, 2007; Gruber et al., 2008; Mineka et al., 1998). Moreover, these constructs can account for the overlap between discrete anxiety disorders and depression (Brown, 2007). Specifically, Brown et al. (1998) found that virtually all temporal covariance among latent variables corresponding to DSM-IV constructs of depression, social anxiety disorder, GAD, OCD, and panic disorder (with or without agoraphobia) could be explained by higher order dimensions of neuroticism and extraversion (see Figure 3.2).

Brown and Barlow (2009) also acknowledged that an exclusive focus on temperament may be "overly reductionist" (p. 264) given that there is still variation in how clinical disorders manifest (e.g., social anxiety presents differently from generalized anxiety), despite etiological overlap, as described in Chapter 2. Thus they proposed several additional constructs that represent lower order phenotypes; although they are typically associated with a particular disorder, these dimensions may also be present transdiagnostically. First, the *depressed mood* and *mania* dimensions capture excessive sadness and positive affect and are useful to assess for the purposes of risk management. The *autonomic arousal* dimension is defined by the experience of physiological symptoms due to sympathetic nervous system activation often observed in panic disorder, though it can occur in the context of any disorder, as panic attacks are ubiquitous. *Somatic anxiety* reflects distress over somatic symptoms and is associated with worry about health; although somatic anxiety represents a distinct DSM category, it is also observed in GAD (Lee, Ma, & Tsang, 2011), panic disorder (Hiller, Leibbrand, Rief, & Fichter, 2005), and obsessive–compulsive disorders (Abramowitz et al.,

1999). The *social anxiety* dimension indicates fear of negative evaluation in interaction and performance situations. *Intrusive cognitions* reflect the experience of uncontrollable thoughts, images, and impulses that are the hallmark feature of OCD, though there is evidence that they are present across the emotional disorders (Brewin, Gregory, Lipton, & Burgess, 2010). The *traumatic reexperiencing* dimension refers to the dissociative and flashback experiences associated with past traumatic events. Finally, the *avoidance dimension* represents behavioral and cognitive strategies to prevent or reduce the intensity of emotional experiences (both negative and positive). Here, the neurotic and positive temperament dimensions represent the generalized biological and psychological vulnerabilities for emotional disorders (described in Chapter 2), and the domains representing the specific foci of distress correspond to the specific psychological vulnerability described in Chapter 4.

A dimensional system that includes not only higher order dimensions of temperament that confer broad risk but also more specific features that may be present transdiagnostically paints a more comprehensive clinical picture than a categorical (yes–no) diagnosis. Specific examples of disorder profiles gleaned from the Brown and Barlow (2009) proposal highlight the heuristic clinical value associated with dimensional classification of emotional disorders. For example, individuals with a principal diagnosis of panic disorder would likely display profiles with high levels of neuroticism, avoidance, and preoccupation with panic/autonomic arousal and other somatic symptoms. In contrast, patients presenting with PTSD might display high neuroticism and preoccupation with panic/autonomic arousal (flashbacks) and past trauma. Although each diagnostic category is linked to a prototypical dimensional profile, this classification system would allow clinicians to determine the extent to which other key features are present that would potentially affect treatment planning.

Assessment

Recently, a new measure, the Multidimensional Emotional Disorder Inventory (MEDI; Rosellini & Brown, 2019), was developed to assess the vulnerabilities and characteristics of emotional disorders included in Brown and Barlow's (2009) proposal with a single assessment tool. Factor analysis of the 49-item measure yielded a 9-factor solution (representing the dimensions described above), with each item loading most strongly on its intended subscale. To illustrate the information that can be gleaned from a MEDI profile, we present a case example. The patient depicted in this profile, a 28-year-old Latinx female, had been assigned a DSM-5 diagnosis of OCD to reflect the significant interference and distress associated with her intrusive thoughts (e.g., doubting, contamination and germs, unwanted sexual thoughts) and their accompanying compulsive behaviors (e.g., checking locks and appliances, excessive cleaning, and rigid adherence to time-consuming routines, such as grooming). She also met diagnostic criteria for social anxiety disorder, GAD, and persistent depressive disorder with intermittent MDD. The patient reported panic attacks cued by both intrusive thoughts and social situations. With regard to her MEDI profile, the patient displayed elevations on all subscales ranging from mild to severe symptoms, with the exception of the Positive Temperament (Extraversion) subscale. The most severe elevations were exhibited on the Neurotic Temperament, Intrusive Cognitions, and Social Concerns subscales, followed by moderate elevation on Somatic Anxiety, Depressed Mood, and Avoidance and mild elevation on Autonomic Anxiety and Traumatic Re-experiencing. A dimensional measure such as the MEDI has promise for clinical utility, given its ability to characterize a number of transdiagnostic signs and symptoms that may not be readily apparent with a DSM diagnostic label.

Research Domain Criteria (RDoC)

Another proposal for understanding the full range of psychopathology from a more dimensional point of view, and in response to the limitations of the DSM's categorical approach, was created by NIMH: the Research Domain Criteria (RDoC; Insel et al., 2010).* Instead of determining whether an individual meets criteria for a psychiatric diagnosis based on presenting signs and symptoms, RDoC anchor psychiatric classification and diagnosis into a dimensional matrix system. The RDoC matrix consists of five broad domains thought to be important for a range of psychopathology, including the negative valence system, positive valence system, cognitive systems, systems for social processes, and arousal/modulatory systems. These domains are then crossed with various levels of analysis such as genes, molecules, cells, circuits, physiology, behavior, and self-reports. RDoC are not currently envisioned as a system of psychiatric classification in their own right (Insel, 2014); instead, they are viewed as a facilitator of long-term research that may ultimately yield the outlines of such a system (Macdonald & Krueger, 2013).

RDoC share features with the dimensional proposals for classification that we have previously described. For example, the RDoC approach is consistent with a dimensional understanding of psychopathology, though it does allow for the possibility of threshold effects ("tipping points") whereby some psychopathological phenomena may differ qualitatively rather than

---

*The name of this proposal, Research Domain Criteria, bears striking similarity to another paradigm-shifting NIMH initiative, the Research Diagnostic Criteria (RDC; Spitzer et al., 1978), which paved the way for the (once revolutionary) DSM-III classification system.

quantitatively from normality (i.e., categorical effects; Cuthbert & Insel, 2013). Additionally, more than the previous proposals, RDoC explicitly strive to be truly translational in emphasis, encouraging researchers to relate the basic science of brain systems to the behaviors and symptoms that represent mental disorders. Applying the burgeoning literature created by clinical neuroscience research to the classification and etiology of psychopathology continues the pioneering work of Eysenck and Gray that aimed to connect self-report and behavioral manifestations of temperament to underlying brain structures.

Though RDoC ostensibly ascribe equal weight to the different levels of analysis (Cuthbert & Insel, 2013), some have argued that, in practice (i.e., how NIMH funding is allocated), biological mechanisms have been overemphasized (e.g., Lilienfeld, 2014; Lilienfeld & Treadway, 2016; Persson, 2019). Although all mental disorders have some neural input, it is reductionist to assume, as some think RDoC do, that biological mediation is synonymous with biological etiology. As we describe in Chapter 2, a mental disorder may have etiological roots in environmental factors that subsequently influence neural structures, and a classification system that solely focuses on biology would miss this information. Additionally, likely motivated by their prioritization of biological mechanisms, RDoC discourage drawing conclusions solely on the basis of self-report data. This, too, may be shortsighted, as "there are no biomarkers that can be used to clinically confirm a diagnosis or identify a given individual as at risk, and it is not clear that the candidate biomarkers that exist do a better job identifying cases than existing interview methods" (Iacono, Malone, & Vrieze, 2017, p. 117). Despite the imbalance of emphasis placed on biological and behavioral mechanisms in the RDoC system, the charge to connect these constructs remains necessary, particularly for understanding the relationship between personality/temperament and psychopathology.

With regard to personality variables within this classification scheme, RDoC's negative valence system is most closely aligned with neuroticism and is further divided into five constructs: responses to acute threat (fear), responses to potential harm (anxiety), responses to sustained threat, frustrative nonreward, and loss. The first construct, *responses to acute threat* (fear), refers to activation of the defensive motivational system to promote behaviors that protect the organism from perceived danger. Next, *responses to potential harm* (anxiety) are characterized by activation of a brain system in which harm may potentially occur but is distant, or ambiguous, along with behavioral responses that include heightened vigilance. *Responses to sustained threat* describes an aversive emotional state caused by prolonged exposure to internal or external conditions or stimuli that would be adaptive to escape from or avoid. *Frustrated nonreward* occurs in response to withdrawal or prevention of reward (i.e., the inability to obtain positive rewards following repeated or sustained efforts). Finally, *loss* refers to a state of deprivation of a motivationally significant event, object, or situation; loss may be social or nonsocial and may include permanent or sustained loss of shelter, behavioral control, status, loved ones, or relationships.

Assessment

Given that the RDoC matrix spans multiple units of analysis (i.e., genes, neurotransmitters, behaviors), there are no comprehensive assessment tools to measure its negative valence system. Of course, as noted previously, one advantage of RDoC's conceptualization of neuroticism is its translational view of this trait ("Negative Valence System"). Thus relevant genes (e.g., *BDNF, 5HT*), molecules (e.g., serotonin, gamma-aminobutyric acid [GABA]), circuits (e.g., sustained amygdala reactivity), and physiology (e.g., HPA axis dysregulation) are represented within its purview. (See our review of these biological mechanisms in Chapter 2.) Although understanding the biological underpinnings of common mental health conditions may provide new insights that inform intervention, it is unlikely that assessment of these constructs will ever routinely occur in clinical practice settings. Instead, behavioral indicators and self-report measures (that will hopefully be correlated with neurological/physiological vulnerabilities) are likely to remain the norm given their feasibility to administer and interpret; in fact, considerable progress has already been made toward a personality neuroscience, particularly for neuroticism (DeYoung et al., 2010).

The NIMH website lists several self-report measures to assess constructs within the RDoC negative valence system. In a recent study, Gore and Widiger (2018) explored relationships between neuroticism and selected self-report measures suggested in the RDoC matrix. For example, in this study, the Beck Anxiety Inventory (Beck & Steer, 1993) was used to measure RDoC's acute threat construct, whereas the Hopelessness Depression Symptom Questionnaire (Uliaszek, Al-Dajani, & Bagby, 2015) provided coverage for loss, and the Buss–Durkee Hostility Index (Buss & Durkee, 1957) assessed frustrative nonreward. Of note, no specific measures for acute threat (fear) and potential threat (anxiety) are currently included in the RDoC matrix; the Negative Affect subscale of the Positive and Negative Affect Schedule (PANAS; Watson & Clark, 1994a), however, was also used as a general measure of the negative valence system. In order to create a composite variable to reflect the negative valence system of the RDoC, Gore and Widiger (2018) utilized z-scores, which transform and average the total score from each measure. The negative valence system demonstrated substantial convergence not only with FFM neuroticism (measured with the NEO-PI-R [Costa & McCrae, 1992] and the Big Five Aspects Scale [DeYoung et al., 2007]), but also with the negative affectivity domain of the DSM-5 AMPD (assessed with the PID-5; Krueger et al., 2012). This consistency across two proposed models of psychopathology (i.e., RDoC and the AMPD), along with their alignment with conceptions of normal personality functioning (i.e., FFM), continues to underscore the importance of including neuroticism in any dimensional classification system for psychopathology.

Hierarchical Taxonomy of Psychopathology

Similar to early factor analytic work in which symptoms of common mental disorders were reduced to high-order dimensions resembling temperament (e.g., Tellegen, 1985; Achenbach, 1966; see Chapter 1), the hierarchical taxonomy of psychopathology (HiTOP) represents a more recent quantitative approach to understanding psychopathology (Kotov et al., 2017). It was developed by a "consortium of clinical researchers who aim to develop an empirically-driven classification system based on advances in quantitative research on the organization of psychopathology" (Kotov et al., 2017, p. 456). Consortium members describe their model as an evolving system that is updated as new data emerge, with the core assumption that a more valid nosological system can be developed on the basis of empirical clustering of phenotypes (e.g., symptoms of mental disorders).

HiTOP conceptualizes psychopathology as dimensional and, as the name suggests, organized hierarchically such that it can be described at various levels. At the top of the hierarchy is a *superfactor* of General Psychopathology, often referred to as the p factor (Caspi et al., 2014; Kotov et al., 2017). This p factor is analogous to the g (i.e., General Intelligence) factor that has been proposed to explain the covariation among cognitive ability tasks (see Neisser et al., 1996). The p factor has emerged in studies examining psychopathology categorically and dimensionally (Caspi et al., 2014; Laceulle, Vollebergh, & Ormel, 2015; Olino, Dougherty, Bufferd, Carlson, & Klein, 2014; Tackett et al., 2013).

Organized beneath p, the HiTOP model also contains broad factors, called *spectra*, that distinguish between major forms of psychopathology. Spectra are defined as the most basic factors of psychopathology that can be distinguished from a general predisposition to mental disorder (Kotov et al., 2017). As introduced briefly in Chapter 1, Achenbach (1966) was the first to uncover clinical spectra in his seminal factor analytic studies. Specifically, his work yielded two primary dimensions: *Internalizing*, which subsumed anxiety, depressive, and somatic symptoms, and *Externalizing*, to capture aggressive and rule-breaking forms of psychopathology. More recently, Krueger and Markon (2006a) added a third factor, labeled *Thought Problems*, and HiTOP expands this to six proposed spectra: Internalizing, Disinhibited Externalizing, Antagonistic Externalizing, Thought Disorder, Detachment, and Somatoform.

The next level of the HiTOP model, beneath spectra, is referred to as "subfactors," which disaggregates Internalizing into Sexual Problems, Eating Problems, Fear, and Distress and breaks Externalizing into Substance Abuse and Antisocial Behavior (Kotov et al., 2017). Next, subfactors are further broken down into syndromes/disorders that roughly correspond to DSM categories (e.g., the Fear subfactor comprises agoraphobia, OCD, panic disorder, social anxiety disorder, and specific phobia). The HiTOP consortium notes that research establishing these levels within their model is provisional (Kotov et al., 2017; Brandes & Tackett, 2019).

A large literature exists with studies describing relationships between the dimensions included in HiTOP and neuroticism. Given that p confers risk for the broadest range of psychopathology, research suggests that it consists predominantly of neuroticism and, to a lesser degree, extraversion and conscientiousness (Uliaszek et al., 2015). Indeed, there is robust support for the strong association between p and neuroticism (Brandes & Tackett, 2019; Caspi et al., 2014; Olino et al., 2014; Tackett et al., 2013). With regard to spectra, the strongest research literature links neuroticism to internalizing problems; indeed, studies with varied methods (longitudinal, cross-sectional) and samples (children, adolescents, adults; e.g., Clark & Watson, 1991; Griffith et al., 2010), have demonstrated that neuroticism is a key vulnerability for internalizing disorders (see Barlow et al., 2014b). There is, however, some specificity within this broad relationship; for example, withdrawal and anxiety-related facets of (FFM) neuroticism demonstrate the greatest associations with internalizing disorders, whereas the anger-related facet of this trait is a less robust predictor of this class of conditions (Zinbarg et al., 2016). Beyond Internalizing, there is also evidence that the propensity to experience negative emotions is associated with the Somatoform and Thought Disorder spectra. With regard to the relationship between an overall neuroticism factor and somatoform disorders, meta-analytic work suggests a strong association between these constructs (Malouff, Thorsteinsson, & Schutte, 2005). The Thought Disorder spectrum in the HiTOP model consists of both psychosis- and bipolar-related conditions and has only recently been studied alongside personality traits (Brandes & Tackett, 2019). Neuroticism is strongly related to the severity of bipolar disorder (both manic and depressive symptoms; Quilty, Sellbom, Tackett, & Bagby, 2009), as well as prospectively predicting schizophrenia and psychosis (Drvaric, Bagby, Kiang, & Mizrahi, 2018; Myin-Germeys & van Os, 2007). Moreover, when Caspi and colleagues (2014) created a Thought Disorder factor consisting of bipolar, psychotic, and obsessive–compulsive symptoms, its association with neuroticism was quite strong ($r = .41$). Of course, with the exception of Caspi et al.'s (2014) work, support for the relationships between neuroticism and HiTOP spectra has largely come from studies associating this trait to the DSM disorders that fall within each spectrum. More research is needed to fully understand how the broad dimension of neuroticism, as well as its lower order facets, relates to HiTOP spectra.

Relationships between neuroticism and externalizing psychopathology have also been explored (e.g., Eisenberg et al., 2009; Kotov, Gamez, Schmidt, & Watson, 2010; Tackett & Lahey, 2017). Indeed, neuroticism demonstrates moderate to large correlations with conditions that fall within the Disinhibited Externalizing spectrum (i.e., substance use disorders; Kotov et al., 2010; Malouff et al., 2005; Ruiz, Pincus, & Schinka, 2008). In the context of Antagonistic Externalizing (primarily operationalized as antisocial behavior and narcissism), correlations with neuroticism have been moderate and negative (e.g., grandiose narcissism; Miller, Lynam, Hyatt, & Campbell, 2017), small and positive (e.g., antisocial behavior; Ruiz et al., 2008), and moderate/large and positive (e.g., vulnerable narcissism; Miller et al., 2017). Additionally, after accounting for the general relationship between Externalizing and the propensity for negative affect, neuroticism facets display specific associations within this spectrum. For example, anger and irritability facets are strongly correlated with Externalizing (Brandes & Tackett, 2019), while anxiety facets are not (Brandes & Tackett, 2019; Zinbarg et al., 2016). Finally, the relationship between neuroticism and the HiTOP spectrum of Detachment, conceptualized as the interpersonal symptoms of social withdrawal and low expressiveness, is less well established. Indeed, the FFM trait that best captures detachment appears to be low extraversion (Wright & Simms, 2015). Taken together, this body of work suggests that neuroticism conveys risk for a broad range of psychopathology, though externalizing disorders are also characterized by low agreeableness (antagonistic externalizing) and low conscientiousness (disinhibited externalizing).

In terms of HiTOP subfactor relationships with neuroticism, there is evidence to suggest that there may be predictive utility in considering lower order facets of neuroticism when examining psychopathology at the subfactor or syndrome level. For example, several studies have shown that psychopathology that falls into the Distress category (e.g., GAD, depression) is best accounted for by distress and depression facets over and above the contribution of the other facets (Naragon-Gainey, Watson, & Markon, 2009; Naragon-Gainey & Watson, 2018). Other research, however, has not found this predictive specificity (Bagby, Quilty, & Ryder, 2008; Walton, Pantoja, & McDermut, 2018). For Eating Problems, meta-analytic work shows strong associations between a higher order neuroticism factor and this class of conditions (Malouff et al., 2005), as well as significant relationships between eating difficulties and several neuroticism facets (anxiety, depression, vulnerability, and impulsivity; Terracciano et al., 2009b), though the depression facet appears to explain the most variance (Ellickson-Larew, Naragon-Gainey, & Watson, 2013). Finally, Sexual Problems also shows strong prospective and concurrent associations with neuroticism (Forbes, Baillie, Eaton, & Krueger, 2017), though limited research has been conducted at the facet level.

Assessment

Similar to RDoC, a comprehensive assessment tool that can simultaneously assess all levels in the HiTOP system has not been developed. On their website, the members of the HiTOP Measures Development Workgroup have listed a number of instruments that are relevant for at least some of the spectra, subfactors, syndromes, and components. For example, at the spectra level, they suggest using the Achenbach System of Empirically Based Assessment (Achenbach & Rescorla, 2004) and the Child and Adolescent Psychopathology Scale (Reynolds, 1993) for Internalizing and Disinhibited Externalizing. The Externalizing Spectrum Inventory (Krueger et al., 2007a) is recommended to specifically assess Disinhibited Externalizing, whereas the Inventory for Depression and Anxiety Symptoms (Watson et al., 2007) represents a specific measure of Internalizing. Additionally, the Scale for the Assessment of Negative Symptoms (Andreasen, 1989) and the Scale for the Assessment of Positive Symptoms (Andreasen, 1984) can be used to measure the Thought Disorder spectrum of HiTOP. Finally, the HiTOP Measures Development Workgroup note that the Personality Assessment Inventory (Morey, 1991) is equipped to capture five of six spectra (Somatoform is not accounted for by this measure), making it the most comprehensive tool listed. Given that the HiTOP system is relatively new, considerably more research is needed to understand its clinical utility.

Summary

We have described four dimensional alternatives to the DSM's categorical classification system. In each model, a domain that captures an individual's tendency to experience negative emotions is featured prominently: negative affectivity in the AMPD, neurotic temperament in Brown and Barlow's (2009) proposal for emotional disorders, negative valence system in the RDoC matrix, and Internalizing in HiTOP. This makes sense given that prior research has repeatedly shown that the propensity to experience negative emotions is strongly linked to the development, maintenance, and severity of symptoms across anxiety and depressive disorders and has demonstrated substantial explanatory power as higher order variables (see Barlow et al., 2014b; Brown & Barlow, 2009; Clark, 2005). Similarly, within the child literature, the tendency to express distress inward or to "internalize" has similarly been shown to account for the co-occurrence of anxiety and depressive disorders (e.g., Kovacs & Devlin, 1998; Krueger, 1999). Though this research has been paramount in advancing our understanding of co-occurring psychological disorders, these higher order descriptive variables alone may lack clinical utility as intervention targets. Indeed, HiTOP and RDoC conceptions of negative affectivity represent a composite of heterogeneous symptoms that hang together statistically. Even models that feature neuroticism as a personality trait more specifically (i.e., the AMPD and Brown and Barlow's proposal for emotional disorders) may not translate easily to clinical practice, as it is unclear what it means to "treat" neuroticism. Thus a classification that includes functional, intermediate transdiagnostic mechanisms that are more proximally related to clinical phenotypes may provide more useful information regarding putative intervention targets.

> We need a classification that includes mechanisms closely related to clinical phenotypes.

A FUNCTIONAL MODEL AS A BRIDGE BETWEEN PERSONALITY AND PSYCHOPATHOLOGY

Despite a large body of literature supporting the strong association between personality features and psychopathology, as well as initiatives to incorporate temperamental factors into nosological schemes, this research has had little influence on day-to-day therapeutic practice, particularly in cognitive-behavioral traditions that focus primarily on addressing DSM disorder symptoms. This lack of integration is unfortunate, as there are numerous advantages to adopting a personality-informed model of psychopathology (e.g., HiTOP, AMPD). The prevailing categorical-prototypical approach, in which patients are assigned diagnoses and treated with the associated intervention protocol(s), creates an enormous training burden for clinicians who must learn numerous discrete treatments in order to provide empirically supported care. Moreover, patients do not fit neatly within our nosological categories (due to subthreshold symptoms or diagnostic comorbidity, for example), leading to diagnosis-specific treatments that do not align with real-world clinical presentations. Thus, a limited number of personality-informed dimensions (e.g., neuroticism, extraversion) has the potential to significantly streamline care.

Despite the promise of a hierarchical system in which psychopathology is organized beneath shared dimensions of personality, clinicians may be hesitant to adopt such an approach because they simply don't know what it means to treat "neuroticism," "internalizing," or "disinhibition." Recently, however, there has been an increased focus on understanding cognitive and behavioral treatment techniques that address intermediate dimensional mechanisms that may functionally link psychopathology and personality. These transdiagnostic constructs include anxiety sensitivity, experiential avoidance, distress intolerance, and intolerance of uncertainty, each of which refers to the tendency to find emotional experiences aversive. As reviewed in Chapter 4, there is ample evidence linking these processes to DSM disorder severity, and they may *also* provide a functional link between personality, specifically internalizing/neuroticism (i.e., the tendency to experience negative emotions), and the typical diagnostic categories (e.g., GAD, OCD) addressed in psychotherapy.

Treatment techniques under development will target mechanisms that link psychopathology and personality.

In our model, individuals with a trait-like propensity for negative affect (personality), who find these emotional experiences aversive (intermediate dimensional mechanism), engage in behavioral strategies to escape or avoid these experiences (e.g., leaving a feared situation; engaging in nonsuicidal self-injury; DSM disorder symptoms such as checking and worry). Focusing on the functional mechanisms (i.e., aversive reactivity to emotion as experiences) that connect personality vulnerabilities and symptoms may shed light on treatment targets that are naturally amenable to change, increasing the acceptability of personality-based classification systems. Indeed, our work with neuroticism suggests that interventions specifically targeting aversive reactions to emotional experiences lead to improvement in both symptoms of psychopathology and the trait itself (see Chapter 6).

The incorporation of functional elements into a system of mental health classification is not inconsistent with the dimensional proposals described previously. In fact, understanding the mechanisms through which an individual's symptoms are functionally related to higher order dimensions of psychopathology provides valuable information to inform treatment approaches. This is particularly the case for disorders/symptoms that load onto multiple higher order dimensions/spectra. For example, borderline personality disorder (BPD) is captured on both the Internalizing and Antagonistic Externalizing spectra in the HiTOP system. Similarly, this condition, in the AMPD, is composed of facets from negative affectivity, disinhibition, and psychoticism. If an individual patient's interpersonal difficulties, for example, are the result of internalizing psychopathology, the treatment approach would be different than it would be if this symptom were mediated by Antagonistic Externalizing. In the following section, we demonstrate how a functional understanding of the relationship between symptoms and higher order dimensions can paint a more comprehensive picture of an individual's difficulties that can be used to inform treatment. In particular, we focus on disorders/symptoms that may result from more than one higher order input (i.e., neuroticism, externalizing) in order to highlight the importance of differential functional assessment. Additionally, given the focus on neuroticism in this book, our discussion prioritizes constructs that represent aversive reactivity to emotional experiences as the bridge between this trait and symptoms (see Chapter 4); however, we note that similar functional constructs can be identified to link psychopathology to other broad domains of personality (see Chapter 7).

Determining Functional Relationships between Personality and Symptoms

For a full review of psychopathology that results from neuroticism coupled with aversive reactivity to emotional experiences, see Bullis and colleagues (2019). To illustrate how focusing on the intermediate, functional mechanism between neuroticism and symptoms (i.e., constructs representing aversive reactions to emotions) can inform treatment, we turn to eating disorders as our exemplar. Eating disorders are clearly located on the Internalizing spectrum in the HiTOP model; indeed, individuals with anorexia nervosa and bulimia nervosa score higher than healthy controls on measures of neuroticism (Cassin & von Ranson, 2005; Forbush & Watson, 2006), and this trait prospectively predicts disordered eating (Fox & Froom, 2009; Wildes & Ringham, 2010). With regard to aversive reactivity, individuals with eating disorders report strong negative beliefs about emotions and less acceptance of their emotional experiences (Brockmeyer et al., 2014; Harrison, Sullivan, Tchanturia, & Treasure, 2009, 2010; Ioannou & Fox, 2009; Lawson, Emanuelli, Sines, & Waller, 2008; Svaldi, Griepenstroh, Tuschen-Caffier, & Ehring, 2012), which are associated with anorexia symptom severity (Hambrook et al., 2011) and can even differentiate between individuals with current symptoms and those in recovery (Oldershaw et al., 2012).

Characteristic behaviors seen in individuals with eating disorders include restriction, bingeing and purging, mirror checking, and excessive exercise, which have recently been conceptualized as efforts to escape aversive emotional experiences (Kolar, Hammerle, Jenetzky, Huss, & Bürger, 2016; Wildes, Ringham, & Marcus, 2010). Studies with longitudinal designs and frequent assessment have shown that acute increases in negative affect predict ritualized eating, purging, and weighing behaviors in women with anorexia and that engaging in these behaviors led to significant decreases in emotional intensity (Engel et al., 2013). Similarly, for individuals high in self-reported neuroticism, greater lability in negative affect predicted frequency of binge-eating episodes (De Young, Zander, & Anderson, 2014). With regard to aversive reactions to emotions, daily fluctuations in patients' willingness to tolerate unpleasant emotions predicted anorexia-related cognitions and behaviors, and improvements in emotion regulation are associated with treatment gains for patients with eating disorders (Racine & Wildes, 2015; Rowsell, MacDonald, & Carter, 2016).

Thus typically cited etiological factors for eating disorders (e.g., idealization of thinness and body dissatisfaction; Stice & Shaw, 2002; Thompson & Stice, 2001) may serve as triggers for acute emotional experiences against the backdrop of the neurotic temperament. Aversive reactions to these emotions and maladaptive attempts to regulate them function to maintain eating psychopathology and represent targets for treatment. Although we discuss treatment for aversive/avoidant responses to emotional experiences in the next chapter, it is worth noting preliminary evidence that recently developed intervention approaches designed explicitly to address aversive reactivity to negative emotional experiences result in significant improvements in eating-disorder symptoms (Thompson-Brenner et al., 2018a).

There are also instances in which psychopathology does not fit so neatly within a spectrum/dimension of the proposed classification systems. Thus, in these cases, it is necessary to conduct a functional analysis of an individual's symptoms to better understand the factors maintaining them. For example, substance use disorders represent a diagnostic category for which treatment approaches may differ based on a functional examination. For individuals who find the experience of negative affect intolerable and use substances as a means to escape or avoid their emotions, it is likely that their substance use disorders can be conceptualized within the neurotic/internalizing spectrum. Indeed, substance use disorders are often associated with elevated levels of neuroticism/negative emotionality (Kotov et al., 2007; Swendsen, Conway, Rounsaville, & Merikangas, 2002) and are highly comorbid with anxiety and depressive disorders (Grant et al., 2008; Trull, Sher, Minks-Brown, Durbin, & Burr, 2000). Moreover, there is evidence to suggest that many individuals engage in substance use to dampen or reduce unwanted emotional experiences, such as worry or depressed mood (Bolton, Robinson, & Sareen, 2009; Cooper, Frone, Russell, & Mudar, 1995; Robinson, Sareen, Cox, & Bolton, 2009), and that low distress tolerance may mediate this relationship (Buckner et al., 2007; Bujarski, Norberg, & Copeland, 2012). Finally, there is evidence to suggest that psychological treatments that target how individuals interpret and relate to their emotions may be effective in reducing heavy drinking among patients with alcohol use disorders (Ciraulo et al., 2013).

Of course, it's worth noting that, in the HiTOP model, substance abuse is formally listed as falling within the Disinhibited Externalizing spectrum. Possible intermediate mechanisms that may connect substance use with its higher order dimension of personality include various forms of impulsivity (e.g., sensation seeking, lack of planning; Crawford, Pentz, Chou, Li, & Dwyer, 2003). If an individual patient's substance use falls within the Externalizing spectra, maintained by impulsive mechanisms, targeting aversive reactivity to emotional experiences should not lead to significant improvements in this target. Thus a functional analysis is necessary to determine whether the presentation is consistent with a pattern of emotion intolerance and avoidance or driven by other factors in order to select the appropriate treatment. Of course, in some patients, both spectra might be contributory.

To take another example of how functional assessment can better elucidate the intermediate mechanisms that link specific disorders to their higher order vulnerabilities, we use BPD, which (as noted previously) is formally listed within the Internalizing and Antagonistic Externalizing spectra of HiTOP. With regard to internalizing, there is ample evidence to suggest that symptoms of BPD can be explained by the functional model delineated above (see Sauer-Zavala & Barlow, 2014). In sum, individuals with BPD indeed experience frequent and intense negative emotions (Henry et al., 2001; Koenigsberg et al., 2002; Levine, Marziali, & Hood, 1997), and this emotional intensity has been linked to the severity of BPD symptoms (Cheavens et al., 2005; Rosenthal, Cheavens, Lejuez, & Lynch, 2005; Yen, Zlotnick, & Costello, 2002). Additional studies utilizing physiological measures also indicate heightened emotional intensity and reactivity in BPD (Austin, Riniolo, & Porges, 2007; Ebner-Priemer et al., 2005; Ebner-Priemer et al., 2007). Individuals with BPD also demonstrate a negative stance toward emotions. For instance, aversive reactivity accounts for significant incremental variance in predicting BPD symptom severity beyond frequency of negative emotions (Chapman, Specht, & Cellucci, 2005; Iverson, Follette, Pistorello, & Fruzzetti, 2012; Shorey et al., 2016; Wupperman, Neumann, & Axelrod, 2008; Wupperman, Neumann, Whitman, & Axelrod, 2009; Lilienfeld & Penna, 2001; Gratz, Tull, & Gunderson, 2008).

Given that individuals with BPD experience high levels of negative emotions and find these experiences aversive, it is not surprising that they engage in efforts to escape or avoid them (Putnam & Silk, 2005). In fact, there is evidence to suggest that the behavioral difficulties associated with BPD serve to suppress intense negative emotion (see Bijttebier & Vertommen, 1999). For example, nonsuicidal self-injury most often functions to escape unwanted emotional experiences (Bentley, Nock, & Barlow, 2014; Carr, 1977; Chapman, Gratz, & Brown, 2006; Gratz, 2003). Likewise, substance users with BPD more frequently described their drug and alcohol use as serving to escape negative emotions, compared with substance abusers without BPD (Kruedelbach, McCormick, Schulz, & Grueneich, 1993). Further, dissociation and binge eating, also common in BPD, have similarly been associated with avoidance of negative mood states (Deaver, Miltenberger, Smyth, Meidinger, & Crosby, 2003; Paxton & Diggens, 1997; Wagner & Linehan, 1998). Individuals with BPD also engage in cognitive coping motivated by avoidance. For instance, thought suppression has been shown to mediate the relationship between negative emotionality and BPD symptoms (Cheavens et al., 2005; Rosenthal et al., 2005; Sauer & Baer, 2009a). Similarly, rumination is common in BPD (Abela, Payne, & Moussaly, 2003), correlated with symptom severity (Baer & Sauer, 2011; Smith, Grandin, Alloy, & Abramson,

2006), and predicts dysregulated behavior (Sauer & Baer, 2012; Selby et al., 2009). In contrast, when symptoms of BPD are better accounted for by the Antagonistic Externalizing spectra (or domains of disinhibition and/or psychoticism in the AMPD), alternative functional mechanisms likely maintain these symptoms (Hallquist & Pilkonis, 2012; Wright et al., 2013) and alternative treatment modalities should be explored.

Summary

For disorders within the neurotic/internalizing spectrum, the functional assessment incorporated into the Unified Protocol for Transdiagnostic Treatment of Emotional Disorders (UP), discussed in the next chapter, is complementary to hierarchical, dimensional models of personality. In a clinical interview that is practical to administer for professionals in busy practice settings, this assessment distills key information at both the spectrum level, in this case evidence for frequent and intense negative emotions, and at the level of symptom/components (i.e., avoidance of public transportation, checking, rumination). The functional assessment does not encourage clinicians to group symptoms/components into the DSM diagnoses with which they are traditionally associated, instead emphasizing that all of these behaviors function to escape uncomfortable emotional experiences. Of course, such behavioral/cognitive efforts to avoidant emotions result from aversive reactivity to these affective experiences that, as we have noted, represents an intermediate functional mechanism between personality and symptoms that is notably absent from proposed dimensional models of classification. Completion of a functional assessment such as the one included in the UP may help clinicians identify a limited number of transdiagnostic mechanisms that are amenable to change in treatment.

CONCLUSIONS

The construct of neuroticism, and of temperament more generally, exerted varied influence on nosological schemes throughout the course of the 20th century. The propensity to experience negative emotions was part of the formal definition of neurosis, an important class of disorders in early versions of the DSM system. When neurosis as a diagnostic label was removed in 1980 (DSM-III), references to emotional vulnerabilities were also downplayed somewhat. Decades later, at the start of the 21st century, several groups have called for a more dimensional system for classifying psychopathology, owing to dissatisfaction with the DSM's categorical-prototypical approach. We reviewed four prominent proposals, including the DSM's AMPD, Brown and Barlow's (2009) model of emotional disorders, HiTOP, and NIMH's RDoC.

Each of these proposals reflects the importance of temperament generally and neuroticism specifically for psychopathology, as this trait is described as a higher order dimension across all four, albeit referred to by different names (i.e., negative affectivity in the AMPD, negative temperament in Brown and Barlow's [2009] proposal, negative valence system in RDoC, and Internalizing in HiTOP). Dimensional models of psychopathology with a limited number of high-order domains that can become the focus of treatment (rather than their numerous clinical manifestations; i.e., discrete DSM diagnoses) have the potential to significantly streamline care. Unfortunately, despite having demonstrated clinical feasibility in terms of assessment (e.g., Samuel & Widiger, 2006), it may be difficult to translate them into concrete treatment recommendations. Thus we propose complementing personality-based classification with identification of intermediate, functional mechanisms that may be more amenable to direct intervention with existing protocols. Given our focus on neuroticism, we have used our functional model of emotional disorders (see Bullis et al., 2019) to illustrate how aversive reactivity to emotions (i.e., an intermediate mechanism) can serve as a bridge between the neurotic temperament and the emotionally avoidant behavioral coping that, in many cases, constitutes DSM disorder symptoms. In the next chapter, we discuss treatment approaches for aversive reactivity, along with their implications for both psychopathology and neuroticism itself.

6

Treatment of Neuroticism

Neuroticism predicts a range of public health problems (see Chapter 1), including a variety of mental disorders and comorbidity among them (Clark, Watson, & Mineka, 1994; Henriques-Calado, Duarte-Silva, Junqueira, Sacoto, & Keong, 2014; Khan et al., 2005; Krueger & Markon, 2006a; Trull & Sher, 1994; Weinstock & Whisman, 2006). Given its association with psychological difficulties, it is no surprise that neuroticism also predicts treatment seeking (Shipley et al., 2007), prompting consideration of how this trait may best be addressed. For example, can neuroticism be treated directly, rather than separately targeting each of its manifestations in the form of discrete DSM or ICD mental health disorders? Targeting underlying vulnerabilities, such as neuroticism, is consistent with the dimensional approaches to understanding psychopathology described in the previous chapter (e.g., Brown & Barlow, 2009; Insel et al., 2010; Kotov et al., 2007). Indeed, treating neuroticism itself may represent a more efficient and cost-effective means of addressing the wide swath of public health problems associated with this trait.

The goal of this chapter is to delineate treatment elements that may directly target neuroticism. Specifically, we begin by describing the evidence that neuroticism is more malleable than originally believed, both naturalistically and in response to treatment. Next, we propose that neuroticism may be most responsive to pharmacological and behavioral interventions that are designed to explicitly target this trait. With specific regard to behavioral interventions, we outline how the functional model of emotional disorders, described in Chapter 4, can be used to guide the selection of existing treatment elements that may be particularly relevant for neuroticism; specifically, skills/activities that reduce aversive reactivity to emotions may simultaneously affect both neuroticism *and* the discrete DSM disorders accounted for

Treating neuroticism directly is efficient and cost-effective.

by it. Next, we review several treatment packages that have adapted a range of these elements to directly address neuroticism.

MALLEABILITY OF NEUROTICISM

Naturalistic Change

Although personality has long been considered stable and inflexible across time (American Psychiatric Association, 2013), there is increasing evidence that traits do change significantly across the lifespan. For example, several studies support the notion that personality traits fluctuate in young adulthood (e.g., Neyer & Asendorpf, 2001), middle age (e.g., Hill, Turiano, Mroczek, & Roberts, 2012), and among older adults (Mõttus, Johnson, & Deary, 2012; Mroczek & Spiro, 2003; Small, Hertzog, Hultsch, & Dixon, 2003). Specifically with regard to neuroticism, longitudinal studies of the general population show gradual age-related decreases in this trait (Eaton et al., 2011b; Roberts, Walton, & Viechtbauer, 2006; Roberts & Mroczek, 2008). Although, on average, neuroticism decreases with age, there appears to be great variability in the extent of this change (Mroczek & Spiro, 2003), with some people maintaining stable levels and others shifting considerably (Helson, Jones, & Kwan, 2002; Small et al., 2003). Indeed, individuals with higher initial levels of neuroticism demonstrate less change in this dimension over time, and, conversely, individuals with lower initial levels of neuroticism tend to show greater change (Brown, 2007).

Change in Response to Treatment

Change in neuroticism has also been explored in the context of treatment-seeking individuals. It is worth noting, however, that personality change is rarely the focus of the interventions under study in treatment outcome trials; instead, the protocols being tested are typically aimed at reducing the symptoms of specific DSM disorders, with measures of neuroticism included as an additional metric by which to evaluate a treatment's effects (Roberts, Hill, & Davis, 2017a). That said, there are numerous studies that explore the extent to which personality features, particularly neuroticism, change during the course of therapeutic intervention for DSM disorders.

When evaluating the degree of trait change that occurs over the course of therapy, it is important to consider that any given personality measure captures some amount of state and trait variance. Some authors contend that *any* change in neuroticism that appears as a result of therapy can be attributed to state-level variance in the measure used to assess this trait (Du, Bakish, Ravindran, & Hrdina, 2002; Gracious, 1999). In other words, the *state-artifact position* suggests that fluctuations in DSM disorder severity account for inflections in scores obtained on measures of neuroticism and that what looks like personality trait change is really only a temporary state change resulting from the fact that our personality measures are imperfect and capture both state and trait variance.

In contrast, the *cause-correction hypothesis* (Soskin, Carl, Alpert, & Fava, 2012) indicates that changes in symptoms are, in fact, the result of changes in the trait component of the personality domain measured. In support of the cause-correction hypothesis, there is increasing evidence that personality change and symptom change are not isomorphic. Indeed, results from a recent study indicate that measures of neuroticism primarily capture true temperamental variance, even in individuals with emotional disorders (Naragon-Gainey et al., 2013). Moreover, a number of longitudinal studies have controlled for the periodic occurrence of anxious or depressive symptoms and still found neuroticism to act independently in predicting DSM disorder onset (Lahey, 2009; Spijker, de Graaf, Oldehinkel, Nolen, & Ormel, 2007). Additionally, although neuroticism predicts the course of DSM disorders, with higher levels of this trait reflecting less change in symptoms across time, the converse does not appear to occur; that is, initial levels of DSM disorder severity do not predict changes in temperament over time (Brown & Rosellini, 2011; Gershuny & Sher, 1998; Kasch, Rottenberg, Arnow, & Gotlib, 2002; Meyer, Johnson, & Winters, 2001). Taken together, this body of work suggests that neuroticism is distinct from DSM disorder severity, and thus measurement error is unlikely to entirely account for changes that occur in this trait across treatment studies.

Further, evidence that neuroticism and DSM symptom severity can be evaluated separately is also available in the context of clinical samples seeking treatment for DSM disorders. For example, Eaton and colleagues (2011a) found that neuroticism remained stable across 8 months in a small sample of individuals with MDD (most of whom received some kind of treatment), despite changes in clinical state. In other words, neuroticism displayed the same high level of temporal stability in individuals who no longer met criteria for MDD as it did in the subgroup of patients who were depressed at both assessment points, suggesting that trait and disorder constructs can shift independently. Additionally, Brown (2007) evaluated a large sample (N = 606) of individuals with DSM depressive and anxiety disorders at intake, along with 1-year and 2-year follow-ups, with the majority (76%) of patients receiving some kind of treatment (of varying quality and duration) throughout the study. As expected, DSM disorders improved significantly over time, and most temperamental variables (e.g., extraversion) remained stable; however, contrary to Eaton et al.'s (2011a) results, neuroticism evidenced the greatest amount of temporal change and was the dimension associated with the largest treatment effect.

Beyond examining fluctuations in neuroticism in samples that participated in varied, unspecified treatments, change in this trait has also been explored in the context of trials evaluating specific interventions. In a large randomized controlled trial (RCT), Tang and colleagues (2009) compared the effects of cognitive therapy (CT), SSRIs, and placebo on neuroticism in adults with MDD. Both CT and SSRIs resulted in significantly larger improvements in neuroticism than placebo, an effect that remained after controlling for changes in depressive symptoms for individuals in the SSRI condition but not for those receiving CT. In contrast, the advantage of SSRIs over placebo on improvement for depressive symptoms was not maintained after controlling for neuroticism. These results suggest that SSRIs produce a specific effect on neuroticism and provide additional support for the notion that temperament and psychopathology can change independently. Additionally, these findings also suggest that whereas depressive symptoms are responsive to placebo, neuroticism is not.

With regard to the magnitude of change in neuroticism observed in individuals receiving treatment, Roberts and colleagues (2017b) recently completed a meta-analysis of 199 treatment studies that included a measure of this trait. The authors found a moderate pre- to posttreatment effect (i.e., 0.59) on neuroticism, which they note is nearly half of the amount of change typically observed from young adulthood to old age in naturalist studies (e.g., Roberts et al., 2006). Additionally, moderate between-group effects comparing various forms of active treatment, including cognitive-behavioral therapy (CBT), with a no-treatment control were also observed. The authors of this study contend that greater change in neuroticism in the treatment group suggests the presence of intervention-specific effects not attributable to changes in generalized distress or specific symptoms that are apt to fluctuate naturalistically in the control group (Widiger, Verheul, & van den Brink, 1999; Clark, Vittengl, Kraft, & Jarrett, 2003; Jylhä & Isometsä, 2006).

Although a meta-analysis (i.e., Roberts et al., 2017b) can provide information about the average effect of a certain type of treatment (e.g., CBT), these methods ignore potentially important differences across studies. For example, when change in neuroticism has been examined in the context of cognitive-behavioral interventions, results have been quite mixed. For example, some authors have found significant decreases in neuroticism following a course of CBT (e.g., Kring, Persons, & Thomas, 2007), whereas others have not observed such improvements (Davenport, Bore, & Campbell, 2010). It is possible that inconsistency regarding the degree to which neuroticism is responsive to treatment may be due to the fact that the studies described above examined changes in neuroticism in the context of naturalistic treatments or treatments targeting DSM disorder-specific symptoms. Indeed, the research reviewed raises questions about the mechanisms through which neuroticism changes and whether *directly* targeting this trait in treatment would lead to more definitive results.

EXISTING TREATMENTS WITH RELEVANCE FOR NEUROTICISM

Attempts to treat mental health difficulties date back millennia, including interventions related to the four-humors theory described in Chapter 1. Owing to increased sophistication in clinical trial research, considerable empirical support for the efficacy of a variety of strategies in addressing disorder symptoms has been amassed over the last decade. In the following section, we review treatment elements that, although developed to address DSM disorders, may have particular relevance for neuroticism.

Pharmacological Approaches

There is emerging literature to suggest that specific pharmacological agents are particularly adept at treating certain domains of personality (i.e., neuroticism, extraversion). For example, given that neuroticism has been shown to reflect stable differences in the serotonergic system (Frokjaer et al., 2008; Hirvonen, Tuominen, Någren, & Hietala, 2015), it is not surprising that serotonergic agents appear to exert the strongest effects on neuroticism (Quilty, Meusel, & Bagby, 2008; Tang et al., 2009).

As noted previously, the RCT conducted by Tang and colleagues (2009) provides compelling evidence for the specific effect of SSRIs on neuroticism. In this study, patients with MDD were randomly assigned to receive 16 weeks of CT, 16 weeks of an SSRI (i.e., paroxetine, flexibly dosed, mean 38.8 mg), or 8 weeks of matched placebo. All three groups (i.e., paroxetine, CT, placebo) showed substantial improvement in depressive symptoms over the first 8 weeks of treatment, yet changes in neuroticism were 8 times greater with paroxetine than placebo. Moreover, in support of the cause-correction hypothesis, when changes in neuroticism were statistically controlled, the antidepressant advantage for paroxetine over placebo was no longer significant. Tang and colleagues (2009) also performed a within-participants analyses of 31 patients who completed 8 weeks of placebo, followed by a crossover to another 8 weeks of paroxetine. Depressive symptoms changed more during the placebo phase than the paroxetine phase, whereas neuroticism was relatively unchanged during the placebo phase but improved significantly during the paroxetine phase. This pattern of results suggests SSRI-specific effects on temperament (relative to CT and placebo) that are independent from depressive symptom severity.

Several additional studies provide more evidence for the specific effect of the SSRIs on neuroticism. For example, Quilty and colleagues (2008) performed structural equation modeling on data from patients with MDD who were receiving varied pharmacological interventions. They found that patients who received SSRIs demonstrated greater change in neuroticism than those taking noradrenergic and dopamine reuptake blockers or reversible monoamine oxide inhibitors. Additionally, they found support for a mediation model in which SSRIs produced an antidepressant effect through decreases in neuroticism. Here, results suggest that SSRIs produce specific effects on neuroticism relative to other antidepressant medications.

In another study, Knutson and colleagues (1998) conducted a double-blind RCT in which healthy individuals were randomized to receive either the SSRI paroxetine (20 mg/day) or placebo for 4 weeks; consistent with other studies, they observed significantly greater decreases in neuroticism for those in the paroxetine condition relative to the placebo condition. They also included a measure of extraversion in their trial, which did not change as a function of treatment in either condition. Additionally, two case-control studies have explored the unique effects of serotonergic agents and norepinephrine dopamine reuptake inhibitors (i.e., bupropion) on depressive symptoms (Andrews, Parker, & Barrett, 1998; Bodkin, Lasser, Wines, Gardner, & Baldessarini, 1997). Although these studies did not include measures of neuroticism and extraversion, the authors contend that the symptoms addressed by the serotonergic agent (anxiety, rumination, compulsions) most closely align with a high neuroticism presentation, whereas the symptoms affected by bupropion (fatigue, anergia) represent deficits in positive affectivity. Taken together, this pattern of results suggests that SSRIs may be particularly relevant for neuroticism, whereas agents that act on alternative neurotransmitters (e.g., norepinephrine, dopamine) may exert effects on other domains of personality relevant for depression (e.g., extraversion).

Of course, it is worth noting that other researchers have found nonspecific effects of SSRIs, suggesting that these drugs can produce improvements on both neuroticism and extraversion (Bagby, Levitan, Kennedy, Levitt, & Joffe, 1999; Du et al., 2002). In a study exploring the combined effect of serotonergic and noradrenergic agents, Dichter, Tomarken, Freid, Addington, and Shelton (2005) randomized patients with MDD to receive fixed doses of either venlafaxine XR (225 mg/day; combined serotonin and norepinephrine reuptake inhibitor) or paroxetine (30 mg/day; SSRI) for a duration of 12 weeks. Both conditions demonstrated decreases in neuroticism and depressive symptoms, and, contrary to expectations, venlafaxine did not produce greater effects on positive affectivity relative to paroxetine. Overall, these results suggest that serotonergic antidepressants produce a dampening effect on neuroticism, with mixed support for their impact on other domains of personality (i.e., extraversion). More work is needed to better understand the effects of antidepressant medication on temperament, along with the mechanisms through which these effects are exerted.

With regard to understanding the neural pathways involved in antidepressant effects on temperament, Harmer and colleagues have conducted a number of studies in healthy samples. In one study (i.e., McCabe, Mishor, Cowen, & Harmer, 2010), they randomized healthy participants to receive 7 days of citalopram (SSRI), reboxetine (norepinephrine reuptake inhibitor), or placebo, and they used functional MRI to assess neural responses to aversive and rewarding stimuli. They found that the SSRI reduced neural processing of rewarding stimuli in the ventral striatum and the ventral medial/orbitofrontal cortex and of aversive stimuli in the lateral orbitofrontal cortex. The norepinephrine reuptake inhibitor increased neural responses to reward within the medial orbitofrontal cortex and weakened effects on the processing of aversive stimuli. The results of this study suggest that SSRIs may exhibit an antidepressant/anti-anxiolytic effect through the dampening of neural responses to aversive stimuli, though simultaneous dampening of reward processing may underscore why patients taking these agents also report flattening of positive affect (i.e., Opbroek et al., 2002; Price, Cole, & Goodwin, 2009). In another study of healthy volunteers, Harmer and colleagues assessed the neural effects of citalopram (2 mg) on emotional processing of facial expressions. Functional MRI performed 3 hours after administration demonstrated a significantly reduced amygdala response to fearful facial expression compared with placebo (Murphy, Norbury, O'Sullivan, Cowen, & Harmer, 2009). Similar reductions in limbic reactivity have been found in healthy individuals treated with citalopram over 7 days (Harmer, Mackay, Reid, Cowen, & Goodwin, 2006).

More recently, Harmer and colleagues have extended their work with healthy individuals to include studies of nonclinical participants with elevated levels of neuroticism. In one study (i.e., Di Simplicio, Norbury, Reinecke, & Harmer, 2014), they aimed to explore the neural effects of SSRIs on implicit processing of fearful facial expressions in individuals high in neuroticism. Participants were randomized to receive citalopram (20 mg/day) or placebo for 7 days, and, on the last day, they completed a gender discrimination task that included fearful and happy faces while functional magnetic resonance imaging (fMRI) was conducted. A 7-day course of SSRIs was associated with elevated resting perfusion in the right amygdala, increased amygdala activation to all facial expressions (regardless of valence), and increased activation in the occipital, parietal, temporal, and prefrontal cortical areas in response to fearful (but not happy) facial expressions. This pattern of results is in contrast to the amygdala dampening observed in healthy samples. The authors postulate that SSRIs may acutely increase neural markers of fear reactivity for individuals at the high end of the neuroticism distribution, which corresponds to increases in agitation and anxiety observed in the early stages of treatment with a serotonergic agent (e.g., Burghardt, Sullivan, McEwen, Gorman, & LeDoux, 2004). Future work is needed to assess the effects of longer term SSRI administration on neural responses to aversive stimuli in high-risk (i.e., high neuroticism) populations, particularly Di Simplicio et al.'s (2014) assertion that these early increases in amygdala activation are likely to reverse when the course of care is longer.

Summary

There is increasing evidence that serotonergic agents (e.g., SSRIs) exhibit a preferential effect on neuroticism relative to additional dimensions of personality and other antidepressant medications (see Soskin et al., 2012). There is also support for the notion that SSRIs exert their effects via decreased hyperreactivity of the amygdala in response to fear-inducing stimuli (for reviews, see Ilieva, 2015; Soskin et al., 2012). In other words, SSRIs seem to act directly on the frequency/intensity of emotion component of the emotional-disorders functional model described in Chapter 4 (see Figure 4.1); although decreased emotional intensity may reduce aversive/avoidant reactions (i.e., emotions are less aversive if they weaker), this would likely occur without any substantial "learning" or extinction of distress mediated via frontal lobe or higher cognitive process changes (more likely to be achieved in the behavioral interventions described in the subsequent section). Indeed, although SSRI administration is associated with immediate reductions in cognitive biases (e.g., Harmer et al., 2006), antidepressant effects often take weeks to manifest (e.g., Stassen, Angst, & Delini-Stula, 1996). It is possible that this lag in symptom improvement is due to the time it takes individuals to create their own new learning via natural interactions with the world that allow them to see that their emotional reactions in response to stressors have changed. Behavioral interventions, described in detail in the next section, often include opportunities for learning, underscoring the finding that the combination of psychopharmacological and behavioral approaches is most robust (Van Apeldoorn et al., 2008), at least immediately posttreatment (e.g., Barlow et al., 2000).

Behavioral Approaches

Behavioral approaches may also have promise in addressing neuroticism. By emphasizing the functional mechanisms through which this trait confers risk for psychopathology, we may be able to identify treatment elements that can be used to address both disorder symptoms and underlying personality vulnerabilities. Specifically, interventions that target aversive reactions to a wide variety of negative emotions when they occur may reduce reliance on the avoidant emotion-regulation strategies that, paradoxically, have been shown to lead to more frequent and intense emotional experiences (Wegner et al., 1987; Rassin et al., 2000a). Moreover, when negative emotions become less frequent over time, and when these changes are sustained, this may constitute decreases in neuroticism (for a description of what constitutes trait change, see Magidson, Roberts, Collado-Rodriguez, & Lejuez, 2014). Although the treatment elements described in this section were originally designed to alleviate DSM disorder symptoms, there is support for the notion that they indeed address aversive reactivity and preliminary support for their impact on neuroticism.

Mindfulness

Mindfulness has been described as intentionally focusing one's attention on experiences occurring in the present moment in a nonjudgmental or accepting way (Kabat-Zinn, 1982). Mindfulness, and its cultivation through meditation practice, has its roots in Eastern spiritual traditions, primarily Buddhism (Linehan, 1993); these traditions describe mindfulness meditation as a way of reducing suffering and encouraging the development of positive qualities such as awareness, insight, and compassion (Goldstein, 2002; Kabat-Zinn, 2003). Mindfulness practices have been secularized for empirical study and are now included in interventions that target depression and anxiety (Eifert & Forsyth, 2005; Segal, Teasdale, Williams, & Gemar, 2002); BPD (Linehan, 2015); chronic pain, illness, and stress (Kabat-Zinn, 1982); substance abuse (Witkiewitz, Marlatt, & Walker, 2005); and eating disorders (Kristeller & Hallett, 1999; Leahey, Crowther, & Irwin, 2008). A growing body of literature supports the efficacy of mindfulness-based interventions for the range of common mental health conditions (Baer, 2003; Grossman, Niemann, Schmidt, & Walach, 2004; Hayes et al., 2006; Lynch, Trost, Salsman, & Linehan, 2007; Robins & Chapman, 2004).

Participants in mindfulness training are encouraged to focus their attention on particular stimuli that can be observed in the present moment, such as the sensations of breathing or sounds in the environment. Often this attentional focus is accomplished through guided meditation, though present-focused awareness can also be applied to everyday activities, such as washing the dishes, eating, walking, and taking a shower. If cognitions, emotions, urges, or other experiences arise during these practices, participants are encouraged to observe them closely. Brief mental labeling of observed internal or external experiences is often suggested. For example, participants may silently say "anger," "planning," or "aching" as they observe internal and external phenomena (Hayes et al., 1999; Linehan, 1993). In addition to bringing awareness to the present moment, participants are also asked to cultivate an attitude of acceptance, openness, willingness, kindness, compassion, and friendly curiosity to all observed experiences, regardless of how pleasant or unpleasant they may be, and to refrain from efforts to judge, evaluate, change, or terminate them.

Although mindful attention can be applied to any activity (e.g., walking, washing dishes), when nonjudgmental, present-focused awareness is consistently brought to bear on the thoughts, physical sensations, and behavioral urges that constitute emotional experiences, this therapeutic element may engage the aversive reactivity that maintains emotional-disorder symptoms and neuroticism itself. Indeed, sustained, nonjudgmental/nonreactive observation of internal experience, some of which may be quite unpleasant, represents a form of exposure (Sauer & Baer, 2009c). In other words, when emotions are experienced without escape or avoidance (i.e., observed with nonjudgmental attention) and in the absence of dire consequences, distress over emotional experiences themselves may be extinguished. In support of the view that mindfulness practice can facilitate extinction processes, Lykins and Baer (2009) demonstrated that meditation experience (the length of time an individual had been practicing meditation) was associated with lower self-reported fear of emotion. In another study, Brake and colleagues (2016) found that when participants were encouraged to mindfully approach any emotions that arose in the context of exposure to anxiety-provoking activities, these practices resulted in higher initial emotion intensity with steeper between-trial reductions in distress, relative to exposures in which participants were instructed to distract from their emotional experiences.

Given these proposed mechanisms, it is not surprising that mindfulness practice is associated with reductions in various forms of aversive reactivity. For example, several authors have proposed that reduced experiential avoidance represents a key mechanism through which mindfulness training exerts its beneficial effects on psychopathology (Brown, Bravo, Roos, & Pearson, 2015; Shapiro, 2009). Cross-sectional data suggest that experienced meditators exhibit lower levels of experiential avoidance relative to healthy, matched nonmeditators (Alda et al., 2016). Moreover, meta-analytic results indicate that experiential avoidance mediates improvements in anxiety and depressive symptoms during the course of treatment with acceptance and commitment therapy (ACT), a manualized intervention that includes a large proportion of mindfulness training (Ruiz, 2012). Similarly, mindfulness-based interventions have been shown reduce anxiety sensitivity and intolerance of uncertainty in adult outpatients (Alimehdi, Ehteshamzadeh, Naderi, Eftekharsaadi, & Pasha, 2016; Kim et al., 2010; McCracken & Keogh, 2009), and mindfulness training is also associated with persistence on distressing laboratory tasks (Feldman, Dunn, Stemke, Bell, & Greeson, 2014; Sauer & Baer, 2012) and self-report distress tolerance measures (Nila, Holt, Ditzen, & Aguilar-Raab, 2016).

Meta-analytic findings indicate a strong negative association between dispositional mindfulness and neuroticism (Giluk, 2009; Hanley, Garland, & Tedeschi, 2017). In fact, neuroticism is more strongly associated with dispositional mindfulness than any other Big Five personality domain (Giluk, 2009; Hanley et al., 2017; van den Hurk et al., 2011). Yet, despite established cross-sectional relations between these two constructs, the impact of mindfulness training on neuroticism has only been reported in a few studies. For example, Jacobs and colleagues (2013) found that individuals randomized to attend a mindfulness meditation retreat, compared with a wait-list control group, demonstrated decreases in self-reported neuroticism. Similarly, Krasner et al. (2009) observed decreased neuroticism after an 8-week mindfulness program in a sample of primary care physicians. In another RCT, Hanley, de Vibe, Solhaug, Gonzalez-Pons, and Garland (2019) found that Norwegian medical students who participated in a 7-week mindfulness-based stress reduction (MBSR) program showed decreases in neuroticism that persisted at a 6-year follow-up relative to students who did not receive this intervention. Taken together, these studies suggest that mindfulness practice may be a useful therapeutic mechanism to engage the aversive reactivity that maintains symptoms of emotional disorders, as well as the neurotic temperament. In order to observe robust changes in neuroticism, more research is needed to clarify whether the focus of mindful attention (i.e., specifically on emotional experiences versus other stimuli; e.g., walking, eating) affects the extent to which this trait changes in response to this intervention strategy.

Cognitive Interventions

CT is described as the process of collaboration between therapist and patient, leading to the identification of distorted thoughts, along with subsequent logical analysis and empirical hypothesis testing that results in the realignment of the patient's cognitions with reality (DeRubeis, Webb, Tang, & Beck, 2019). Techniques considered within the purview of CT include thought monitoring, thought challenging, and the generation of alternative interpretations. The goal of these strategies is to identify unhelpful cognitions and to test their validity by providing the patient with an opportunity to examine evidence from their own experience, often leading to revision of the original cognition. An advantage of CT is that it emphasizes relatively easily accessed mental events (i.e., thoughts) that patients can be trained to report.

The cognitive model of emotional disorders focuses on the content of one's thoughts in response to stressors (real or imagined). Indeed, the domains typically included in what has been called the "cognitive triad" (e.g., negative views about the self, the future, and the world; Beck, Kovacs, & Weissman, 1979) are largely consistent with the cognitive elements included in our definition of neuroticism. Specifically, perceptions that the world is a dangerous and unpredictable place, along with the belief that one is ill equipped to cope with challenges that arise, are a key part of the neurotic temperament (Barlow et al., 2014b) and perhaps most apt to change with cognitive interventions. This model of treatment was originally designed to address symptoms of depression (Beck, 1963) but has been successfully applied to a range of other emotional disorders (Beck & Haigh, 2014). Indeed, there is strong evidence to suggest that CT is effective in reducing symptoms across multiple diagnoses (e.g., Butler, Chapman, Forman, & Beck, 2006; Dobson, 1989; Gaffan, Tsaousis, & Kemp-Wheeler, 1995).

Given that CT may address beliefs about one's ability to cope with challenging situations, increasing perceived self-efficacy to manage negative emotional experiences, it is possible that this therapeutic element could affect aversive reactivity to emotion. There is some empirical support for this notion. For example, in a meta-analytic review, Smits and colleagues (Smits, Berry, Tart, & Powers, 2008) found that, across 24 RCTs with a total of 1,851 patients, CT was associated with significant reductions in anxiety sensitivity that were large in magnitude. Similarly, increases in distress tolerance have been observed following a course of CT (Azizi, Borjali, & Golzari, 2010). Reductions in intolerance of uncertainty and experiential avoidance have also been reported in the context of studies evaluating cognitive-behavioral interventions, though the multicomponent nature of these treatments makes it difficult to evaluate the unique effects of cognitive elements (Belloch et al., 2011; Dugas & Ladouceur, 2000; Eustis et al., 2020; Goldman, Dugas, Sexton, & Gervais, 2007; Ladouceur et al., 2000; Overton & Menzies, 2005). Thus, despite the conceptual relevance of CT for ameliorating aversive reactivity to emotions, more research is needed to better understand the unique contributions of this therapeutic element.

There is also some evidence that cognitive strategies may affect neuroticism. Specifically, if an individual can change the content of their thoughts in a way that becomes habitual, they may be less likely to experience negative emotions in response to stressors over time. With regard to the empirical evidence supporting the use of cognitive elements to address neuroticism, CT produced greater reductions in neuroticism than placebo in the Tang et al. (2009) study described previously, though the effect of treatment condition was not significant after controlling for fluctuations in depressive symptoms. More research is necessary to clarify the unique and specific effects cognitive interventions have on this trait.

Behavior Change Elements

An additional technique commonly used in the treatment of emotional disorders involves encouraging patients to change their emotionally avoidant behavior, a key component of the emotional-disorder functional model described in Chapter 4. Countering behavioral avoidance draws from basic emotion science suggesting that the most fundamental way to change an emotion is to alter the action tendencies associated with it (Barlow, 1988, 2002; Barlow et al., 2014b). For example, opposite action, a skill drawn from the emotion-regulation module of dialectical behavior therapy, encourages patients to consider whether their typical (avoidant) behavioral responses may paradoxically increase the frequency/intensity of negative emotions, despite short-term relief (Selby et al., 2008; Selby et al., 2009); then they are asked to practice approach-oriented alternative actions. Several studies have examined the isolated effect of opposite action. For example, in a within-participants laboratory study, participants were instructed to respond to an induced negative mood by acting either consistently with emotion-driven behavioral urges or opposite to them (Sauer-Zavala, Wilner, Cassiello-Robbins, Saraff, & Pagan, 2019). Results suggest that opposite action leads to steeper reductions in negative emotions relative to acting consistently. In a follow-up multiple-baseline study, Sauer-Zavala and colleagues (2020) demonstrated that a brief treatment module aimed at countering emotional behaviors indeed led to reductions in the frequency of avoidant responding, along with decreased negative emotions. Finally, opposite action has been shown to decrease the intensity of a specific negative emotion: shame (Rizvi & Linehan, 2005). Taken together, there is preliminary evidence that encouraging patients to approach their emotional experiences may break the emotional-disorder cycle in which avoidant coping inadvertently increases the frequency/intensity of negative emotions, maintaining the neurotic temperament.

Exposure Therapy

Exposure therapy represents another technique aimed at altering patient behavior. Exposure refers to the repeated and systematic confrontation of feared stimuli and is a central component of treatment for anxiety and related disorders. Exposure can take various forms, including graduated versus intense, brief versus prolonged, with and without various cognitive coping strategies, and imaginal or *in vivo* (i.e., in real life; see Meuret, Wolitzky-Taylor, Twohig, & Craske, 2012). Extinction learning is thought to be a critical process in the long-term reductions of patient fear (Craske et al., 2014). Extinction occurs when the feared stimulus (e.g., making small talk, dogs, dirty doorknobs) is presented without its predicted negative consequences (e.g., appearing awkward, getting bitten, getting sick). It is important to note that the original relationship that paired feared stimuli with undesirable outcomes is not erased during extinction; instead, a secondary relationship wherein a given stimulus no longer predicts the negative consequence develops and inhibits the fear response (Bouton, 1993).

Meta-analytic work suggests that exposure, whether alone or combined with other common techniques (i.e., cognitive reappraisal), exerts large effects on symptoms of anxiety disorders (Cuijpers, Cristea, Karyotaki, Reijnders, & Huibers, 2016). Given that the goal of exposure is to reduce distress in response to emotion-eliciting stimuli, it makes conceptual sense that this therapeutic procedure would result in the sustained decreases in negative affect that constitute change in neuroticism. Data on the isolated effect of this technique on temperament, or aversive reactivity to emotions, is more limited, however. In one study, Brake and colleagues (2016) demonstrated that exposures (both imaginal and *in vivo*) resulted in decreases in experiential avoidance. Moreover, results from a trial comparing an Internet-based CBT that was largely composed of exposure practices to a wait-list condition suggest that exposures result in significantly larger reductions in neuroticism (Hedman et al., 2014). More research is needed to better understand the effect that exposure has on temperament and the functional mechanisms that maintain it.

Interoceptive Exposure

Interoceptive exposure, which entails repeatedly inducing the physical sensations associated with an individual's emotional experience (e.g., shortness of breath, heart palpitations, dizziness), represents a specific form of exposure that may be particularly relevant for addressing anxiety sensitivity. As described extensively in Chapter 4, anxiety sensitivity refers to aversive reactions to the physiological changes that accompany emotions, typically based on the belief that these symptoms will have negative somatic, cognitive, and social consequences (Reiss et al., 1986). Examples of common interoceptive exposures include running in place to provoke increased heart rate, body temperature, and sweating; spinning in circles to provoke dizziness and nausea; hyperventilating to prompt lightheadedness, blurred vision, and numbness/tingling; and straw breathing (i.e., breathing through a coffee stirrer while stopping airflow through the nose) to prompt shortness of breath (see Meuret, Ritz, Wilhelm, & Roth, 2005). The goal of these exercises is to reduce aversive reactivity associated with emotion-related physiological sensations (i.e., anxiety sensitivity). Similar to traditional exposure, interoceptive exposure likely leads to reduced distress through the extinction of conditioned associations between previously neutral physical sensations and frightening experiences, such as an unexpected panic attack (Bouton, 2002; Bouton et al., 2001). Indeed, inducing physical symptoms that do not escalate to panic attacks is thought to eventually lead to the extinction of the acquired fear response that had developed from this pairing.

Though interoceptive exposure has been most associated with treatment for patients with panic disorder, heightened physiological arousal is a core component of many disorders falling along the neurotic spectrum (Barlow, 2002). Specifically, cued panic attacks are common in social anxiety disorder, OCD, and GAD (Baillie & Rapee, 2005; Craske et al., 2010; Goodwin & Hamilton, 2001). Moreover, strong physiological reactions in the context of emotional experiences may exacerbate hallmark features of these DSM disorders. For example, many individuals with social anxiety disorder report concerns about appearing anxious to others, causing them to be hypervigilant to changes in physiology (Hope, Heimberg, & Turk, 2010). Similarly, muscle tension is an important diagnostic feature of GAD, which contributes to the frequency and intensity of worry episodes (Borkovec, Grayson, & Cooper, 1978). Additionally, Wald, Taylor, Chiri, and Sica (2010) report that many patients with PTSD do not reap the full benefit of treatment because they are unable to tolerate the physical sensations that arise as a function of completing recommended trauma-related imaginal exposures. Beyond anxiety disorders, patients with depression report physiological changes, such as lethargy and heaviness in the limbs, that provoke distress and behavior change (i.e., limited activity, social withdrawal). Indeed, we have theorized that aversive reactions to the physical sensations associated with emotional experiences may contribute to the maintenance of any disorder in which strong emotions are present (Boettcher, Brake, & Barlow, 2016; Boswell et al., 2013a), suggesting that interoceptive exposure may be a useful transdiagnostic intervention.

Unfortunately, research on the specific effects of interoceptive exposure has been sparse, as this element is typically tested within the context of a larger treatment packages or with nonclinical samples. In the 1980s and 1990s, several studies demonstrated that repeated inhalation of a 35% CO_2 mixture, which produces autonomic arousal and panic symptoms, reduced anxiety sensitivity in individuals who were high in this particular form of aversive reactivity (e.g., Beck, Shipherd, & Zebb, 1997; Beck & Shipherd, 1997; Griez & van Den Hout, 1986). More recently, other researchers have found that high-intensity aerobic exercise (which ostensibly produces physiological cues similar to interoceptive exposure) also decreased anxiety sensitivity in nonclinical participants. In a transdiagnostic clinical sample, Boswell and colleagues (2013a) examined patterns of change in anxiety sensitivity in the context of a treatment package that included interoceptive exposure; they found that anxiety sensitivity decreased to a similar degree from pre- to posttreatment across different anxiety disorder diagnoses (i.e., panic disorder, social anxiety disorder, GAD, and OCD), with the largest decrease appearing to coincide with the introduction of interoceptive exposure.

More recently, Boettcher and Barlow (2019) isolated the effects of interoceptive exposures in a clinical samples of patients with panic disorder and claustrophobia. Using a single-case experimental design, their findings suggest that engaging in interoceptive exposure resulted in habituation and extinction of distress associated with anxiety-related physical sensations for the majority of patients included in the study. They did not, however, find that reductions in anxiety sensitivity systematically coincided with the introduction of interoceptive exposure, and they speculated that this treatment element may be particularly useful for individuals who are specifically fearful of the physical consequences of somatic sensations (e.g., heart attack) versus other feared outcomes (e.g., embarrassment).

Although interoceptive exposures are typically used to provoke the physiological sensations associated with anxiety, there is no reason that they couldn't be applied to the other negative emotional experiences encompassed within the neurotic spectrum. For example, muscle tension, jaw clenching, and increased body temperature can be induced via interoceptive exposure and could lead to greater tolerance of anger. Similarly, lying beneath a weighted blanket may reduce aversive reactivity to the heaviness that accompanies sadness/depression. Thus, when applied broadly to the physical sensations associated with the full range of negative emotions, interoceptive exposure may represent a useful treatment element for neuroticism itself, along with the wide swath of psychopathology that can be accounted for by this trait. Although the strong association between anxiety sensitivity and neuroticism has been established (e.g., Naragon-Gainey, 2010), future research is needed to determine whether interoceptive exposure leads to improvements in this trait.

TREATMENTS SPECIFICALLY DEVELOPED FOR NEUROTICISM

Although the cognitive-behavioral treatment elements described above have theoretical relevance for neuroticism, they were originally conceived to target symptoms of DSM disorders and, in many cases, have not been tested with regard to their efficacy in addressing this trait. Several research groups, however, have adapted these interventions to directly target the temperamental vulnerability to experience negative emotions (i.e., neuroticism).

Rapee's Work with Behaviorally Inhibited Children

Rapee and colleagues' (Rapee, Kennedy, Ingram, Edwards, & Sweeney, 2005) intervention for behaviorally inhibited children represents an early attempt to intervene in temperament with the goal of preventing the onset of future anxiety disorders. The authors indicate that a withdrawn/inhibited temperament in young children is a precursor to high levels of neuroticism in adults; thus the program focused on parent training in order to minimize further kindling of the child's biological propensity to experience negative emotions. Parents were provided with psychoeducation about the nature of anxiety, traditional cognitive-behavioral strategies (i.e., exposure and cognitive restructuring) directed toward personal concerns, and training in behavior management techniques to prevent an overprotective parenting style that may confer negative reactions to emotions and patterns of emotional avoidance to their children. To maximize sustainability, this intervention was designed to be brief (six sessions) and conducted in groups.

Following promising results from early pilot work (Rapee & Jacobs, 2002), Rapee's Parent Education Program was tested in the context of an RCT (Rapee et al., 2005). Families were eligible to participate if their children were deemed behaviorally inhibited following a laboratory assessment. The assessment for each child included a 15-minute interaction with a same-age peer, contact with two strangers wearing a cloak and a gas mask, the opportunity to play with an unusual-looking toy, and acceptance of simple medical procedures (e.g., chest electrodes, blood pressure cuff). During these interactions, the researchers recorded the total amount of time the child spent talking, the duration of time spent within arm's length of the parent, the time spent staring at the peer, and the frequency of approach behaviors related to the strangers and peer. To be defined as behaviorally inhibited, a child had to score above the cutoff on three of these five behaviors. Of note, 90% of eligible children also met criteria for an anxiety disorder, despite the fact that a DSM condition was not necessary for inclusion. Eligible families were then randomized to the Parent Education Program or to a monitoring (assessment only) control condition. At the 1-year follow-up assessment, there were no discernible differences between conditions on temperamental variables, though the intervention produced a significantly greater decrease in anxiety disorders over this period compared with the monitoring control condition. This pattern of results was largely maintained at the 3-year follow-up assessment (Rapee, Kennedy, Ingram, Edwards, & Sweeney, 2010).

Although the brief version of Rapee's Parent Education Program (Rapee et al., 2005, 2010) did not appear to produce significant changes in the withdrawn/inhibited temperament, higher risk children (i.e., with a more stringent cutoff on behavioral assessment of inhibition *and* at least one parent with a DSM anxiety disorder) who participated in a more intensive version of the intervention (i.e., eight sessions instead of six) demonstrated significantly greater reductions in this trait compared with those who did not receive the treatment (Kennedy, Rapee, & Edwards, 2009). Moreover, differences among groups increased over time, suggesting that directly targeting the behaviorally inhibited temperament (i.e., neuroticism) might produce an increasing trajectory of change compared with addressing more surface-level disorder symptoms (Rapee et al., 2010).

Mindfulness-Based Approaches

More recently, Armstrong and Rimes (2016) developed a modified version of mindfulness-based cognitive therapy (MBCT; Segal et al., 2002) to directly target levels of neuroticism. In their rationale for developing this approach, the authors describe increased reactivity to emotional provocations, along with behavioral avoidance, as mechanisms through which neuroticism confers risk for emotional disorders and which mindfulness-based interventions may be particularly adept at addressing. Of course, these targets closely align with the functional model maintaining neuroticism (and emotional-disorder symptoms) described in Chapter 4. Specifically, this version of MBCT, delivered in a group format, includes references to neuroticism-related constructs, rather than depression-related themes. For example, Session 1 covers stress reactivity by introducing the fight-or-flight response, the role of the HPA axis, and unhelpful ways of responding to stress (i.e., cognitive and behavioral avoidance). Session 2 involves discussion of the relationship between thoughts and feelings, as well as common interpretation biases, and in Session 3, genetic and environmental contributions that make an individual susceptible to experiencing strong emotional reactions are discussed. In Sessions 4 and 5, patients learn about the long- and short-term consequences of avoiding emotions. Sessions 6 and 7 cover additional maladaptive responses to stress, including overthinking and self-criticism. Finally, Session 8 ties together the skills for "stress management" that had been learned previously in the treatment. Sessions included a combination of guided meditation practice and group discussion focused on experiences during the meditation, along with troubleshooting difficulties that arose during home practice.

In a small, pilot RCT, 34 individuals were randomized to receive eight sessions of neuroticism-focused MBCT or Internet-based self-help; the self-help control condition included cognitive-behavioral strategies applicable to a range of common mental health problems and was freely available in the United Kingdom. Notably, rather than recruiting for individuals with emotional-disorder diagnoses, participants were eligible for this study if their self-reported neuroticism (using the Eysenck Personality Questionnaire) was above a clinically significant cutoff. With regard to feasibility, 15 of 17 patients assigned to the MBSR condition completed the intervention, and 100% of the participants rated the intervention material as "useful" or "very useful." Between-group analyses suggest that neuroticism-focused MBSR demonstrated significantly greater reductions in this trait relative to the Internet-based self-help control condition.

Unified Protocol

The Unified Protocol for Transdiagnostic Treatment of Emotional Disorders (UP; Barlow et al., 2017b, 2017c) represents the best-known example of an intervention explicitly designed to address neuroticism. The UP was developed by our group to target features of the emotional-disorders functional model described in Chapter 4. Specifically, in order to address the aversive, avoidant responses to emotions that maintain both emotional-disorder symptoms and neuroticism itself, the UP consists of five core treatment modules aimed at extinguishing distress in response to the experience of strong emotions (see Figure 6.1). By reducing aversive reactions to negative emotions when they occur, reliance on avoidant emotion-regulation strategies that exacerbate symptoms is reduced, which in turn leads to less frequent and intense negative emotions over time.

The modules of the UP have been described in detail elsewhere (Payne, Ellard, Farchione, Fairholme, & Barlow, 2014); however, a summary of how the five core modules extinguish the distress associated with emotional experiences that maintains neuroticism is provided below. First, by providing information about the adaptive, functional nature of emotions in the Understanding Emotions module, patients begin to cultivate the stance that emotions provide useful information and should not be avoided. Additionally, in order to make overwhelming emotional experiences more manageable, patients are taught to break them down into their component parts—thoughts, physical sensations, and behavioral urges. This exercise is thought to increase the perception that emotions are under patients' control, perhaps decreasing aversive reactivity to these experiences when they occur. The final exercise in this module encourages patients to explore the short- and long-term consequences of avoidant responses to emotions, highlighting

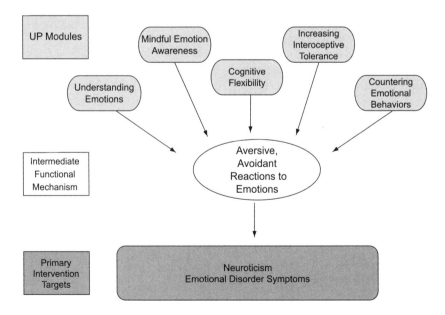

FIGURE 6.1. The five core Unified Protocol modules and their targets.

patterns in which avoidance brings immediate relief yet sets patients up to experience increasing negative emotions in the future.

> *Reducing aversive reactions to negative emotions reduces reliance on avoidant strategies, leading to less frequent and intense negative emotions.*

Next, patients receive instruction on *how* to engage willingly, rather than with avoidance, with their emotional experiences via the Mindful Emotion Awareness module; specifically, patients are taught the benefits of a present-focused, nonjudgmental attitude toward their emotions through three complementary experiential exercises. First, patients are encouraged to practice a brief guided sitting meditation in the context of a neutral mood in order to gain experience with a nonjudgmental and present-focused quality of attention. Next, using a personally relevant piece of music to induce an emotional experience, patients are asked to apply mindful awareness under more challenging circumstances (i.e., in the context of strong emotions). Finally, the UP's exercise in anchoring in the present is used when emotional experiences organically arise in patients' daily lives. Specifically, when they notice an emotion beginning to build, patients are asked to "anchor" their attention to the present moment, using a physical cue (e.g., a deep breath, the feeling of their feet on the floor); subsequently, they are encouraged to take stock of their emotion-related thoughts, physical sensations, and behaviors and to evaluate whether these components are relevant to the demands of the present moment or whether they are exacerbated by ruminations about the past or worries about the future.

Patients are then taught specific skills that map onto three interacting components of an emotional experience (i.e., thoughts, behaviors, and physical sensations). First, patients are encouraged to be more flexible in the way they appraise emotion-eliciting situations (Cognitive Flexibility module). This goal is first accomplished through an in-session exercise in which patients are asked to generate interpretations of an ambiguous picture; often, patients have difficulty producing alternative appraisals beyond their initial assessment, illustrating the tendency to trust our first impressions. Next, patients are introduced to the ways in which negative automatic interpretations can become habitual, referred to as "thinking traps"; specifically, the UP encourages patients to evaluate whether their initial impressions inflate the likelihood of a negative outcome (probability overestimation/jumping to conclusions) or underestimate their ability to cope (catastrophizing/thinking the worst). A list of challenging questions (e.g., "Do you know for certain this will happen? How could you cope if it did?") is then provided to help patients identify ways in which alternative interpretations of a given situation may be viable; specifically, they are encouraged to practice flexibility in their thinking, rather than to change maladaptive cognitions outright—in line with the UP's emphasis on acceptance.

The following module, Countering Emotional Behaviors, involves the identification of patient-specific avoidance behaviors that serve to dampen the experience of strong emotions. Several forms of avoidant behaviors (described in detail in Chapter 4) are introduced, including overt situational avoidance, subtle behavioral avoidance, safety signals, and emotion-driven behaviors. Next, patients are instructed to act counter to their emotion-driven behavioral urges by engaging in activities that may put them in contact with strong emotions in the short term. Here, patients begin to accumulate evidence that, despite immediate increases in emotional intensity, they are setting themselves up for less interfering emotional experiences in the long term.

Finally, treatment culminates with two exposure-based modules. First, patients cultivate a greater tolerance of physical sensations through interoceptive exercises (e.g., hyperventilation, breathing through a thin straw) that deliberately provoke the physiological feelings associated with strong emotions (Tolerating Physical Sensations module). Finally, the Emotion Exposures module encourages patients to engage in a series of activities that elicit strong or uncomfortable emotions. Through this practice, patients' aversive reactions to emotions are gradually extinguished via new learning that emotions are temporary and can be tolerated.

Empirical Support for the UP

Since the publication of its first edition (Barlow et al., 2011a, 2011b), the UP has amassed considerable support for its use with a wide range of emotional-disorder presentations. Moreover, because this intervention is principle-focused (i.e., including common cognitive-behavioral elements with a clear focus on aversive reactivity to emotions), the UP has been tested in a variety of formats (i.e., group, individual) and settings (i.e., outpatient, intensive outpatient, inpatient). In a recent review, Cassiello-Robbins, Southward, Tirpak, and Sauer-Zavala (2020) report that 77 treatment outcome trials have been conducted using the UP as the study intervention; over half of these studies were published between 2017 and 2019, suggesting increasing interest in mechanism-focused transdiagnostic interventions. Given the field's focus on categorical diagnoses, rather than underlying temperament/personality–based syndromes, most of the results reported relate to improvements on symptoms.

The majority of UP outcome studies have focused on patients diagnosed with a primary anxiety disorder or closely related condition (i.e., OCD), though individuals with comorbid diagnoses (e.g., depression) are often included in these samples. Effects of an early version of the UP were first evaluated in the context of a case study of a patient with OCD, panic disorder, and agoraphobia (Boisseau, Farchione, Fairholme, Ellard, & Barlow,

2010). This patient reported improvements in anxiety, depressive, and panic symptoms, time spent on obsessions and compulsions, and interpersonal functioning. Additionally, results from five open trials conducted in three countries (United States, Japan, Spain) suggest that the UP demonstrates preliminary efficacy in treating anxiety disorders with or without comorbid mood disorders, in both individual (Ellard, Fairholme, Boisseau, Farchione, & Barlow, 2010; Ito et al., 2016; Osma, Castellano, Crespo, & García-Palacios, 2015) and group (Bullis et al., 2015) formats.

In RCTs with anxiety disorder samples, the UP has demonstrated significant improvements in anxiety and depressive symptoms relative to wait-list conditions (Farchione et al., 2012; Khakpoor et al., 2019; Mohajerin, Bakhtiyar, Olesnycky, Dolatshahi, & Motabi, 2019; Zemestani, Imani, & Ottaviani, 2017). For example, Farchione et al. (2012) reported that the UP resulted in greater improvements in diagnostic severity and functioning compared with a wait-list/delayed-treatment condition in a transdiagnostic anxiety disorder sample; these improvements were generally maintained for 18 months after treatment concluded (Bullis, Fortune, Farchione, & Barlow, 2014). Beyond anxiety and depression outcomes, the UP was associated with decreases in anxiety sensitivity that, in turn, were related to lower posttreatment clinical severity (Boswell et al., 2013a). In another study, conducted in Iran, that specifically examined patients with primary body dysmorphic disorder (BDD; Khakpoor et al., 2019), individuals in the UP condition demonstrated greater decreases in BDD and depressive symptoms, appearance anxiety, emotion dysregulation, and delusional beliefs relative to individuals in the wait-list condition, and these improvements were generally maintained at 3-month follow-up.

Finally, the UP's effects on patients with primary anxiety disorders have been compared with other active treatments. In the largest RCT in the United States to date, Barlow et al. (2017a) compared the UP with four single-disorder CBT protocols (SDPs) and a wait-list control condition. Relative to SDPs, the UP led to similar improvements in diagnostic severity, anxiety and depressive symptoms, work/social adjustment, hope, quality of life, positive affect, and number of comorbid disorders (Barlow et al., 2017a; Gallagher et al., 2020; Steele et al., 2018; Wilner Tirpak et al., 2019). A similar percentage of patients no longer met criteria for their primary diagnosis in the UP (63.6%) and SDP (57.1%) conditions at the end of treatment, and these gains tended to be maintained at 6-month follow-up (Barlow et al., 2017a). Consistent with previous work, the UP led to greater improvements on all these measures compared with wait-list control. In another study comparing the UP with various SDPs, Lofti, Bakhtiyari, Asgharnezhad-Farid, and Amini (2014) found that the UP led to greater decreases in anxiety symptoms but similar improvements in depressive symptoms and quality of life. Finally, in a study conducted in Brazil in which the UP was compared with a psychotropic-medication-only condition, the UP led to significantly larger decreases in anxiety and depressive symptoms (de Ornelas Maia, Nardi, & Cardoso, 2015).

Several modified versions of the UP have been tested among people with anxiety disorders. For example, Sauer-Zavala, Cassiello-Robbins, Ametaj, Wilner, and Pagan (2019b) varied the sequence of UP modules according to patients' pretreatment skill strengths and weaknesses; they found that capitalizing on existing strengths was associated with earlier improvement in anxiety and depressive symptoms, along with reduced experiential avoidance. In two additional studies, adjunctive interventions were added to the UP. First, in one study with a sample of patients with GAD, mantra-based meditation was added to the standard UP (Roxbury, 2017). Although all patients remitted from GAD at posttreatment and both conditions led to similar improvements in worry, anxiety, sleep impairment, work/social adjustment, negative affect, self-compassion, and mindfulness, the UP plus mantra meditation led to steeper improvements in depressive symptoms, quality of life, emotion dysregulation, and positive affect. Finally, a case report described the treatment of one patient using the standard UP with behavioral activation strategies incorporated (Boswell, Iles, Gallagher, & Farchione, 2017); this individual reported decreases in anxiety and depressive symptoms, worry, and stress.

With regard to the UP's efficacy among individuals diagnosed with primary depressive disorders, two RCTs, one open trial, and three case studies have been conducted. The RCTs, which took place in the United Kingdom and Iran, compared the UP with a wait-list control (Marnoch, 2014) and English-language training (Bameshgi, Kimiaei, & Mashhadi, 2019), respectively. Similar to outcomes in samples consisting primarily of patients with anxiety disorders, both studies suggest that UP produces greater improvements in anxiety and depressive symptoms compared with a wait list. Additionally, in an open trial of a UP group for depressive disorders in Brazil, patients reported large improvements from pre- to posttreatment in depression and anxiety symptoms, quality of life, physical health and sexuality, and social relationships (de Ornelas Maia, Braga, Nunes, Nardi, & Silva, 2013). Finally, three case studies, each describing outcomes from a single-patient treatment with the UP, found improvements in symptoms of depression and anxiety from pre- to posttreatment (Boswell, Anderson, & Barlow, 2014; Hague, Scott, & Kellett, 2015; Osma, Sánchez-Gómez, & Peris-Baquero, 2018).

Additionally, several studies have tested modified versions of the UP in patient samples primarily comprising individuals with depressive disorders. First, two case studies describe making relatively minor modifications to the UP. For example, a patient with MDD and GAD received the UP, modified to include assertiveness training and grief processing (Donahue, Hormes,

Gordis, & Anderson, 2019), and demonstrated improvements in depressive symptoms that were small in magnitude, whereas anxiety symptoms remained in the clinical range. Additionally, in Colombia, Castro-Camacho and colleagues (2019) describe treating a patient with MDD, PTSD, GAD, and panic disorder with a version of the UP that was adapted to better match the patient's cultural context (e.g., including an orientation session, focusing on difficulties functioning instead of diagnoses); this patient reported large reductions in depressive, anxiety, and PTSD symptoms, as well as headaches, sleep difficulties, and uncomfortable physical sensations, which were generally maintained for 2 years following treatment. Finally, the UP has also been modified to treat suicidal thoughts and behaviors among inpatients with MDD and anxiety disorders (Bentley et al., 2017). In this study, the UP was shortened to five sessions focusing on core modules. Compared with treatment as usual (TAU), the UP led to similar improvements in depressive and anxiety symptoms, hopelessness, and overall psychopathology from pre- to posttreatment.

Beyond anxiety and depressive disorders, the UP has also been tested in the context of other disorders that fall within the emotional-disorder functional model. For example, individuals with bipolar disorder also report the frequent experience of negative emotions, along with aversive reactions to these affective experiences. In order to understand the UP's effects among patients with bipolar disorder, Ellard and colleagues have conducted several studies. First, in a case series that included individuals diagnosed with bipolar I and II, the UP was associated with significant improvements in symptoms of depression and anxiety (Ellard, Deckersbach, Sylvia, Nierenberg, & Barlow, 2012). In an RCT in which patients with bipolar I and II were randomized to either standard individual UP with psychiatric TAU ($n = 8$) or psychiatric TAU alone (Ellard et al., 2017), patients in the UP condition demonstrated significantly greater improvements compared with TAU. Of course, bipolar disorder is also characterized by excesses in positive emotionality (i.e., extraversion), which may necessitate additional intervention (a topic we return to in Chapter 7).

The UP has also been evaluated in the context of eating disorders. Indeed, individuals suffering from anorexia nervosa and bulimia nervosa score higher than healthy controls on measures of neuroticism and negative emotionality (Cassin & von Ranson, 2005; Forbush & Watson, 2006), and these traits have been shown to be prospective risk factors for eating psychopathology (Fox & Froom, 2009; Wildes, Ringham, & Marcus, 2010). Empirical research has reliably demonstrated that compared with healthy controls, individuals with eating disorders report more negative beliefs about emotions and less acceptance of their emotional experiences (Brockmeyer et al., 2014; Harrison et al., 2009, 2010; Ioannou & Fox, 2009; Lawson et al., 2008; Svaldi et al., 2012). With regard to empirical support for using the

UP with this population, two large-scale implementation studies have been conducted incorporating this intervention into a residential eating-disorders treatment facility. The UP was modified in several ways to better match this setting, including designing modules to be delivered independently of each other to accommodate rolling admission, incorporating more eating-disorder-relevant examples, and incorporating more active, standardized patient exercises (e.g., eating and mirror exposures; Thompson-Brenner et al., 2018b). Additionally, the UP modules were split into phases of treatment for patients—that is, early (Understanding Emotions, Mindful Emotion Awareness), middle (Cognitive Flexibility, Countering Emotional Behaviors), and late (Exposure)—with assessments to determine when patients would move on to the next phase; this adaptation was possible given long average length of stay in this residential program. In an initial proof of concept evaluation, patients demonstrated small to medium-sized preadmission to postdischarge improvements in experiential avoidance, mindfulness, and anxiety sensitivity, along with medium-sized improvements in eating-disorder symptoms (Thompson-Brenner et al., 2018a). Among a larger sample of patients completing the UP at this site, the UP led to greater pre- to posthospitalization improvements in experiential avoidance, mindfulness, and anxiety sensitivity, but not depressive or eating-disorder symptoms, relative to the treatment used in this setting prior to the UP's implementation (Thompson-Brenner et al., 2018a).

The UP has also been applied to BPD. With regard to the emotional-disorders functional model, the experience of heightened negative affect is considered a core component of BPD (Carpenter & Trull, 2013; Crowell, Beauchaine, & Linehan, 2009), and studies have consistently shown that individuals with BPD experience their emotions more intensely than do those from nonclinical populations (Nica & Links, 2009; Yen et al., 2002). BPD is also associated with heightened emotional reactivity, particularly in the context of interpersonal stress (Chapman, Walters, & Gordon, 2014), along with emotionally avoidant coping. In terms of empirical support for using the UP to treat individuals with BPD, four single-case experiments have been conducted. Specifically, in a multiple-baseline design with 8 participants, Lopez and colleagues (2019) found that 5 patients no longer met criteria for BPD following treatment with the UP. Moreover, half of the patients in their study demonstrated reliable decreases in anxiety and depressive symptoms. Similarly, in another study conducted by this group, half the patients with BPD and comorbid disorders reported lower BPD features during treatment than during the baseline phase (Lopez et al., 2015). In a third single-case experiment, 3 of 5 patients with BPD showed large reductions in BPD features, anxiety and depressive symptoms, and emotion dysregulation (Sauer-Zavala, Bentley, & Wilner, 2016). Finally, in a study conducted in Iran, all patients with BPD and comorbid disorders reported some reductions in emotion dysregulation and BPD features from baseline to posttreatment and/ or follow-up (Mohammadi, Bakhtiari, Masjedi Arani, Dolatshahi, & Habibi, 2018). Relatedly, Bentley and colleagues (2017) describe a case study of an 18-year-old patient who frequently engaged in nonsuicidal self-injury, a characteristic feature of BPD (though this patient did not meet full criteria for this condition). By the end of treatment, the patient had refrained from any self-injurious behaviors for 5 months, maintained low depressive and anxiety symptoms, and reported reductions in GAD symptoms and social anxiety.

Some authors have described insomnia as a condition that, in specific circumstances, may be described as an emotional disorder (Bullis & Sauer-Zavala, 2018), particularly when sleep-related behaviors (e.g., spending too much time in bed, overreliance on sleep aids) function to escape from negative emotional experiences. Two studies, both conducted in Iran, have explored the use of UP for patients with insomnia disorder (i.e., Doos Ali Vand, Banafsheh, Asghar, Farhad, & Mojtaba, 2018a; Doos Ali Vand, Gharraee, Asgharnejad Farid, Ghaleh Bandi, & Habibi, 2018b). Results suggest that the UP was associated with improvements in sleep-related variables (e.g., onset latency, quality, beliefs), along with decreases in emotion dysregulation, anxiety sensitivity, and neuroticism.

Similarly, when substance use functions primarily to escape negative emotional experiences, substance use disorders may be successfully treated from an emotional-disorders framework (see Bullis et al., 2019). In one open trial conducted in a substance use specialty clinic serving individuals experiencing homelessness (Sauer-Zavala et al., 2019a), delivery of the UP was modified (based on provider feedback) to include only its five core modules, which could be delivered in any order. In this study, all patients were diagnosed with opioid use disorder and MDD, though most had additional comorbid conditions; group-based effects suggest that treatment with the UP was associated with medium to large improvements in anxiety, though a worsening of depressive symptoms that was small in magnitude was also observed. In another study, among patients with comorbid anxiety and alcohol use disorder, the UP was provided with venlafaxine or placebo and compared with a relaxation condition with venlafaxine or placebo. The UP-plus-placebo group reported a greater decrease in the percentage of heavy drinking days compared with the relaxation-plus-placebo group (Ciraulo et al., 2013).

In addition to studies comprising patients with specific DSM classes (i.e., anxiety, depressive, eating) or disorders (e.g., BPD, insomnia), several studies have recruited samples with an array of diagnoses. Specifically, one RCT, conducted in Hong Kong, included patients with depressive, anxiety, adjustment, eating, and/or insomnia disorders who were randomized to receive 15 weeks of group UP or disorder-specific CBT (Ling, 2018). The UP group led to greater improvements in depressive and anxiety symptoms and clinical severity at posttreatment. Additionally, three open trials (i.e., Alatiq & Modayfer, 2019; Reinholt et al., 2017; Varkovitzky, Sherrill, & Reger, 2018) have been conducted that included patients with PTSD, depressive disorders, sleep–wake disorders, substance use disorders, anxiety disorders, bipolar disorder, schizophrenia, OCD, panic disorder, social anxiety disorder, conversion disorder, specific phobia, and complicated grief, somatic, eating, personality, and attention-deficit/hyperactivity disorders. Overall, these studies indicated that the UP led to improvements in symptoms of depression and anxiety, as well as emotion regulation (Varkovitzky et al., 2018), functioning, and quality of life (Alatiq & Modayfer, 2019; Reinholt et al., 2017).

Finally, given that neuroticism is also associated with a range of physical health outcomes, the UP has been applied to patients experiencing several physical complaints, including irritable bowel syndrome (IBS), chronic pain, infertility, and Parkinson's disease. Indeed, treatment with the UP, relative to a wait-list control condition, was associated with greater improvement in symptoms of IBS (Johari-Fard & Ghafourpour, 2015; Mohsenabadi, Zanjani, Shabani, & Arj, 2018). With regard to chronic pain, results from a single-case experiment suggest that the UP may not be efficacious for treating chronic pain, though it must be noted that a self-guided Internet-delivered version of the UP was used in these studies (Wurm et al., 2017). One RCT that compared treatments for women struggling with anxiety and depression secondary to infertility found that the UP resulted in similar improvements in these symptoms compared with eight sessions of MBSR (Mousavi et al., 2019). Finally, results from a single-case experiment in which 12 sessions of the UP were provided to patients with Parkinson's disease suggest that this intervention is associated with improvement in anxiety and depressive symptoms compared with baseline (Reynolds, Saint-Hilaire, Thomas, Barlow, & Cronin-Golomb, 2019).

The UP has been applied to gay and bisexual men in the context of an open RCT. Specifically, patients engaged in 10 individual sessions of Effective Skills to Empower Effective Men (ESTEEM), a modification of the UP designed to address the effects of sexual-minority stress on HIV-related stressors, sexual compulsivity, substance use, and HIV transmission risk behaviors (Pachankis, Hatzenbuehler, Rendina, Safren, & Parsons, 2015; Parsons et al., 2017). Results from the RCT suggest that, compared with a wait-list condition, the UP significantly reduced depressive symptoms, alcohol use problems, sexual compulsivity, and past-90-day condomless sex with casual partners and improved condom use self-efficacy. Effects were generally maintained at follow-up.

Taken together, there is considerable empirical support for using the UP, a treatment designed to target neuroticism by addressing the aversive avoidant reactions that maintain this trait, to treat the full range of emotional disorder. Indeed, in a recent meta-analysis that included 15 studies and 1,244 participants conducted by Sakiris and Berle (2019), large effect-size reductions were found across symptoms of depression, GAD, OCD, panic disorder with and without agoraphobia, social anxiety disorder, and BPD.

Of course, given the premise of the UP as a treatment for neuroticism itself, it is also important to consider the effects of this intervention on this trait. First, there is some evidence that the UP addresses the broader range of emotional experiences, beyond anxiety and sadness, that neuroticism comprises. For example, in a subsample of patients from the large equivalence trial described earlier (Barlow et al., 2017a), the UP led to small nonsignificant decreases in anger, whereas SDPs led to moderate nonsignificant increases in anger (Cassiello-Robbins et al., 2018). Moreover, using data from the same study, Sauer-Zavala and colleagues (2020) examined whether the UP led to greater reductions in neuroticism relative to gold-standard, symptom-focused CBT protocols (i.e., SDPs) and a wait-list control condition. Results suggest that patients in the UP condition demonstrated greater reductions in neuroticism than did those in the SDP and wait-list conditions. Further, no differences were observed between the SDP and wait-list conditions on neuroticism scores at the end of the treatment window, indicating that gold-standard, symptom-focused approaches may not provide an advantage over no treatment at all (i.e., wait list) when targeting this temperamental dimension (Barlow et al., 2017a). It is also worth noting that fluctuations in depression and anxiety do not appear to account for changes in neuroticism in this sample, despite significant symptom improvement observed across both active treatment conditions.

Of note, the greatest divergence among UP and SDP patients with regard to the average trajectory of change in neuroticism occurred during the final four sessions of this study. At this point in treatment, all patients (regardless of condition) were engaging in exposures. The goal of exposure in the SDPs, however, is to extinguish distress in response to specific emotion-eliciting situations (e.g., public speaking, contamination), whereas in the UP condition, the focus is on facilitating new learning about emotions themselves (e.g., emotions are temporary and tolerable) regardless of situation. The UP may reduce neuroticism to a greater extent due to its focus on exposure to a broad array of negative emotions across situations, as opposed to the situation-specific focus of SDPs. But future research would be necessary to clarify the mechanisms underlying the unique effect of specific UP treatment components on neuroticism.

Summary

Together, these findings provide evidence that neuroticism may be most apt to change in treatment when it is directly targeted in specific ways. For example, Rapee's work with the parents of behaviorally inhibited children suggests that more intensive early intervention is necessary to produce long-lasting changes in temperament, whereas symptoms of anxiety disorders were equally apt to change with or without the intervention. Here, the intervention was at the caregiver level, likely affecting parent contributions to the specific psychological vulnerability (i.e., learning experiences that contribute to perceptions of the world as dangerous/uncontrollable) described in detail in Chapter 2.

Two interventions that were developed to address neuroticism in adults with emotional disorders have also been tested. First, a version of MBSR specifically focused on neuroticism demonstrated an advantage in targeting this trait relative to an Internet-delivered cognitive-behavioral self-help program, though both interventions produced improvements in anxiety and depressive symptoms. Next, the UP also produced significantly larger decreases in neuroticism compared with gold-standard SDPs, though symptoms improved similarly in both active treatment conditions. Both neuroticism-focused treatments directly address the aversive reactivity to emotions that maintains both the neuroticism temperament and symptoms of emotional disorders. Whereas psychopharmacological treatments (i.e., SSRIs) appear to dampen neuroticism by affecting emotion-generating neural structures (i.e., limbic arousal), these behavioral treatments likely engage higher order learning processes. Indeed, in a recent study, Ellard and colleagues (2017) demonstrated that a selection of modules from the UP resulted in increased dorsal anterior cingulate cortex (dACC) activation and increased ventrolateral prefrontal cortex–amygdala functional connectivity, which are also regions associated with extinction learning (in this case, perhaps, extinguishing distress related to emotions themselves).

These findings add to the existing body of literature aimed at addressing whether temperamental variables, such as neuroticism, are responsive to treatment. First, consistent with Tang and colleagues' (2009) results, results from these studies indicate that neuroticism and psychopathology (i.e., depression and anxiety) are not isomorphic and can change independently. Additionally, though evidence of neuroticism's sensitivity to change in the context of previous treatment outcome trials has been mixed (Eaton et al., 2011a; Kring et al., 2007; Tang et al., 2009), by comparing active CBT approaches (i.e., Armstrong & Rimes, 2016; Sauer-Zavala et al., 2020), there is preliminary evidence that more robust effects are demonstrated when neuroticism is targeted more directly. We contend that engaging the intermediate functional mechanism of aversive reactivity to emotions is necessary for addressing both neuroticism and the emotional disorders related to it. Future research should explore whether change in neuroticism leads to functional improvements related to a wide range of emotional experience (i.e., tolerating anger in a romantic relationship) beyond the circumscribed

> *Engaging aversive reactivity to emotions is necessary for addressing neuroticism and the emotional disorders related to it.*

emotional/situational impairments that abate in disorder-specific CBT in the short term. Additional work can examine whether reductions in neuroticism prevent the emergence of future emotional disorders that are also characterized by aversive, avoidant responses to strong emotions.

PREVENTION OF NEUROTICISM

Directly addressing neuroticism with psychological treatments represents an efficient means to create lasting improvement across a wide swath of DSM disorders (e.g., Armstrong & Rimes, 2016; Barlow et al., 2017a), as well as to prevent them entirely (e.g., Rapee et al., 2005, 2010; Kennedy et al., 2009). Although temperament is often considered a "biological" vulnerability, the literature suggests that environmental variables indeed contribute to its development (see Chapter 2). In other words, a transactional relationship clearly exists between genetic and environmental inputs for the expression of personality, setting genetic contributions up as a predisposition that may not have to be fully realized, as described in some detail in Chapter 2.

In order to prevent the development of neuroticism, early identification of those at risk is paramount. Fortunately, evidence of neuroticism at age 2, which has been associated with emotional-disorder onset in later childhood and adulthood, can be predicted from crying in response to novel stimuli in infants as young as 4 months old (Moehler et al., 2008). Moreover, exposure to stress during pregnancy, as well as maternal diagnosis of a postpartum anxiety disorder, have been shown to predict infant salivary cortisol reactivity in response to novel stimuli (Möhler, Parzer, Brunner, Wiebel, & Resch, 2006; Reck, Müller, Tietz, & Möhler, 2013). Additionally, maternal sensitivity to infant needs predicts asymmetrical electroencephalogram in 6-month-old children that, in turn, protects against negative emotionality at 12 months (Wen et al., 2017). Taken together, this emerging literature suggests that a number of factors may be used to identify those at risk for developing a neurotic temperament, including parental stress level, parental diagnostic status, and biological, physiological, and behavioral measures in infants.

In addition to identifying risk factors that suggest the likely development of a neurotic temperament, it is also necessary to identify early interventions that may prevent its emergence. There is evidence from the animal literature suggesting strategies that may be useful in preventing further kindling of neuroticism in humans (see Barlow et al., 2014a); for example, newborn rats that were exposed to relatively novel environments for 3 minutes a day displayed less behavioral inhibition (defined as time spent in exploration after weaning) compared with newborn rats that stayed in their home cage (Tang, Reeb-Sutherland, Romeo, & McEwen, 2012). Interestingly, these results were moderated by maternal rat HPA-axis reactivity, suggesting that interventions should target both children and parents. Continued investigation into early biological and behavioral markers that may denote the presence of a vulnerability for neuroticism and could conceivably serve as targets for intervention is necessary, as is investigation into efficacy of the preventive interventions themselves.

CONCLUSIONS

Despite characterizations of temperament and personality as stable over time, neuroticism may be more malleable than originally believed. Naturalistic, longitudinal studies suggest that this trait declines across the lifespan, though the evidence is mixed with regard to whether it is responsive to direct intervention. However, most of the studies included in this chapter examined change in neuroticism following treatments developed to address DSM disorders; when neuroticism itself is the focus, improvement on this trait appears more robust and reliable than previously assumed. Indeed, treatments that directly target neuroticism may represent an efficient approach to treating a range of DSM disorders (e.g., Armstrong & Rimes, 2016; Barlow et al., 2017a) and possibly preventing them entirely (e.g., Rapee et al., 2005). These promising results are likely due to the fact that the three interventions for neuroticism described above each include strategies that address components of the functional model maintaining this temperament described in Chapter 4. Although an attractive prospect for many reasons, much remains to be done to fully confirm the functional model of neuroticism, as well as the efficacy and efficiency of targeting aversive/avoidant reactions in the context of emotional disorders thought to reflect the common underlying trait of neuroticism. Additionally, although the functional pairing of neuroticism and aversive reactivity can account for the development of the range of emotional disorders (and can become efficient targets of treatment), they do not explain the full breadth of psychopathology. Thus, in Chapter 7, we review the additional broad dimensions of personality (e.g., extraversion, antagonism, disinhibition) included in dimensional models of psychopathology (see Chapter 5) and propose functional mechanisms that can become the focus of care.

7

Personality as a Basis for Treating Mental Disorders

The previous chapters have largely focused on the role of neuroticism in the development of a wide array of mental health conditions, along with delineating a functional model to account for the path from this trait to the clinical impairment that constitutes emotional-disorder diagnoses. In Chapter 6, we discussed how targeting functional mechanisms in treatment can lead to improvement in the tendency to experience negative emotions (i.e., neuroticism), as well as the symptoms traditionally associated with DSM conditions. Specifically, we described how the unified protocol (UP; Barlow et al., 2017c), a transdiagnostic intervention developed to address common vulnerabilities associated with the broad range of emotional disorders, leads to symptom remission (e.g., Barlow et al., 2017a) and decreased neuroticism (Carl, Soskin, Kerns, & Barlow, 2013; Sauer-Zavala et al., 2020). The UP does this by targeting aversive reactivity to emotions, the putative mechanism maintaining both trait and symptoms.

In Chapter 5, though our main focus was to highlight the role of neuroticism in various approaches to mental health nosology (e.g., DSM/ICD system, dimensional models of psychopathology), we also introduced additional domains of personality that appear to confer unique risk for various forms of psychopathology. For example, considering the well-known five-factor model of personality (FFM), low levels of extraversion account for additional risk beyond neuroticism in predicting depressive disorders, social anxiety, and agoraphobia (e.g., Brown, Chorpita, & Barlow, 1998; Rosellini et al., 2010), whereas high levels of this trait are associated with bipolar disorder (Bagby et al., 1996; Quilty et al., 2009). Similarly, maladaptive variants of agreeableness, conscientiousness, and openness have each been linked to specific forms of psychopathology (Widiger, Lynam, Miller, & Oltmanns,

2012). Indeed, these five broad dimensions (neuroticism, extraversion, conscientiousness, agreeableness, and openness) are clearly represented in prominent dimensional proposals for understanding the broad range of mental health conditions, including the DSM-5 alternative model of personality disorders (AMPD; American Psychiatric Association, 2013) and the hierarchical taxonomy of psychopathology (HiTOP; Kotov et al., 2017).

The use of a dimensional, personality-based scheme to classify the majority of the psychopathology included in the DSM system has many advantages (described in detail in Chapter 5). In summary, instead of numerous categories with overlapping symptoms and high rates of comorbidity (as is the case for the current DSM system), a trait-based approach may allow for greater specificity in communicating the deficits that drive symptoms (Brown & Barlow, 2005, 2009; Hopwood et al., 2012). Indeed, dimensional models provide the ability to determine whether clinically relevant elevations exist on a range of features (e.g., hostility, mistrust) that may then become idiographic treatment targets, rather than relying on a categorical diagnosis and applying a one-size-fits-all treatment.

Several researchers have provided accounts of how an individual's personality profile could be used to select treatment components, though there are limitations to this work. First, the majority of the personality-based treatment recommendations, in which existing interventions (e.g., interpersonal effectiveness in dialectical behavior therapy) are matched to particular traits (e.g., antagonism), lack empirical support; more research is needed to determine whether the suggested treatment components indeed engage these personality domains. Additionally, most of these theoretical accounts have been applied only to personality disorders (i.e., Hopwood, 2018; Mullins-Sweatt et al., 2020), with limited relevance for more prevalent conditions that are also clearly mediated by higher order temperamental domains (e.g., emotional disorders). Finally, within this literature, including more comprehensive accounts that apply to a broader range of psychopathology (i.e., Bach & Presnall-Shvorin, 2020), treatment recommendations are made at the facet level of the FFM; in other words, given that each of the five broad domains of personality consists of six facets (e.g., neuroticism comprises anxiety, depression, anger, self-consciousness, impulsiveness, and vulnerability), this approach yields 30 distinct treatment approaches. Although this number of interventions is far fewer than the number of protocols required to address each DSM diagnosis, it may still result in significant therapist burden (i.e., time and costs associated with learning a large number of treatments). Additionally, it is not clear that the facets organized beneath a broad personality domain are functionally distinct, warranting discrete treatment approaches.

We contend that generally focusing treatment at the broad domain level of personality, as we have done with neuroticism, has the potential to lead to a more manageable number of evidence-based treatment components, reducing therapist training burden, while also providing coverage to the full range of DSM disorders. We also acknowledge that, for many researchers and clinicians, the notion of altering broad dimensions of personality may seem abstract, particularly as these factors were long thought to be inflexible. We argue that the functional mechanisms that link personality to the clinical phenomena associated with them represent more actionable targets of treatment (e.g., Hayes & Hofmann, 2018). Thus the goal of this chapter is to review the literature on the functional processes that account for how other traits beyond neuroticism unfold into the distress and impairment that characterize a mental disorder, along with treatment approaches that have been suggested to address these processes. Figure 7.1 depicts the putative functional mechanisms that have been described in the literature for each domain of the FFM. Of course, the bulk of this work has been conducted in the context of neuroticism, though extraversion has recently received increasing attention. For a truly streamlined approach to personality-based treatment, we argue that the intensive study applied to neuroticism (reviewed in this book) is necessary for the remaining four domains. To illustrate our view of the future of treatment planning based on the broad dimensions of the FFM, case illustrations are used to frame this discussion.

TREATING SYMPTOMS AND TEMPERAMENT: CASE EXAMPLES

In this section, we return to the case vignettes introduced in the preface of this book. Our goal is to illustrate how targeting the higher order dimension of neuroticism, via the functional mechanism of aversive reactivity, is

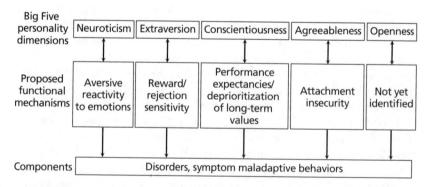

FIGURE 7.1. Intermediate functional mechanisms that connect broad domains of personality to psychopathology.

sufficient for the treatment of some, but not all, psychopathology. First, we describe two cases, a young woman diagnosed with GAD and a middle-aged man with panic disorder and agoraphobia, who were successfully treated with a neuroticism-focused intervention (i.e., the unified protocol [UP], described in detail in Chapter 6). Then we discuss two additional cases (one with social anxiety and depression, another with BPD) who remained symptomatic following treatment with UP. Of course, neuroticism and aversive reactivity to emotions are relevant for these conditions; however, we speculate that additional domains of personality, untreated by the UP, may account for the remaining symptoms these individuals experienced. Following each case description, we summarize the literature on the work conducted to date to identify the functional mechanisms that connect relevant personality domains (i.e., extraversion, conscientiousness, agreeableness) to the remaining symptoms experienced by our patients. Given the limited clinical research on openness to experience, we do not frame our discussion of this trait in the context of a case vignette; instead, a brief summary on what is known about this trait is included. As noted, the majority of this work is largely theoretical, so the purpose of this section is to illustrate areas of necessary future research in order to realize a streamlined, personality-based approach to treatment.

Worry and Irritability (Case 1)

Beth is a 28-year-old married white female who presented for psychological treatment for the first time. She is an international student from an Eastern European country pursuing a graduate degree in a social science field. Beth was referred to our Center by a professor who was concerned about her anxiety, which appeared to be interfering with her schoolwork; she had taken incompletes in two of her classes during her previous spring semester. We began our work together during the following summer, and Beth reported great difficulty finishing the delinquent assignments due to strong feelings of anxiety regarding her capabilities, along with subsequent procrastination. This issue with her schoolwork, as well as irritability with and anger outbursts at her husband, represented Beth's primary concerns, for which she sought treatment.

The initial session was focused on conducting a thorough diagnostic interview. Based on the assessment, Beth met criteria for GAD, describing excessive, uncontrollable worry more days than not over the previous 6 months about her school and work performance, minor matters (e.g., running errands, preparing meals), her husband's health, her family's finances, and her personal safety. She reported that, during her spring semester, she spent approximately 90% of the day engaged in worry. She also reported avoidance behaviors, such as procrastination of school assignments and refusing to enter crowded places that might be more susceptible to terrorist attacks. Additionally, she reported checking behaviors (e.g., going to the doctor frequently) in response to persistent concerns about her own health. Accompanying these worries, Beth described associated symptoms of restlessness, difficulty concentrating, irritability, and muscle tension. She noted that hearing noises triggered her to worry about her safety often cued panic attacks.

Figure 7.2 presents a functional assessment of Beth's symptoms. Here, rather than determining whether Beth does or does not have the categorical criteria necessary for various DSM diagnoses, the focus of this effort is to identify evidence that she experiences her emotions strongly, that she finds these emotional experiences aversive, and that she responds with avoidant coping. Specifically, Beth reported a range of negative affect consistent with a neurotic temperament, including frequent and intense anxiety, considerable irritability, and some sadness. With regard to aversive reactivity, even during the initial assessment visit, Beth made clear her strong negative

Patient: _Beth_

Presenting Problems
- _Trouble finishing school assignments on time_
- _Relationship difficulties with husband_
- _Excessive worry about health of self and family, personal safety_

Strong, Uncomfortable Emotions
- _Anxiety_
- _Irritability/anger_

Aversive Reactivity
- _"It is weak to get so upset"_
- _"My emotions only get me in trouble"_

Avoidant Coping

Situational avoidance: _Avoids attending office hours, school functions, crowded public spaces that may be susceptible to terrorist attacks_
Subtle behavioral avoidance: _Procrastinate on work assignments, overschedule her time, frequent checking in on family_
Cognitive avoidance: _Excessively research medical conditions, watch TV_
Safety signals: _Only visit certain public spaces with husband present_
Emotion-driven behaviors: _Snapping at husband_

FIGURE 7.2. Case conceptualization worksheet for Beth.

views about her own emotional experiences, describing them as weaknesses that only cause problems in her life. Finally, she described various attempts to gain control of her strong emotions via avoidant behavioral responses. These included procrastinating, overscheduling her time (rather than actually working), snapping at her husband, repeatedly checking on her loved ones, excessive Internet research of medical symptoms, and avoiding public spaces.

Neuroticism-Focused Treatment

Given Beth's tendency to experience strong negative affect when faced with stressors, her aversive reactions to these emotional responses, and her propensity to address them using avoidant coping, the UP was selected to target these difficulties. She completed 20 sessions. Early sessions were focused on exploring the adaptive function and nature of emotions (Module 2: Understanding Emotions) and learning to adopt a nonjudgmental, present-focused stance toward this experience (Module 3: Mindful Emotion Awareness). Beth struggled initially with identifying the adaptive function of each emotion, as she described a deeply held belief that her emotions had only caused problems for her in the past. Psychoeducation regarding differentiation between initial, adaptively triggered emotions and maladaptive responses to these emotions were discussed, and ultimately Beth was able to articulate why experience of the full range of emotions is necessary. We further explored maladaptive responses to her emotions by discussing a recent argument between Beth and her husband within the context of the three-component model of emotion; this allowed her to examine how the interaction of her thoughts, physical sensations, and behaviors that followed her initial emotional trigger may have escalated the intensity of the experience. Beth described a frequently occurring disagreement in which her husband asked her to help him prepare dinner despite their having previously agreed to take turns with the cooking. She identified automatic thoughts ("I will not be able to complete my school work if I help with dinner"; "My husband does not respect my time") and how such appraisals led to physical sensations of increased heart rate and muscle tension. This escalation of emotion was reportedly followed by Beth's snapping at her husband and storming out of the room. We highlighted the long- and short-term consequences of Beth's emotion-driven behavioral response by engaging in a functional analysis of these actions; in the short term, snapping at her husband led to a decrease in anxiety, as she was able to return to her schoolwork rather than helping with dinner; however, Beth reported subsequent guilt over her reaction and increased anxiety on following evenings in which her husband is preparing dinner for fear that he might ask her again to help.

Adopting a more mindful approach to her emotional experiences in order to facilitate emotion exposures was achieved through formal meditation practice and mindfully informed coping techniques (anchoring in the present). Beth reported that the rationale for this module, developing a present-focused and nonjudgmental stance toward emotions, mapped onto her tendencies to be self-critical for her strong emotions and to engage in a great deal of future-themed cognition. Despite her initial enthusiasm, Beth struggled with completing the formal meditation task outside of session, only attempting the task three times during the week, though it had been assigned twice daily. She cited concerns about her ability to complete the exercise correctly and whether the task was taking too much time away from her studies. In the following session, we discussed how engaging in the mindfulness meditation represents a first exposure activity; by objectively observing all stimuli without responding to it, including thoughts about completing the task correctly, patients learn what happens when they do not engage in attempts to avoid or dampen emotions. Beth subsequently reported greater success in completing the exercise during the next week, stating that she was better able to label her worries as thoughts that may not represent the truth. Beth also indicated that using her breath or other sensory cues to anchor herself in the present moment was particularly helpful in terms of future-oriented worries. For example, she described a situation in which she was walking to a potluck at her school and noticed herself making negative predictions about the event (e.g., "It will be awkward, no one will talk to me"); Beth stated that she was able to pull herself away from these cognitions by focusing on the feeling of her feet hitting the sidewalk, reminding her that the awful consequences she was forecasting were not yet happening in the present moment and might not happen at all. She noted that taking this "space" to objectively observe and label her future-oriented thoughts allowed her to overcome her behavioral urge to avoid the potluck.

The next three sessions were spent going into greater depth, exploring the contributions of the three components of an emotional response described above (thoughts, behaviors, and physical sensations). We began with the role of negative automatic appraisal in generating strong emotions (Module 4: Cognitive Flexibility), and Beth was able to identify thinking patterns that contributed to her anxiety and irritability. In-session activities and homework exercises provided an opportunity to identify "thinking traps," such as overestimating the likelihood that a negative prediction would occur and discounting one's ability to cope with it if it did. Beth described a situation in which one of her professors did not call on her during class and identified automatic thoughts regarding the professor's opinion of her ("She doesn't like me") and her ability to tolerate future classes ("It will be too uncomfortable for me to raise my hand again" and "If she doesn't call on me, I'll confirm my suspicion that she doesn't like me"). During session, we were able to increase Beth's cognitive flexibility by generating alternate possibilities with regard to her professor's behavior. Additionally, this experience also provided an opportunity to explore the role of behaviors during her emotional experiences (Module 5: Countering Emotional Behaviors). In general, Beth was asked to monitor and record behavioral urges associated with certain emotions or automatic thoughts. With regard to the situation with her professor, Beth described the urge to sit in the back of the class and to refrain from participating for the rest of the semester. Following an exploration of the short- and long-term consequences of these behaviors, she was willing to act inconsistently with these urges. Not only was she able to successfully participate in the subsequent class, but her professor also praised her contribution, disconfirming her negative automatic appraisals. Finally, we attended to how Beth's physical sensations (racing heart, muscle tension) contributed to her negative automatic appraisals and urges to engage in avoidant behaviors (Module 6). Beth was encouraged to complete interoceptive exposures, including hyperventilation and breathing through a thin straw, to practice relating to these sensations in a mindful manner, thereby facilitating interoceptive exposure.

The final phase of treatment was focused on utilizing the skills Beth had learned thus far through emotion exposure tasks (Module 7). Specifically for Beth, exposures were designed to elicit anxiety about personal safety (taking public transportation in the evening), health (going to the doctor), and completing schoolwork (starting and continuing assignments without distraction). Throughout this phase of treatment, Beth became concerned about a medical issue and was able to address this concern with her exposure practices by making and attending medical appointments. In preparation for these activities, she challenged automatic thoughts (e.g., "The doctor will think I'm stupid for seeking treatment if this turns out to be nothing" and "It will be horrible if I find out I am really sick") and identified and devised alternatives to likely behavioral urges (e.g., the urge to refrain from asking questions in order to shorten the appointment). In addition, she described successfully using her mindful anchoring skills (i.e., nonjudgmentally acknowledging her anxiety and allowing it to be present while attending to daily tasks) throughout the week that she was waiting for test results.

At the time of treatment termination (Module 8: Relapse Prevention), Beth reported significant improvement in her ability to tolerate and respond to strong emotions and that this had had a positive effect on her relationship with her husband. She completed several self-report measures at baseline and again at posttreatment that corroborated her verbal assessment of treatment gains. Specifically, Beth demonstrated reductions in self-reported symptoms of anxiety and depression that were large in magnitude, along with increases in her ability to regulate her emotions. Finally, Beth expressed confidence in her ability to maintain treatment gains and did not request additional services at the time of termination.

Although the UP shares many therapeutic techniques with traditional, symptom-focused cognitive-behavioral therapy, the goal of this intervention is to apply these skills to the experience of one's emotions, rather than the circumscribed symptoms and situations that apply within specific diagnostic contexts (e.g., GAD, panic disorder). Here, the UP, a neuroticism-focused treatment, adequately addressed the patient's symptoms by targeting her aversive reactions to her emotions.

> *The UP applies the skills learned in therapy to the experience of one's emotions, rather than to specific diagnoses.*

Panic and Agoraphobic Avoidance (Case 2)

Marty is a married white man in his mid-50s who sought treatment from our Center for frequent panic attacks, along with excessive worry about having a future attack. In our first visit, he indicated that he had had his first panic attack several months prior while driving to work and reportedly felt terrified that he would lose control of the car. Following that initial attack, he endorsed having panic attacks several times a month, along with significant changes to his behavior. Indeed, Marty described avoiding driving (particularly on the highway, over bridges, or through tunnels), riding in elevators, attending work or social events where escape might be difficult, or going anywhere (stores, theaters) without the anxiolytic medications his primary care physician had prescribed. Marty also noted that when he couldn't "get out of" visiting an unfamiliar place (e.g., a mandatory work meeting in a remote location), he would extensively research these settings to gain a sense of control over the unknown; for instance, he reported looking up whether he would have to take elevators in the building (vs. being able to use the stairs) and how easily he could the leave the building if he felt the beginning of a panic attack. Our first session was focused on conducting a thorough diagnostic interview, after which Marty was assigned diagnoses of panic disorder and agoraphobia. Beyond categorical classification, his case formulation worksheet, conceptualizing his difficulties from the emotional-disorder functional model, can be viewed in Figure 7.3.

Neuroticism-Focused Treatment

Following his diagnostic and functional assessment, Marty completed 12 sessions of treatment with the UP. During the decisional balance exercise conducted in Module 1, which examines ambivalence associated with making changes in therapy by encouraging patients to explore pros and cons of engaging with treatment, Marty identified two potential costs. First, he noted that "change is scary," elaborating that avoiding driving and enclosed

Patient: _Marty_

> **Presenting Problems**
> - _Frequent panic attacks_
> - _Work and relationship interference_
> - _Excessive worry about (and planning to avoid) future attacks_

> **Strong, Uncomfortable Emotions**
> - _Anxiety_
> - _Panic_

> **Aversive Reactivity**
> - _"These feelings are so uncomfortable"_
> - _"I'm going to die or go crazy"_

> **Avoidant Coping**
>
> Situational avoidance: _Avoids elevators, driving on highways, through tunnels, or under bridges, unfamiliar places_
> Subtle behavioral avoidance: _Excessive planning for unavoidable work trips to new locations_
> Cognitive avoidance: _Worry, distraction_
> Safety signals: _Carrying cell phone, Xanax_
> Emotion-driven behaviors: _Escaping a situation if feeling panicky_

FIGURE 7.3. Case conceptualization worksheet for Marty.

spaces made him feel less anxious. Second, Marty articulated that his "hopes [may be] dashed" by failing to achieve full remission after putting forth the effort to change. Despite these powerful sources of ambivalence, Marty indicated that the potential benefits of changing (i.e., continued professional success, being a better partner and father) outweighed the costs. He then described two primary goals for treatment: (1) to reduce his avoidance of important work and family events and (2) to have greater spontaneity by being more "carefree" in his decisions (i.e., to think less about the potential consequences of various actions and to refrain from planning activities extensively before completing them).

Next, in Module 2, Marty was introduced to the three-component model of emotion (i.e., thoughts, feelings, behaviors) as a method for better understanding the trajectory of his panic attacks. He noted that escalating emotional experiences typically began with a slight shift in his physiological sensations (i.e., mild increase in heart rate, slightly more shallow breathing). These sensations produced negative appraisals (e.g., "This is so uncomfortable"; "This is going to escalate to a panic attack"; "I will pass out or otherwise lose control"), which, in turn, exacerbated his physical sensations—sometimes culminating in a full-blown panic attack. To explain why thoughts and physiological sensations compound each other to produce increasingly intense emotional experiences, we discussed how the sympathetic nervous system responds to *thoughts* about dangerous outcomes in the same way it views *in vivo* threats—by producing a flight, fight, or freeze response made up of strong physiological sensations. Thus Marty's aversive reactivity to his physical sensations, highlighted by his negative thoughts, played a strong role in increasing the frequency and intensity of his negative emotions. The role of aversive reactivity was also reinforced using Module 2's antecedent–response–consequence (ARC) exercise. Here, we focused on how avoidant behaviors factored into Marty's panic cycle; specifically, his attempts to escape or prevent the fluctuations in his physiological symptoms, driven by his negative appraisals about them, functioned in the short term to provide relief from unwanted emotional experiences. However, in the long term, these behaviors reinforced the notion that emotion-related physical sensations are dangerous, maintaining the aversive reactivity that actually backfires and exacerbates them when they occur.

In Module 3, Mindful Emotion Awareness, we capitalized on Marty's willingness to consider that his avoidant behaviors were actually increasing the likelihood of experiencing a panic attack following mild fluctuations in physiological symptoms. We used the UP's sitting meditation to practice a present-focused, nonjudgmental stance toward emotional stimuli. Given Marty's panic disorder diagnosis, it was not surprising that he demonstrated future-oriented concerns related to the physical sensations that arose during the meditation exercise; for example, he observed thoughts such as "this is going to get worse" and "I am going to panic." We discussed ways to relate to his physiological changes in a more present-focused and nonjudgmental manner (e.g., "I'm noticing that my cheeks feel warm right now" instead of "I am so flush and this is going to turn into a full-blown attack").

In order for Marty to practice maintaining a mindful stance in the context of emotional experiences, we also conducted an in-session mood induction using a piece of music; specifically, we chose an improvisational jazz song that reliably produces anxiety symptoms and an urge to avoid (e.g., covering ears, pressing a stop button) in our patients. After listening to the song, Marty made the powerful observation that his anxiety was worse at the beginning while he was "fighting against the song" (i.e., saying to himself "this is so terrible"; "I wish this would follow a more predictable pattern"; "I don't really have to listen to this, I can ask to turn it off"). However, he also noted that he recommitted to applying a nonjudgmental/present-focused stance about halfway through the exercise by "trying to take each part of the song as it came," regardless of how it made him feel. Marty expressed surprise at how quickly his anxiety abated after he stopped trying to fight against it. Here, the goal of mindful emotion awareness is to notice internal experiences (i.e., physical sensations, thoughts, and emotions) without the aversive reactivity that prolongs and intensifies them.

As described above, the next three UP modules zero in on the three components of an emotional experience (i.e., thoughts, physical sensations, and behaviors). First, given that Marty had been readily able to identify the negative thoughts that contributed to the escalation of his panic symptoms, as well as his anxiety about having future attacks, during previous modules, he was quickly able to extend this awareness by generating alternative appraisals. For example, he was able to address his fears of dying, passing out, or losing control during a panic attack by reminding himself that the physiological sensations associated with panic, while uncomfortable, are designed for survival (i.e., are not likely to result in death). With regard to his concern that he would panic in unfamiliar, difficult-to-escape situations, Marty was able to recall the numerous times when he had experienced increased physiological sensations that did not result in a full-blown attack; however, he was also able to note that "it wouldn't kill [him]" if he did experience panic. Here again, aversive reactivity is explicitly discussed in the Cognitive Flexibility module. Indeed, Marty adopted the alternative appraisal, "it is human to have feelings," anytime he noticed an emotion building in response to day-to-day stressors (i.e., frustration with coworkers, running late).

Perhaps the most powerful way for patients to address aversive reactivity is to deliberately approach situations and activities that bring up emotional experiences. This process allows patients who may have previously avoided their emotions at all costs to learn that emotions are temporary (even without avoidant coping) and can be tolerated. In UP Module 5, Marty identified a variety of avoidant behaviors that were likely reinforcing his belief that emotions, particularly their associated physical sensations, are dangerous. For example, he indicated that he completely avoided driving on highways, over bridges, or through tunnels, as well as elevators, work or social events in unfamiliar settings, and crowded spaces. With regard to subtle behavioral avoidance, Marty stated that he had switched to decaffeinated coffee and would excessively research escape routes if he was forced to visit a new location. He also endorsed blasting music when driving as a form of cognitive avoidance to distract from any physiological changes he might experience, as well as always having his anxiolytic medication on hand as a safety signal. After generating this list of diverse ways he engaged in emotional avoidance, Marty was encouraged to brainstorm alternative actions that might put him in closer contact with his emotions. For instance, when a mandatory work meeting arose at an offsite location, Marty agreed to simply follow the directions provided by his GPS, rather than researching routes that would avoid his triggers (i.e., bridges, tunnels, highways).

Next, in Module 6, patients are encouraged to engage in activities that provoke emotion-related physical sensations, including hyperventilation, breathing through a thin straw, running in place, and spinning in circles. As described in detail in Chapter 6, the purpose of these interoceptive exposures is to demonstrate to patients that uncomfortable physiological sensations are not dangerous, thus over time decreasing aversive responses to them. Although Marty readily understood the rationale for these exercises, he was reluctant to begin. We discussed how this apprehension may have been the result of the lingering suspicion that emotion-related physiological sensations are indeed dangerous. We agreed to test these exercises in session together; in fact, UP therapists typically engage in interoceptive exposures alongside their patients in order to reinforce the notion that these sensations are safe. Marty indicated that hyperventilation and spinning in circles produced the sensations most similar to his panic symptoms; he agreed to repeatedly practice these exercises for homework and noted, in the subsequent session, that his distress over the sensations decreased significantly across the week.

Finally, Marty's treatment culminated in Module 7 with emotion exposures. The purpose of these exercises is to provoke emotional experiences in order to facilitate new learning that emotions are temporary and that patients are adequately equipped to cope with them. In session, we created a hierarchy of activities and situations that Marty was currently avoiding. Although he had made several changes to his behavior (e.g., no longer carrying his anxiolytic or excessively planning visits to unfamiliar locations) over the course of the previous sessions, he still had not ridden in an elevator, nor had he driven on a highway, over a bridge, or through a tunnel. Again, by facing situations that provoked these sensations, Marty sent an important message to himself—that he believed he could tolerate all aspects of the emotions he had been avoiding.

Indeed, at the time treatment ended, Marty reported significant improvement in his ability to tolerate the physiological sensations associated with strong emotions. He was better able to notice his aversive reactions to these experiences that had previously served to escalate them, often culminating in a panic attack. He reported that simply telling himself "it's normal to feel nervous in this situation" and "these feelings are not dangerous" interrupted his cycle of intensifying emotion. With regard to functional improvements in Marty's life, he reported that he had encouraged his wife to plan several outings for them without his input, in line with his goal of being more spontaneous. Additionally, Marty stated that he was trying to be a "yes man" at work such that he would agree to whatever meetings and tasks were asked of him. Marty was no longer experiencing panic attacks at the time of termination and no longer met criteria for panic disorder or agoraphobia. Again, in Marty's case, a neuroticism-focused treatment was sufficient to address his difficulties.

Depression and Social Anxiety (Case 3)

Amira is an 18-year-old Somali-American freshman at a large, private university located 2 hours away from her hometown. During our initial intake appointment, Amira's mood appeared depressed, and her affect was flat; she had difficulty maintaining eye contact, was slow to respond verbally, and her responses were brief. She was, however, able to communicate her history and current symptoms. Amira noted that she "always" felt awkward and uncomfortable in social situations for "as far back as [she] could remember"; although she acknowledged that she had a few close friends, Amira reported that she had known them since kindergarten and couldn't remember how the relationships were formed (i.e., "They've just always been with me"). She further indicated that her difficulties with social anxiety became more apparent in middle school, as her classes became larger and were populated with more unfamiliar people. She reportedly refrained from participating in class for fear that others, particularly her peers, would view her as weird or stupid. Since transitioning to college (about 4 months prior to our initial appointment), Amira indicated that she had been feeling increasingly isolated; she noted that she seldom interacted with other students living in her dorm and drove home on the weekends, which made it difficult to make friends. With regard to her academics, Amira regularly attended class at the start of her first semester but did not participate. As the material became more difficult, her anxiety prevented her from going to her professors' office hours, and, as she struggled to follow along with the lectures, Amira began to skip class more frequently. She reported that, by the end of her first semester, she rarely left her dorm room, spending the majority of the time napping, surfing the Internet, or "staring at the wall." When asked whether she had lost interest in activities she used to enjoy, Amira confirmed that she had stopped engaging in several hobbies, though she mentioned that she never really enjoyed them; she further clarified that, unlike her peers, she rarely felt happy or excited about anything.

After our initial assessment, we determined that Amira met criteria for social anxiety disorder and MDD. In terms of the emotional-disorders functional model (see Figure 7.4), Amira reported strong feelings of anxiety, guilt, and sadness, which were recorded as evidence of her tendency to experience strong negative emotions. Additionally, she expressed a great deal of embarrassment over having these symptoms (i.e., "No one else seems to react like this"; "I should just be able to get over it"; "If other people see that I'm upset, they'll think I'm weak or stupid"), which we classified as aversive reactivity

Patient: _Amira_

> **Presenting Problems**
> - Social isolation
> - Skipping class
> - Low motivation due to depression

> **Strong, Uncomfortable Emotions**
> - Anxiety
> - Sadness/depression
> - Guilt

> **Aversive Reactivity**
> - "I'm the only one that reacts like this"
> - "People will think I'm ridiculous"

> **Avoidant Coping**
>
> Situational avoidance: Avoids attending class, office hours, school functions
>
> Subtle behavioral avoidance: Procrastinate on assignments, refrain from class participation, wait until roommate leaves to get up
>
> Cognitive avoidance: "Space out", watch TV
>
> Safety signals: Carry cell phone to avoid looking awkward
>
> Emotion-driven behaviors: Napping, leaving a room if people come in

FIGURE 7.4. Case conceptualization worksheet for Amira.

toward emotions. Amira's presentation also involved a great deal of emotional avoidance. For example, in terms of overt avoidance, she refrained from attending socials in her dorm, informational meetings about clubs, and, ultimately, her classes. She also engaged in more subtle forms of avoidance, including making limited eye contact, apologizing if she needed to speak to anyone, napping, and refraining from participating in class. For cognitive avoidance, Amira endorsed distracting herself with the Internet or television, along with "spacing out." Given this functional pattern of difficulties, we agreed to move forward with the UP.

Neuroticism-Focused Treatment

We began by discussing the adaptive nature of emotions (Module 2); in particular, we focused on sadness. Initially, Amira struggled with understanding how sadness and guilt could be useful to her, rather than simply an unnecessary painful experience. We discussed how sadness often occurs after a loss or setback, prompting withdrawal to temporarily process the loss or consider ways to resolve the setback. In Amira's case, she felt sadness related to the loss of her close friend group upon her transition to college, as well as in response to the poor grades she received after her first semester. These feelings let her know that her established relationships and her school performance were important to her and that the purpose of these emotions was to motivate her to reach out to her friends or seek help for her academic difficulties. Although Amira was able to acknowledge the logic behind the adaptive function of emotions, she noted that the intensity with which she felt her emotions made it difficult to harness the information these feelings provided. In response to this feedback, we then discussed the three-component model of emotions as a strategy to break overwhelming affective experiences down into thoughts, physical sensations, and behaviors. Here, aversive reactivity was addressed by fostering Amira's understanding that emotions are important sources of information, as well as by increasing her self-efficacy to cope with these experiences when they occurred by breaking them down into more manageable parts. Next, Mindful Emotion Awareness (Module 3) focused on helping Amira to combat her tendency to judge herself harshly for responding to stressors with strong emotions, though she found the meditation exercise unpleasant and rarely practiced it.

In the Cognitive Flexibility module (Module 4), we explored the automatic thoughts that were contributing to Amira's anxiety in social situations and overall depressed mood. Specifically, we identified circumstances in which she tended to overestimate the likelihood of a negative outcome ("I'm going to fail this test"; "They'll think I'm awkward if I try to initiate a conversation"), to inflate the probability that she would experience little pleasure when engaging in activities ("What's the point of going, anyway? I won't have fun"), and to underestimate her ability to cope with feeling down ("I can't handle feeling depressed for another week"; "It will be awful if I'm depressed when I go home for spring break"). We also observed Amira's tendency to inflate the veracity of negative thoughts about herself ("I'm such a loser"). For each of these types of thoughts, Amira was able to use the challenging questions (e.g., "Do you know for certain this thought is true? If it were true, how would you cope?") provided in the UP workbook (Barlow et al., 2017c) to create some flexibility around her initial automatic thoughts in order to generate alternative appraisals. In addition, we used the downward-arrow technique to delve deeper into the negative beliefs. The downward arrow is a strategy drawn from cognitive therapy (Beck, 2021) to elucidate core beliefs that may underlie and promote surface-level negative thoughts. For example, we asked Amira what it would mean to her if the thought "I'm a loser" were true. Amira speculated that this line of thinking was so provoking because, for her, it signaled that she wouldn't amount to anything in her life. Of course, this thought (i.e., "I'm a total failure") can also be disputed; however, given the tendency to focus on information that confirms existing beliefs, Amira felt she did not have enough evidence to support alternative appraisals (e.g., "I have had some success").

Although Amira was engaged during session and attempted to integrate the strategies we had discussed in her daily life, she did not report any reliable change in symptoms up until this point in treatment. However, the modules associated with behavior change (i.e., Module 5: Countering Emotional Behaviors, and Module 7: Emotion Exposures) appeared to have more of an impact on her difficulties. Amira was readily able to conceptualize the behaviors she used to cope with her anxiety and depression (i.e., skipping class, refraining from participation, limiting contact with her dormitory mates, napping, spacing out, distracting herself with television and the Internet) as functioning to avoid emotional experiences. Moreover, she acknowledged that these behaviors were likely increasing her anxiety in the long term, despite providing immediate relief. With regard to exposure exercises, Amira engaged in a number of activities that brought her in contact with emotional stimuli. For instance, she agreed to raise her hand to participate once per class period, attend information meetings about clubs, and ask her roommate to join her for dinner. When she returned to session after completing these tasks, Amira reported that these activities had gone better than expected (i.e., feared outcomes of being rejected did not occur) and that her anxiety about continuing to pursue social contact was decreasing (slightly). We also expanded our discussion to include new learning about the anxiety itself, and Amira confirmed that she had been able to perform despite high levels of distress and that these feelings had been temporary. Amira also completed several exposures related to her depressive symptoms. For instance, she was encouraged to write a vivid narrative account of what it means to be "a failure," record herself reading it, and listen to it over and over. Amira wrote about getting kicked out of her university and continuing to rely on her parents' support indefinitely. At first, listening to this script provoked strong feelings of sadness and guilt; however, the intensity of these feelings decreased over time, and Amira noted that when intrusive thoughts related to this topic came up while she was studying, she was able to notice them without responding (rather than immediately engaging in cognitive avoidance such as distraction).

Finally, in addition to the standard interoceptive exposures described in the previous cases (relevant for Amira's social anxiety), we used several alternative strategies to address the physiological experiences associated with Amira's depression (UP Module 6). For example, Amira was encouraged to use ankle and wrist weights to approximate the feelings of heaviness that can accompany depression. She was also asked to swallow several times in quick succession in order to replicate the feeling of having a lump in her throat that occurred when she felt guilty or embarrassed. Amira noted that these sensations were not particularly provoking for her, though she understood their rationale and agreed to repeated practice of them throughout the week.

Amira's treatment concluded after 16 sessions with the UP. Although she demonstrated improvement on her symptoms of social anxiety disorder and MDD (clinical severity ratings on the ADIS decreased for both diagnoses from 6 to 4 on an 8-point scale), Amira's level of interference remained at a clinical level. It was possible that her initial level of severity precluded full recovery during the standard length of treatment provided with the UP, and additional sessions were needed. Another possibility, however, was that risk for the symptoms Amira displayed was only partially conferred via neuroticism/aversive reactivity and that addressing additional higher order domains of personality (i.e., extraversion) might be relevant for her treatment plan.

Treatment for Extraversion

Extraversion is defined as the tendency to be talkative, warm, assertive, active, and excitement seeking and to generally experience positive affect (Costa & McCrae, 1992). Indeed, Amira demonstrated deficits in these qualities. Disturbances in extraversion (i.e., low and high levels of this trait) are associated with various psychopathology (see Seligman, Steen, Park, & Peterson, 2005). Specifically, research studies employing structural models have revealed specific core deficits in positive affectivity in individuals with depressive disorders, social anxiety (Brown et al., 1998; Brown, 2007), and agoraphobia (Rosellini et al., 2010). Thus, in Amira's case, her limited experience of positive emotions may have accounted for her residual social anxiety and depressive symptoms. Although not relevant for this case, excessively high levels of positive affectivity have also been well documented as a risk fact for mania in bipolar disorder (Gruber et al., 2008).

Several related theories (e.g., Depue & Iacono, 1989; Gray, 1987) have conceptualized positive emotions as important for approach-oriented, goal-driven behavior, likely due to the fact that the experience of positive emotions following successful pursuit of goals is reinforcing (e.g., Berridge & Robinson, 1998). Furthermore, Fredrickson (1998, 2001) suggests that, over time, healthy amounts of positive emotions help individuals "broaden and build" personal and social resources that enhance functioning and well-being (Fredrickson, 1998, 2001). In a recent review, Carl and colleagues (2013) provide a theoretical account, based on Gross's (2015) process model of emotion regulation, for how deficits in positive emotionality can evolve into DSM disorder symptoms. Briefly, this model delineates five categories of emotion-regulation processes corresponding to the temporal points at which an emotion can be generated or modified: (1) situation selection, (2) situation modification, (3) attentional deployment, (4) cognitive change, and (5) response modulation. Individuals with a temperamental vulnerability to experience fewer positive emotions may systematically engage with fewer positive-emotion-eliciting situations or activities, resulting in less incentive (in the form of reinforcing positive emotions) to approach such situations in the future; over time, this may lead to fewer attentional resources being allocated to positive stimuli (including emotions) and the belief that these experiences do not matter. In contrast, those with excessively high levels of trait extraversion (e.g., individuals at risk for bipolar disorder) may overemphasize the importance of positive-emotion-eliciting activities and seek them out, to their detriment. At both extremes, patterns of reinforcement (or lack thereof) lead to a kindling effect in which temperamental vulnerabilities grow into disorder symptoms (see Figure 7.1).

Recent work by Craske and colleagues (2019) provides support for the view that deficits in extraversion are mediated by lower levels of reward sensitivity from a neuroscience perspective. They posit that anhedonia, defined as symptomatic deficits in positive affect accompanied by a loss of desire to engage in pleasurable activities, is associated with dysfunction in the appetitive reward system, specifically the anticipation, consumption, and learning of reward (Der-Avakian & Markou, 2012; Pizzagalli, 2014; Treadway & Zald, 2011). Each of these components of the reward system is associated with a distinct neural signature. For instance, the neural regions most strongly linked to the *anticipation* of reward include the ventral tegmental area, the amygdala, and the ventral striatum (Castro & Berridge, 2014; Der-Avakian & Markou, 2012). At the behavioral level, deficits in this area among healthy individuals correlate with choosing easy tasks for a small reward over harder tasks for larger rewards (Treadway, Buckholtz, Schwartzman, Lambert, & Zald, 2009). The *consumption* (liking) of reward appears to be most strongly linked with ventral striatum (representing overlap with the anticipation of reward) and orbitofrontal cortex (Castro & Berridge, 2014; Der-Avakian & Markou, 2012). Finally, various areas of the prefrontal cortex have been implicated in decision making and reward *learning*, and animal research highlights areas such as the anterior cingulate cortex, orbitofrontal cortex (representing overlap with consumption of reward), ventromedial prefrontal cortex, and dorsal lateral prefrontal cortex (Der-Avakian & Markou, 2012).

Recently, some work has been conducted in an effort to identify behavioral strategies specifically aimed at increasing positive affect (extraversion) by augmenting responsivity to rewards. As noted earlier, one factor maintaining low levels of extraversion is difficulty selecting and modifying situations and activities that promote positive emotions (Carl et al., 2013). Indeed, interventions that encourage the selection of specific rewarding activities are associated with short-term increases in positive affect. For example, in an experience sampling study, participants with depression reported increased positive affectivity directly following physical activity (Mata et al., 2012). Additionally, positive psychology interventions in which participants were encouraged to engage in mastery activities or acts of kindness have also been linked to increases in positive emotions, particularly happiness (Seligman et al., 2005; Lyubomirsky, Sheldon, & Schkade, 2005). Moreover, existing treatments for depression have also explored the effect of increased selection of rewarding activities on positive affectivity in clinical samples. For example, behavioral activation (BA; Jacobson, Martell, & Dimidjian, 2001) has been shown to increase the frequency of positive emotions by encouraging patients to select and engage with situations that are more likely to elicit such experiences. BA counters avoidance of pleasant stimuli, resulting in increased positive reinforcement that maintains these activities in the long term (Hopko, Lejuez, Ruggiero, & Eifert, 2003; Syzdek, Addis, & Martell, 2009).

Another approach to augmenting extraversion may be via attentional shifts that allow patients to focus on positive emotions that are already present. Here again, individuals with low levels of this trait may not naturally deploy their limited attentional resources toward positive emotions, as these experiences are not particularly rewarding. With regard to intervention strategies, mindfulness-based treatments cultivate nonjudgmental attention to the present moment, which may facilitate greater awareness of pleasant experiences (Fredrickson & Joiner, 2002; Garland et al., 2010). Preliminary studies have demonstrated that practicing mindfulness, typically using meditation-based strategies, is associated with increases in positive affectivity in the context of treatment for emotional disorders (e.g., Erisman & Roemer, 2012; Jimenez, Niles, & Park, 2010). Additional research from nonclinical samples suggests that a specific type of meditation, loving kindness, may be particularly beneficial for enhancing extraversion (Fredrickson & Joiner, 2002; Hutcherson, Seppala, & Gross, 2008). Similarly, savoring interventions developed in the context of positive psychology also encourage individuals to focus on positive aspects of their sensory (e.g., eating, drinking, touching, smelling, seeing, or listening; Bryant & Veroff, 2007) and nonsensory (e.g., reminiscing or positive memory encoding; Bryant, Smart, & King, 2005) experiences. Finally, preliminary evidence suggests that computer-based approaches (e.g., cognitive bias modification programs) can be effective for retraining attention toward positive stimuli (Grafton, Ang, & MacLeod, 2012; Tamir & Robinson, 2007; Wadlinger & Isaacowitz, 2008).

Strategies explicitly aimed at changing cognitions in order to promote increased positive affect have also been utilized. Of course, cognitive reappraisal has traditionally been used to challenge negative appraisals of situations in order to decrease associated negative emotions; however, this strategy may be adapted to interpret situations in ways that up-regulate positive emotions. In fact, well-being therapy (Fava & Ruini, 2003) addresses cognitive dampening by encouraging patients to identify sources of their well-being and any negative cognitions ("interrupting thoughts") that interfere with its attainment. An additional approach aimed at the cognitive factors that maintain low positive affectivity may be computer-based retraining of interpretation biases. Studies suggest that practice interpreting ambiguous situations positively leads to increased subsequent positive interpretations for both clinical and nonclinical populations (Lothmann, Holmes, Chan, & Lau, 2011; Mathews & Mackintosh, 2000; Murphy, Hirsch, Mathews, Smith, & Clark, 2007).

Recently, Carl, Gallagher, and Barlow (2018) developed a comprehensive intervention for engaging positive emotions that includes the behavioral (i.e., situation selection modification), attentional (i.e., savoring), and cognitive (i.e., reappraisal) strategies described here. This four-session protocol was designed as an adjunctive intervention for individuals with emotional disorders who scored low on measures of extraversion and remained symptomatic following a course of neuroticism-focused treatment (i.e., the UP). Preliminary results suggest that the majority of patients in the study demonstrated significant increases in positive affect following this intervention. Given that Amira had already responded favorably, though not completely, to the UP, this adjunctive intervention might have been well suited to build on the momentum she had already achieved in order to address her deficits in positive affectivity.

Similarly, Craske and colleagues (2019) recently tested a comprehensive cognitive behavioral treatment aimed at addressing reward sensitivity in anhedonia, which they refer to as *positive affect treatment* (PAT). This treatment was developed to target the deficits in reward processing described earlier in this section (i.e., Craske et al., 2019) that serve as a functional link between low levels of extraversion and psychopathology: (1) reward anticipation/wanting/motivation, (2) reward consumption/liking, and (3) reward learning. The first module is described as "augmented behavioral activation training"; it combines planning for pleasurable activities (reward approach motivation) and reinforcement of those activities (reward learning) with "in-session" recounting designed to savor pleasurable moments (reward attainment). The second module includes exercises for identifying positive aspects of experience (approach motivation and attainment), in which participants are encouraged to delineate positive features of recent events that were judged to be neutral or negative (i.e., cognitive training). They were also guided to identify aspects of their own behavior that contributed to positive outcomes (reward learning) and practiced present-tense imagining of details (situations, emotions, physical responses, and thoughts) of future positive events (approach motivation). The third module includes loving kindness, generosity, gratitude, and appreciative joy exercises designed to savor positive experiences (reward attainment). Results from an RCT suggest that PAT resulted in significantly greater improvements in positive affectivity, as well as depressive and anxiety symptoms, relative to more traditional cognitive-behavioral approaches (Craske et al., 2019). This pattern of results further underscores the importance of considering the tendency to experience positive emotions (i.e., extraversion) in treatment planning for some individuals.

Of course, the ability to down-regulate positive emotions may also be important for some individuals, including those at risk for bipolar spectrum disorders or excessive reward-seeking behaviors (e.g., substance use); in these cases, too much up-regulation versus down-regulation can have harmful consequences (Gruber et al., 2008). Interventions that employ strategies encouraging selection of situations that reduce excessive engagement with positive emotions have been used with bipolar samples. For example, interpersonal and social rhythm therapy (Frank et al., 2005) includes monitoring of mood, along with activities that change mood (e.g., sleep and social interactions), with the goal of stabilizing affect. Similarly, GOALS (Johnson & Fulford, 2009), a recently developed treatment to prevent mania, aims to decrease bipolar patients' ambitious goal setting and reduce the pace at which they pursue goals. This intervention also includes a cognitive change component in which thoughts about the importance of achieving lofty goals, along with beliefs that feelings of confidence mean one should increase efforts toward a goal, are reappraised. Finally, mindfulness-based approaches that focus on the present moment as opposed to rumination about positive effects have been shown to stabilize positive affect in patients with bipolar disorder (Gruber et al., 2008).

Borderline Personality Disorder with Pathological Eating and Substance Use (Case 4)

Jami is a 20-year-old single white female who was initially referred for outpatient psychotherapy at our Center by her university's counseling center. The first psychotherapy session included a thorough diagnostic interview, during which we began to consider how aspects of Jami's presentation might be conceptualized within the emotional-disorder functional framework. Jami began by describing frequent and intense shifts in affect (e.g., "It feels like I just go from zero to sixty") that had plagued her for "as long as [she] can remember." She further elaborated that intense anxiety (especially in interpersonal situations), sadness, and "feeling lonely" would often come out of nowhere for her. Jami also reported frequently becoming annoyed or angry at boyfriends, friends, and housemates, leading to rude comments, rolling her eyes, and giving others the silent treatment. These descriptions of negative affect fit within the emotion-dysregulation criteria for BPD (i.e., mood lability, inappropriate anger) but can also be conceptualized as evidence of the neurotic temperament that characterizes emotional disorders. Accordingly, these experiences were noted on the case formulation worksheet (Figure 7.5).

Additionally, Jami demonstrated the tendency to view her emotional experiences negatively (i.e., aversive reactivity). For instance, she stated that after receiving a negative performance review for her angry behavior in her work–study position, she was reportedly "so overwhelmed" that she "couldn't handle how upset [she] was." These appraisals about her emotional experiences prevented her from leaving her dorm for several days straight. Indeed, she called in "sick" to the work–study position (a form of behavioral avoidance, noted in Figure 7.5), which led to more difficulties with her boss. Jami also noted that she "hated" how emotional she could become.

A number of additional examples of emotionally avoidant coping also emerged during our initial assessment. For example, Jami described engaging in "passive–aggressive" behavior toward her friends and family;

Patient: ___Jami___

Presenting Problems
- Unstable relationships
- Poor work performance
- Self-destructive behaviors

Strong, Uncomfortable Emotions
- Anxiety
- Anger
- Sadness
- Jealousy

Aversive Reactivity
- "I hate feeling this way"
- "I will lose control of myself"

Avoidant Coping

Situational avoidance: None

Subtle behavioral avoidance: Picking fights, giving the silent treatment, texting for reassurance, alcohol and marijuana use

Cognitive avoidance: Inability to make a decision, dissociation

Safety signals: Asking friends to accompany her to new situations

Emotion-driven behaviors: Cutting, binge eating

FIGURE 7.5. Case conceptualization worksheet for Jami.

specifically, she reported making remarks to her parents aimed at making them feel guilty for not visiting her more often and frequently sent text messages to her sister and close friends to ensure that they still cared about her. In the short term, these behaviors appeared to provide some relief from her emotions (sadness, anxiety, guilt) and related states (e.g., loneliness), but in the long term, they were likely to maintain the negative emotions that came up in the context of her relationships. Jami further described that this pattern of unstable, intense relationships also extended to friendships (e.g., picking fights and then ignoring people whom she perceived as having wronged her) and romantic partners. Additionally, in response to school and relationship stressors, Jami endorsed a number of impulsive behaviors that also functioned to escape negative emotional experiences. These included engaging in nonsuicidal self-injury off and on since she was a freshman in high school, drinking alcohol and smoking marijuana, and binge eating.

With regard to BPD symptoms of identity disturbance, Jami reported frequently questioning "what [she is] doing with her life" and vacillating between wanting to go to graduate school and dropping out of college to do yoga teacher training. We conceptualized Jami's tendency to fantasize about changing courses in life and frequent doubts about her current path (without making proactive changes or engaging in active problem solving) as forms of cognitive avoidance, serving to escape from her anxiety and insecurity in the moment but maintaining her negative emotions over a longer course of time. Along these lines, she described often feeling jealous (another frequent emotion for Jami) of acquaintances who she perceived as "knowing who they are" and being better able to effectively handle day-to-day stressors.

Neuroticism-Focused Treatment

Across the first several sessions of treatment with the UP, Jami was only minimally compliant with completing worksheets outside of session, which she attributed largely to concerns that her roommate or coworkers would notice her doing so. We brainstormed several possible solutions to this problem, including completing homework on her smartphone instead of a worksheet (less conspicuous) and scheduling time for homework when she was likely to have more privacy. During in-session homework review, when Jami had attempted an assignment, she typically emphasized that she had done a "bad" job or did not understand the workbook readings, despite the fact that her strong grasp of treatment concepts was clear in session. During Session 4 (Module 2: Understanding Emotions), we identified the consequences of this overarching pattern of discounting her capacities across many life areas, including her schoolwork (e.g., doubts that she would be accepted into graduate school preventing her from pursuing this path) and her relationships (e.g., not introducing herself to new people because "they probably wouldn't like [her] anyway"). In the short term, this tendency served to reduce her anxiety about the possibility of future failure or rejection, but in the long term, it strengthened her low self-esteem and prevented her from achieving her goals.

Though she still struggled to complete homework, this functional analysis helped facilitate Jami's use of treatment strategies when she was distressed, including objective recording of upsetting emotional experiences (i.e., "breaking down an emotion" into thoughts, physical sensations, and behavioral urges in UP Module 2), as well as anchoring in the present (UP Module 3: Mindful Emotion Awareness) when an emotion began to build. For example, upon noticing her face flushing and heart beating rapidly after receiving an email from her work–study manager about setting up an individual meeting, Jami described using her breath as a cue to bring her attention back to the present from both past-oriented ruminative thoughts (e.g., "I must have [messed] up yet again") and negative predictions about the future (e.g., "I'm going to get written up"). By anchoring in the present in this situation, Jami was able to tolerate the negative emotions that came up without immediate attempts to push them away by giving in to behavioral urges to send a curt email back or ignore the request for a meeting entirely.

During UP Module 4 (Cognitive Flexibility), Jami learned to identify her common patterns of automatic negative thinking, including jumping to conclusions about others (family, friends) being upset and/or not wanting to spend time with her or having malicious motives toward her (e.g., "I always feel like they're talking about me") in neutral situations with little evidence to support these interpretations. Through the use of a downward-arrow technique, we also explored possible underlying automatic thoughts (i.e., core beliefs) that may have been contributing to her surface-level appraisal patterns and emotional responses in key problem areas. Two themes emerged for Jami: beliefs about her lack of competence and about her worthlessness, both of which played a role in her tendency to catastrophize about "ending up alone" and never finding career or life satisfaction. Jami was tearful when discussing these cognitions in session, yet she was able to acknowledge the potential importance of identifying (rather than avoiding) how these global views about herself might be contributing to her distress across many situations. Jami also practiced generating other possible interpretations of stressful events; for example, when her roommate asked whether she could do Jami a favor by returning a library book for her, Jami's initial automatic thought was "she must think I can't take care of myself," which contributed to irritability and anger toward her roommate, as well as guilt and frustration with herself. Using challenging questions focused on examining the evidence, Jami was able to generate several alternative and more balanced interpretations, including "she's probably just being nice" and "even if she does think I need help, who cares?"

Next, Jami demonstrated a strong ability to identify her idiosyncratic forms of emotion avoidance associated with anxiety (e.g., distracting herself with Netflix shows, seeking reassurance that her close family and friends still cared about her, drinking/smoking, binge eating, cutting/burning her skin), anger (e.g., making "snarky" comments, leaving rude voice mails or sending mean text messages to people she thinks have rejected her), and intense sadness (e.g., withdrawing, ruminating, comparing herself to others, restricting her food intake). Jami was also able to identify a number of more adaptive alternative actions to try when experiencing urges to avoid, including refraining from seeking reassurance from loved ones, delaying sending a text or email when annoyed, and continuing a conversation with someone she didn't know well (rather than making up an excuse to cut it short). Given Jami's pathological eating behaviors, along with cognitions suggesting poor body image (e.g., "I miss being skinny"), we had an in-depth discussion exploring the short-term and long-term consequences of her suggestion to go the gym when feeling sad and unmotivated. Through guided discussion, Jami was able to differentiate between exercising to activate herself when negative emotions might be driving her to withdraw (i.e., an adaptive alternative action) and exercising to avoid distressing thoughts (e.g., "Guys will like me better if I lose weight") and emotions (e.g., guilt, anxiety, sadness; i.e., a maladaptive emotional behavior). The concept that the same behaviors can serve as both avoidance *and* adaptive functions, depending on the situation, appeared to resonate with Jami. However, throughout this module, she remained more motivated to engage in behavioral change related to her school performance (i.e., limiting procrastination) and self-injurious behaviors, rather than patterns of ineffective interpersonal communication and substance use.

Using her previously completed three-component model homework assignments, in Module 6, Jami identified the distressing physical sensations she tended to experience when anxious (fast heartbeat, shortness of breath), angry (feeling hot, muscle tension), sad (weighted down, fatigue), and guilty (knot in stomach). She observed how, for example, when her face began to feel flushed and her fists clenched, her urges to say rude things to her roommates or coworkers seemed to become stronger. Jami was willing to engage in systematic interoceptive exposure exercises, including breathing through a thin straw, sitting in front of a space heater while clenching her fists, and wearing wrist and ankle weights.

During Module 7 (Emotion Exposures), we expanded upon the alternative actions generated during Module 5 to develop a hierarchy of situations and activities that were likely to elicit intense emotion (including anxiety, anger, sadness, guilt, and shame) for her. Over the next four sessions, Jami applied her newly acquired emotion-management strategies during a variety of exposure tasks, which included (1) waiting until the following morning to respond to an email from her manager (when her initial urge was to "fire back immediately"), (2) undergoing a mock interview with a confederate who criticized her qualifications (while a space heater elicited heat-related sensations), (3) complimenting a roommate with whom she had recently had a conflict, and (4) rereading "desperate" Facebook messages she had sent to an ex-boyfriend after their breakup. Over the course of completing these emotion exposures, Jami gained the new knowledge that even emotions she found highly distressing tended to reduce in intensity on their own without her "doing something rash" to relieve them, and she observed that, by repeatedly approaching feared situations, her self-confidence improved.

By the time of treatment termination, after completing 18 sessions of the UP, Jami indicated that she had begun to adopt a less judgmental view of her emotional experiences. She noted that she was also better able to generate alternative appraisals in response to her initial negative thoughts about stressful events. However, she reported still having a great deal of difficulty considering alternative interpretations of others' motives; indeed, she stated that, most of the time, she simply didn't believe that people in her life had good intentions toward her. Jami was also able to generate several adaptive alternative actions to counter her emotion-driven behaviors. For example, she was better able to approach situations that made her anxious and to get herself started on tasks even when feeling down or unmotivated. In contrast, Jami stated that she often struggled to use the alternative actions we had planned when she had the urge to engage in "[her] more impulsive" behaviors (i.e., cutting, binge eating, smoking marijuana, engaging in aggressive interpersonal behavior). These qualitative descriptions of Jami's improvements were consistent with self-report data she provided; specifically, reductions in anxiety and depressive symptoms were large, whereas improvements in BPD symptoms were small in magnitude.

ADDITIONAL RELEVANT PERSONALITY TARGETS

Given that the UP is an intervention that was developed to address the functional mechanisms that maintain neuroticism, it is not surprising that Jami's symptoms related to anxiety and sadness were the most responsive to this treatment approach. Of course, anger and related emotionally avoidant interpersonal behaviors, along with impulsive responses to negative emotions (i.e., urgency), also fit within the emotional-disorders functional model and can be discussed during treatment with the UP (as described earlier). Indeed, as described in the previous chapter, many individuals with BPD are quite responsive to treatment with the UP (e.g., Sauer-Zavala, Bentley, & Wilner, 2016). However, given Jami's limited improvement on these targets (i.e., interpersonal functioning, impulsivity), it is possible that these difficulties might be maintained by additional personality domains beyond neuroticism. In support of this hypothesis, BPD has long been considered both an internalizing *and* an externalizing disorder (Eaton et al., 2011a). In the AMPD in DSM-5 (American Psychiatric Association, 2013), BPD is described as comprising negative affectivity, disinhibition, and antagonism, and, similarly, from a HiTOP perspective (Kotov et al., 2017), this condition loads onto the internalizing and antagonistic externalizing spectra. Thus Jami's treatment may have benefited from consideration of other broad domains of personality.

Here we describe the emerging research that has been conducted on altering conscientiousness and agreeableness; we use the FFM labels for these domains, as they are most widely used and they display considerable conceptual and empirical overlap with other personality-based models of psychopathology.

Conscientiousness and Agreeableness

First, conscientiousness refers to the tendency to be self-controlled, responsible, hardworking, orderly, and rule abiding (Roberts, Lejuez, Krueger, Richards, & Hill, 2014). This trait has been consistently associated with outcomes in most areas of life, including work and school performance, relationship quality, and physical and emotional health (e.g., Dudley, Orvis, Lebiecki, & Cortina, 2006; Hampson, Edmonds, Goldberg, Dubanoski, & Hillier, 2013; Hill, Nickel, & Roberts, 2014; Kotov et al., 2010; Poropat, 2009). Specifically, in the context of psychopathology, low conscientiousness is a risk factor for externalizing conditions, such as substance use disorders and antisocial behavior (Krueger et al., 2007a), and could account for Jami's disinhibition with regard to smoking marijuana and engaging in nonsuicidal self-injury.

Roberts and colleagues have published several theoretical accounts on the development and malleability of conscientiousness, along with proposed mechanisms for altering this trait in response to intervention (Magidson et al., 2014; Roberts et al., 2017a). With regard to development, they note that children vary widely on temperamental precursors to conscientiousness, such as effortful control (Deal, Halverson, Havill, & Martin, 2005), and that these differences are likely due to genetic contributions (Krueger & Johnson, 2008). In concert, the authors view environmental factors, including stability of the family environment and supportive social institutions (e.g., good schools, community services), as another important contributor to the development of this trait (Hill, Roberts, Grogger, Guryan, & Sixkiller, 2011); they suggest that certain environments are more likely to provide positive reinforcement for orderly, rule-abiding behavior (e.g., praise for completing homework on time), increasing the likelihood that these actions will continue over time. Indeed, on average, conscientiousness increases across the lifespan, though the magnitude of this change varies from individual to individual (Roberts et al., 2006). This view of conscientiousness is similar to our conception of neuroticism's developmental trajectory, in which a biologically mediated predisposition can be exacerbated by stressful events or parenting styles, resulting in behaviors that are reinforced (in the case of neuroticism, negatively) over time.

Additionally, Roberts and colleagues have described a theoretical model for changing conscientiousness (i.e., Magidson et al., 2014). With regard to a functional mechanism that may account for the maintenance of current levels of this trait (akin to aversive reactivity and avoidant behaviors for neuroticism), they suggest that individuals' expectancies about their performance on certain tasks, along with how much they value these actions, predicts persistence in conscientious pursuits (e.g., paying bills on time, double-checking one's work, remembering materials needed at work or school, subjugating impulses that would be gratifying in the short term; Eccles, 2009). These authors go on to suggest that, in order to increase positive expectancies about conscientious actions (along with the actions themselves), environmental contingencies that reinforce these beliefs and behaviors must be altered (Roberts et al., 2006).

Although no behavioral interventions have been developed to directly target conscientiousness, Roberts and colleagues suggest that an intervention with a detailed structure that focuses on values and goal setting and provides immediate feedback on progress, clear accountability, and an opportunity for remediation would be potentially useful for this trait (Magidson et al., 2014). In particular, they suggest that BA, an evidence-based approach for addressing depressive symptoms (Jacobson et al., 2001), may be a useful strategy to engage these targets. The goal of BA is to increase engagement in goal-directed activities that are considered important, enjoyable, and in accordance with individual values across numerous domains of life. These researchers contend that many of the components of BA, including monitoring daily activities, setting goals, and optimizing daily schedules, are, in and of themselves, consistent with trait conscientiousness. Using BA to enact change in conscientiousness is, at this point, a promising theoretical proposition, as empirical data on its utility in this context have not yet been collected.

Next, the extreme poles of agreeableness may also reflect an important target of personality-based treatment (e.g., Malouff, Thorsteinsson, & Schutte, 2005), though considerably less work has been conducted for this domain. Agreeableness refers to the tendency to be trusting, cooperative, kind, straightforward, and sympathetic (Bucher, Suzuki, & Samuel, 2019). Low levels of this trait, often referred to as antagonism (e.g., Samuel & Gore, 2012), are characterized by vindictiveness, aggression, or narcissism (Williams & Simms, 2018) and confer risk for externalizing disorders, including conduct disorder, antisocial personality disorder, and substance use disorders, as well as strained interpersonal relationships (Anderson, Tapert, Moadab, Crowley, & Brown, 2007; Kotov et al., 2010; Miller, Lynam, & Leukefeld, 2003). Jami displayed elevated mistrust, a facet of agreeableness in the FFM, which may account for her interpersonal difficulties being less responsive to neuroticism-focused treatment.

With regard to the development of agreeableness, theorists have suggested that this trait is functionally related to attachment styles that result from relationships with parents or other caregivers (Carver, 1997; Young, Klosko, & Weishaar, 2003). Specifically, in these accounts, low levels of agreeableness develop from insecure attachment styles, such as ambivalence (characterized by clinging to caregivers when they leave and then rejecting caregivers upon their return) and avoidance (characterized by a calm response to caregiver departure, followed by avoidance/rejection of caregivers when they return; Bowlby, 1973; Crittenden & Ainsworth, 1989). In adults, insecure attachment is believed to manifest as feeling vulnerable in relationships, leading to the seemingly protective behaviors that characterize externalizing psychopathology, including acting cruelly and selfishly and seeking excessive admiration from others (Young et al., 2003). Thus, as aversive reactivity serves as an intermediate mechanism between neuroticism and internalizing (i.e., emotional) disorders, attachment insecurity represents an actionable functional mechanism linking agreeableness to antagonistic externalizing psychopathology.

With regard to specific interventions that target low agreeableness, some have argued that psychodynamic approaches with a particular focus on the relationship between patient and therapist may be particularly relevant. In particular, schema-focused therapy (SFT) has recently been adapted to explicitly target this trait (Bernstein, Arntz, & Vos, 2007). The primary assumption in SFT is that dysfunctional schemas (i.e., pervasive patterns of thinking and feeling), developed through early experiences with caregivers, drive the behaviors that characterize maladaptively low agreeableness. In SFT, the therapeutic relationship is used to address patients' difficulty forming a secure attachment, and past traumatic experiences are processed. Recently, a modified version of SFT has been developed to purportedly address the severe forms of antagonism seen in antisocial and narcissistic personality disorders (Bernstein et al., 2007). A 3-year, multisite trial is now under way to evaluate this intervention compared with TAU within a sample of criminal offenders with personality disorders. Preliminary reports suggest that administration of SFT is associated with lower recidivism; however, the effects of this approach on personality disorder symptoms, as well as on agreeableness versus antagonism, have not been reported (Bernstein et al., 2012). Finally, others have suggested that treatment for individuals with maladaptively low levels of agreeableness should begin with motivational techniques aimed at illustrating the costs of using antagonistic strategies in interpersonal contexts (Livesley, 2003; Widiger et al., 2012)—specifically, highlighting how components of agreeableness, such as modesty and altruism, may actually result in better achievement of one's goals (e.g., employment).

In contrast, although a high level of agreeableness is typically considered a desirable trait, when taken to an extreme, it can be also quite maladaptive. For instance, trusting may translate to gullibility, altruism may be manifested as self-sacrificing selflessness, compliance may become subservience, and modesty may evolve into self-effacement (Gore, Presnall, Miller, Lynam, & Widiger, 2012; Lowe, Edmundson, & Widiger, 2009). These characteristics have been associated with dependent personality disorder (Widiger & Presnall, 2013). Unfortunately, there is limited literature on treatment approaches for addressing high agreeableness, though some have suggested that assertiveness training might be particularly beneficial to these patients, along with other cognitive-behavioral and interpersonal methods to address their meekness, self-effacement, and self-sacrificing timidity (Bornstein, 2004).

> Agreeableness, when taken to an extreme, can be maladaptive.

Openness to Experience

Finally, factor analysis of personality structure has yielded a fifth domain that has been referred to by various names: openness, unconventionality, oddity, or psychoticism (Chmielewski, Bagby, Markon, Ring, & Ryder, 2014). High levels of openness to experience are associated with having a strong imagination, interest in abstract thinking and idea generation, and appreciation for aesthetics; however, maladaptive variants include cognitive and perceptual dysregulation, eccentricity, and unusual beliefs and experiences. Indeed, in the HiTOP model, the Thought Disorder spectrum is most closely aligned with maladaptively high openness (Kotov et al., 2017). Unlike the other four traits included in the FFM, research on functional mechanisms related to the development and maintenance of this trait is limited. Similarly, research on directly addressing this trait in treatment is quite sparse, though some authors have suggested using established treatments for disorders associated with high openness as a starting point for identifying intervention strategies suited to this domain (Bach & Presnall-Shvorin, 2020).

For example, when unusual beliefs, experiences, and eccentricity occur in the context of schizotypal features, cognitive therapy may adjust distorted thought patterns and give the patient a set of coping skills for anxiety in social situations (Renton & Mankiewiecz, 2015). It may also be valuable to target core beliefs, schemas, and modes related to mistrust, isolation, and alienation that are historically thought to be associated with psychotic or prepsychotic features (Bach, Lee, Mortensen, & Simonsen, 2015; Hopwood et al., 2013a). In cases in which perceptual dysregulation is predominant due to dissociative phenomena or psychotic-like episodes (common in BPD), a trauma-focused approach might be relevant (Kulkarni, 2017). In addition, mindfulness may assist patients in thinking more concretely and reducing emotional vulnerability by engaging in basic self-care skills (i.e., balanced eating, treating physical illness, avoiding mood-altering drugs, balanced sleep, getting exercise, and building mastery) that may reduce the likelihood of perceptual dysregulation (Linehan & Dexter-Mazza, 2008).

Summary

In this chapter, we demonstrated the advantages and limitations associated with neuroticism-focused treatment for a range of common difficulties. In the clinical cases presented, the diverse difficulties experienced by Beth, Marty, Amira, and Jami were all treated, to some extent, by the UP, a neuroticism-focused intervention. These patients demonstrate the various ways in which high levels of neuroticism manifest (i.e., anxiety and irritability in Beth; anxiety and autonomic surges in Marty; anxiety, sadness, and guilt in Amira; anxiety and anger in Jami), along with idiosyncratic presentations of aversive reactivity and emotionally avoidant coping. A single, neuroticism-focused treatment allows the simultaneous treatment of comorbid conditions, as well as reducing therapist burden (i.e., one protocol to address diverse patient concerns).

Of course, the UP as presently constituted is not sufficient to address all psychopathology, even within the emotional disorders; although Amira and Jami demonstrated some improvement following treatment with this intervention, some symptoms remained. Thus we highlighted additional broad domains of personality (i.e., extraversion, conscientiousness, agreeableness, and openness) that may confer risk for psychopathology beyond neuroticism. We also summarized the literature on the functional processes that link maladaptive levels of these processes to clinical dysfunction and illustrated how Amira (low extraversion, residual symptoms of depression, and social anxiety disorder) and Jami (low conscientiousness and agreeableness, residual symptoms of BPD) might have benefited from adjunctive, personality-based treatment components.

CONCLUSIONS

Contrary to some theoretical conceptions of personality, emerging literature suggests that traits may be malleable over time and in response to treatment. The most research in this area has been conducted in the context of neuroticism, and data suggest that interventions explicitly developed to target the functional processes that maintain this trait have the most robust effects (e.g., Rapee et al., 2005; Sauer-Zavala et al., 2020). As noted previously, there are several advantages to shifting the focus of treatment to personality-based dimensions, rather than focusing on disorder-specific symptoms. First, the rates of comorbidity among groups of mental disorders are quite high (e.g., Grant et al., 2008; Kessler et al., 1998), and, rather than prioritizing treatment of one condition over another, an intervention focused on shared vulnerabilities (e.g., neuroticism) could lead to simultaneous improvement across co-occurring conditions. Additionally, separate treatments for each DSM diagnosis places a burden on practitioners to receive costly and time-intensive training to competently provide these interventions; targeting common mechanisms (e.g., aversive reactivity) informed by personality-based functional models may reduce the number of discrete treatments, increasing the likelihood that empirically supported treatments will be more widely disseminated.

Beyond neuroticism, the notion of using a functional model that accounts for the evolution from trait vulnerability to clinical disorder can also be applied to the other domains of the FFM and may facilitate a fresh approach to treatment development that is both broader and deeper than the existing focus on categorical disorders. However, functional models and related treatments are not uniformly well articulated across each FFM trait, necessitating additional study in this area. Indeed, we propose that the research on the development, maintenance, and treatment of neuroticism reviewed in this book may serve as a template for a new approach to treatment development across dimensions of personality. This work has the potential to connect treatment development and dissemination to the robust research literature on dimensional, personality-based classification systems for psychopathology. Nosological systems based on dimensional models of psychopathology not only represent a more valid depiction of mental illness (see Chapter 5) but may also vastly simplify treatment delivery, rendering care available to a greater number of individuals. Functional mechanisms such as aversive reactivity and reward sensitivity represent the bridge between personality and disorder that could possibly change the focus of mental health care substantially.

References

Abela, J. R. Z., Payne, A. V. L., & Moussaly, N. (2003). Cognitive vulnerability to depression in individuals with borderline personality disorder. *Journal of Personality Disorders, 17*(4), 319–329.

Abramowitz, J. S., Brigidi, B. D., & Foa, E. B. (1999). Health concerns in patients with obsessive–compulsive disorder. *Journal of Anxiety Disorders, 13*(5), 529–539.

Abramowitz, J. S., Tolin, D. F., & Street, G. P. (2001). Paradoxical effects of thought suppression: A meta-analysis of controlled studies. *Clinical Psychology Review, 21*(5), 683–703.

Abramson, L. Y., Metalsky, G. I., & Alloy, L. B. (1989). Hopelessness depression: A theory-based subtype of depression. *Psychological Review, 96*(2), 358–372.

Abramson, L. Y., Seligman, M. E., & Teasdale, J. D. (1978). Learned helplessness in humans: Critique and reformulation. *Journal of Abnormal Psychology, 87*(1), 49–74.

Achenbach, T. M. (1966). The classification of children's psychiatric symptoms: A factor-analytic study. *Psychological Monographs: General and Applied, 80*(7), 1–37.

Achenbach, T. M., & Edelbrock, C. S. (1978). The classification of child psychopathology: A review and analysis of empirical efforts. *Psychological Bulletin, 85*(6), 1275–1301.

Achenbach, T. M., & Rescorla, L. (2004). The Achenbach System of Empirically Based Assessment (ASEBA) for ages 1.5 to 18 Years. In M. E. Maruish (Ed.), *The use of psychological testing for treatment planning and outcomes assessment: Instruments for children and adolescents* (Vol. 2, pp. 105–141). New York: Taylor & Francis.

Alatiq, Y., & Modayfer, O. A. (2019). Transdiagnostic CBT for adult emotional disorders: A feasibility open trial from Saudi Arabia. *Cognitive Behaviour Therapist, 12*, Article e30.

Alda, M., Puebla-Guedea, M., Rodero, B., Demarzo, M., Montero-Marin, J., Roca, M., & Garcia-Campayo, J. (2016). Zen meditation, length of telomeres, and the role of experiential avoidance and compassion. *Mindfulness, 7*(3), 651–659.

Aldao, A., Nolen-Hoeksema, S., & Schweizer, S. (2010). Emotion-regulation strategies across psychopathology: A meta-analytic review. *Clinical Psychology Review, 30*(2), 217–237.

Alden, L. E., Wiggins, J. S., & Pincus, A. L. (1990). Construction of circumplex scales for the Inventory of Interpersonal Problems. *Journal of Personality Assessment, 55*(3–4), 521–536.

Alimehdi, M., Ehteshamzadeh, P., Naderi, F., Eftekharsaadi, Z., & Pasha, R. (2016). The effectiveness of mindfulness-based stress reduction on intolerance of uncertainty and anxiety sensitivity among individuals with generalized anxiety disorder. *Asian Social Science, 12*(4), 179–187.

Alloy, L. B., Black, S. K., Young, M. E., Goldstein, K. E., Shapero, B. G., Stange, J. P., . . . Abramson, L. Y. (2012). Cognitive vulnerabilities and depression versus other psychopathology symptoms and diagnoses in early adolescence. *Journal of Clinical Child and Adolescent Psychology, 41*(5), 539–560.

Alloy, L. B., Kelly, K. A., Mineka, S., & Clements, C. M. (1990). Comorbidity of anxiety and depressive disorders: A helplessness–hopelessness perspective. In J. D. Maser & C. R. Cloninger (Eds.), *Comorbidity of mood and anxiety disorders* (pp. 499–543). Washington, DC: American Psychiatric Association.

Allen, L. B., White, K. S., Barlow, D. H., Shear, K. M., Gorman, J. M., & Woods, S. W. (2010). Cognitive-behavior therapy (CBT) for panic disorder: Relationship of anxiety and depression comorbidity with treatment outcome. *Journal of Psychopathology and Behavioral Assessment, 32*(2), 185–192.

Allport, G. (1937). *Personality: A psychological interpretation.* New York: Holt, Rinehart & Winston.

Allport, G. (1961). *Pattern and growth in personality.* New York: Holt, Rinehart & Winston.

Allport, G., & Odbert, H. S. (1936). Trait-names: A psycho-lexical study. *Psychological Monographs, 47*(211), 1–171.

Almagor, M., Tellegen, A., & Waller, N. (1995). The Big Seven model: A cross-cultural replication and further exploration of the basic dimensions of natural language trait descriptors. *Journal of Personality and Social Psychology, 69,* 300–307.

Amat, J., Baratta, M. V., Paul, E., Bland, S. T., Watkins, L. R., & Maier, S. F. (2005). Medial prefrontal cortex determines how stressor controllability affects behavior and dorsal raphe nucleus. *Nature Neuroscience, 8*(3), 365–371.

Ameral, V., Reed, K. P., Cameron, A., & Armstrong, J. (2014). What are measures of distress tolerance really capturing?: A mixed methods analysis. *Psychology of Consciousness: Theory, Research, and Practice, 1*(4), 357–369.

American Psychiatric Association. (1952). *Diagnostic and statistical manual of mental disorders.* Washington, DC: Author.

American Psychiatric Association. (1968). *Diagnostic and statistical manual of mental disorders* (2nd ed.). Washington, DC: Author.

American Psychiatric Association. (1980). *Diagnostic and statistical manual of mental disorders* (3rd ed.). Washington, DC: Author.

American Psychiatric Association. (1987). *Diagnostic and statistical manual of mental disorders* (3rd ed., rev.). Washington, DC: Author.

American Psychiatric Association. (1994). *Diagnostic and statistical manual of mental disorders* (4th ed.). Washington, DC: Author.

American Psychiatric Association. (2013). *Diagnostic and statistical manual of mental disorders* (5th ed.). Arlington, VA: Author.

Amir, N., Cashman, L., & Foa, E. B. (1997). Strategies of thought control in obsessive–compulsive disorder. *Behaviour Research and Therapy, 35*(8), 775–777.

Anacker, C., Scholz, J., O'Donnell, K. J., Allemang-Grand, R., Diorio, J., Bagot, R. C., . . . Meaney, M. J. (2016). Neuroanatomic differences associated with stress susceptibility and resilience. *Biological Psychiatry, 79*(10), 840–849.

Anderson, J. L., Sellbom, M., Bagby, R. M., Quilty, L. C., Veltri, C. O. C., Markon, K. E., & Krueger, R. F. (2013). On the convergence between PSY-5 domains and PID-5 domains and facets: Implications for assessment of DSM-5 personality traits. *Assessment, 20*(3), 286–294.

Anderson, K. G., Tapert, S. F., Moadab, I., Crowley, T. J., & Brown, S. A. (2007). Personality risk profile for conduct disorder and substance use disorders in youth. *Addictive Behaviors, 32*(10), 2377–2382.

Andreasen, N. C. (1984). *The Scale for the Assessment of Positive Symptoms (SAPS).* Iowa City: University of Iowa.

Andreasen, N. C. (1989). The Scale for the Assessment of Negative Symptoms (SANS):

Conceptual and theoretical foundations. *British Journal of Psychiatry, 155*(S7), 49–52.

Andrews, G. (1990). Classification of neurotic disorders. *Journal of the Royal Society of Medicine, 83*(10), 606–607.

Andrews, G. (1996). Comorbidity in neurotic disorders: The similarities are more important than the differences. In R. M. Rapee (Ed.), *Current controversies in the anxiety disorders* (pp. 3–20). New York: Guilford Press.

Andrews, W., Parker, G., & Barrett, E. (1998). The SSRI antidepressants: Exploring their "other" possible properties. *Journal of Affective Disorders, 49*(2), 141–144.

Anestis, M. D., Selby, E. A., Fink, E. L., & Joiner, T. E. (2007). The multifaceted role of distress tolerance in dysregulated eating behaviors. *International Journal of Eating Disorders, 40*(8), 718–726.

Angleitner, A., & Ostendorf, F. (1994). Temperament and the Big Five factors of personality. In C. F. Halverson, G. A. Kohnstamm, & R. P. Martin (Eds.), *The developing structure of temperament and personality from infancy to adulthood* (pp. 69–90). Hillsdale, NJ: Erlbaum.

Anokhin, P. K. (2016). *Biology and neurophysiology of the conditioned reflex and its role in adaptive behavior* (Vol. 3). New York: Elsevier.

Antony, M. M., Purdon, C. L., Huta, V., & Swinson, R. P. (1998). Dimensions of perfectionism across the anxiety disorders. *Behaviour Research and Therapy, 36*(12), 1143–1154.

Armstrong, L., & Rimes, K. A. (2016). Mindfulness-based cognitive therapy for neuroticism (stress vulnerability): A pilot randomized study. *Behavior Therapy, 47*(3), 287–298.

Austin, M. A., Riniolo, T. C., & Porges, S. W. (2007). Borderline personality disorder and emotion regulation: Insights from the polyvagal theory. *Brain and Cognition, 65*(1), 69–76.

Azizi, A., Borjali, A., & Golzari, M. (2010). The effectiveness of emotion regulation training and cognitive therapy on the emotional and addictional problems of substance abusers. *Iranian Journal of Psychiatry, 5*(2), 60–65.

Bach, B., Lee, C., Mortensen, E. L., & Simonsen, E. (2015). How do DSM-5 personality traits align with schema therapy constructs? *Journal of Personality Disorders, 30*(4), 502–529.

Bach, B., & Presnall-Shvorin, J. (2020). Using DSM-5 and ICD-11 personality traits in clinical treatment. In C. W. Lejuez & K. L. Gratz (Eds.), *The Cambridge handbook of personality disorders* (pp. 450–467). New York: Cambridge University Press.

Bach, B., Sellbom, M., Kongerslev, M., Simonsen, E., Krueger, R. F., & Mulder, R. (2017). Deriving ICD-11 personality disorder domains from DSM-5 traits: Initial attempt to harmonize two diagnostic systems. *Acta Psychiatrica Scandinavica, 136*(1), 108–117.

Baer, R. A. (2003). Mindfulness training as a clinical intervention: A conceptual and empirical review. *Clinical Psychology: Science and Practice, 10*(2), 125–143.

Baer, R. A., & Sauer, S. E. (2011). Relationships between depressive rumination, anger rumination, and borderline personality features. *Personality Disorders: Theory, Research, and Treatment, 2*(2), 142–150.

Bagby, R. M., Levitan, R. D., Kennedy, S. H., Levitt, A. J., & Joffe, R. T. (1999). Selective alteration of personality in response to noradrenergic and serotonergic antidepressant medication in depressed sample: Evidence of non-specificity. *Psychiatry Research, 86*(3), 211–216.

Bagby, R. M., Quilty, L. C., & Ryder, A. C. (2008). Personality and depression. *Canadian Journal of Psychiatry, 53*(1), 14–25.

Bagby, R. M., Young, L. T., Schuller, D. R., Bindseil, K. D., Cooke, R. G., Dickens, S. E., . . . Joffe, R. T. (1996). Bipolar disorder, unipolar depression and the five-factor model of personality. *Journal of Affective Disorders, 41*(1), 25–32.

Bailey, H. (1927). *Demonstration of physical signs in clinical surgery.* Bristol, UK: J. Wright & Sons.

Baillie, A. J., & Rapee, R. M. (2005). Panic attacks as risk markers for mental disorders. *Social Psychiatry and Psychiatric Epidemiology, 40*(3), 240–244.

Baker, A. (2001). Crossing the quality chasm: A new health system for the 21st century. *British Medical Journal, 323*(7322), 1192.

Baker, R., Holloway, J., Thomas, P. W., Thomas, S., & Owens, M. (2004). Emotional processing and panic. *Behaviour Research and Therapy, 42*(11), 1271–1287.

Ballash, N. G., Pemble, M. K., Usui, W. M., Buckley, A. F., & Woodruff-Borden, J. (2006). Family functioning, perceived control, and anxiety: A mediational model. *Journal of Anxiety Disorders, 20*(4), 486–497.

Bameshgi, M., Kimiaei, S. A., & Mashhadi, A. (2019). Effectiveness of the Unified Protocol for Transdiagnostic Treatment in reducing depression associated with marital problems. *International Journal of Health and Life Sciences, 5*(2).

Barenbaum, N. B., & Winter, D. G. (2008). History of modern personality theory and research. In O. P. John, R. W. Robins, & L. A. Pervin (Eds.), *Handbook of personality: Theory and research* (3rd ed., pp. 3–27). New York: Guilford Press.

Barger, S. D., & Sydeman, S. J. (2005). Does generalized anxiety disorder predict coronary heart disease risk factors independently of major depressive disorder? *Journal of Affective Disorders, 88*(1), 87–91.

Barlow, D. H. (1982). The death of neurosis: Review of Marks, I. Cure and care of neuroses: Theory and practice of behavioral psychology. *Contemporary Psychology, 27,* 512–514.

Barlow, D. H. (1985). *Clinical handbook of psychological disorders: A step-by-step treatment manual.* New York: Guilford Press.

Barlow, D. H. (1986). Causes of sexual dysfunction: The role of anxiety and cognitive interference. *Journal of Consulting and Clinical Psychology, 54*(2), 140–148.

Barlow, D. H. (1987). The classification of anxiety disorders. In G. L. Tischler (Ed.), *Diagnoses and classification in psychiatry: A critical appraisal of DSM-III* (pp. 223–242). Cambridge, UK: Cambridge University Press.

Barlow, D. H. (1988). *Anxiety and its disorders: The nature and treatment of anxiety and panic.* New York: Guilford Press.

Barlow, D. H. (1991). Disorders of emotion. *Psychological Inquiry, 2*(1), 58–71.

Barlow, D. H. (1996). Health care policy, psychotherapy research, and the future of psychotherapy. *American Psychologist, 51*(10), 1050–1058.

Barlow, D. H. (2000). Unraveling the mysteries of anxiety and its disorders from the perspective of emotion theory. *American Psychologist, 55*(11), 1247–1263.

Barlow, D. H. (2002). *Anxiety and its disorders: The nature and treatment of anxiety and panic* (2nd ed.). New York: Guilford Press.

Barlow, D. H. (2004). Psychological treatments. *American Psychologist, 59*(9), 869–878.

Barlow, D. H., Blanchard, E. B., Vermilyea, J. A., Vermilyea, B. B., & DiNardo, P. A. (1986). Generalized anxiety and generalized anxiety disorder: Description and reconceptualization. *American Journal of Psychiatry, 143*(1), 40–44.

Barlow, D. H., Brown, T. A., & Craske, M. G. (1994). Definitions of panic attacks and panic disorder in the DSM-IV: Implications for research. *Journal of Abnormal Psychology, 103*(3), 553–564.

Barlow, D. H., Bullis, J. R., Comer, J. S., & Ametaj, A. A. (2013). Evidence-based psychological treatments: An update and a way forward. *Annual Review of Clinical Psychology, 9,* 1–27.

Barlow, D. H., Chorpita, B. F., & Turovsky, J. (1995). Fear, panic, anxiety, and disorders of emotion. In D. A. Hope (Ed.), *Nebraska Symposium on Motivation: Vol. 43. Perspectives on anxiety, panic, and fear* (pp. 251–328). Lincoln: University of Nebraska Press.

Barlow, D. H., & Craske, M. G. (1988). The phenomenology of panic. In S. Rachman &

J. D. Maser (Eds.), *Panic: Psychological perspectives* (pp. 11–36). Hillsdale, NJ: Erlbaum.

Barlow, D. H., Ellard, K. K., Fairholme, C., Farchione, T. J., Boisseau, C., Allen, L., & Ehrenreich-May, J. (2011a). *Unified Protocol for the Transdiagnostic Treatment of Emotional Disorders: Therapist guide.* New York: Oxford University Press.

Barlow, D. H., Ellard, K. K., Fairholme, C., Farchione, T. J., Boisseau, C., Allen, L., & Ehrenreich-May, J. (2011b). *Unified Protocol for the Transdiagnostic Treatment of Emotional Disorders: Patient workbook.* New York: Oxford University Press.

Barlow, D. H., Ellard, K. K., Sauer-Zavala, S., Bullis, J. R., & Carl, J. R. (2014a). The origins of neuroticism. *Perspectives on Psychological Science, 9*(5), 481–496.

Barlow, D. H., & Farchione, T. J. (Eds.). (2018). *Applications of the Unified Protocol for the Transdiagnostic Treatment of Emotional Disorders.* New York: Oxford University Press.

Barlow, D. H., Farchione, T. J., Bullis, J. R., Gallagher, M. W., Murray-Latin, H., Sauer-Zavala, S., . . . Cassiello-Robbins, C. (2017a). The Unified Protocol for Transdiagnostic Treatment of Emotional Disorders compared with diagnosis-specific protocols for anxiety disorders: A randomized clinical trial. *JAMA Psychiatry, 74*(9), 875–884.

Barlow, D. H., Farchione, T. J., Sauer-Zavala, S., Latin, H. M., Ellard, K. K., Bullis, J. R., . . . Cassiello-Robbins, C. (2017b). *Unified Protocol for Transdiagnostic Treatment of Emotional Disorders: Therapist guide* (2nd ed.). New York: Oxford University Press.

Barlow, D. H., Gorman, J. M., Shear, M. K., & Woods, S. W. (2000). Cognitive-behavioral therapy, imipramine, or their combination for panic disorder: A randomized controlled trial. *Journal of the American Medical Association, 283*(19), 2529–2536.

Barlow, D. H., & Hersen, M. (1984). *Single case experimental designs: Strategies for studying behavior change* (2nd ed.). New York: Pergamon Press.

Barlow, D. H., Nock, M. K., & Hersen, M. (2009). *Single case experimental designs: Strategies for studying behavior change* (3rd ed.). San Antonio, TX: Pearson.

Barlow, D. H., Rapee, R. M., & Brown, T. A. (1992). Behavioral treatment of generalized anxiety disorder. *Behavior Therapy, 23*(4), 551–570.

Barlow, D. H., Sauer-Zavala, S., Carl, J. R., Bullis, J. R., & Ellard, K. K. (2014b). The nature, diagnosis, and treatment of neuroticism: Back to the future. *Clinical Psychological Science, 2*(3), 344–365.

Barlow, D. H., Sauer-Zavala, S., Farchione, T. J., Latin, H. M., Ellard, K. K., Bullis, J. R., . . . Cassiello-Robbins, C. (2017c). *Unified Protocol for Transdiagnostic Treatment of Emotional Disorders: Patient workbook* (2nd ed.). New York: Oxford University Press.

Barlow, D. H., Vermilyea, J., Blanchard, E. B., Vermilyea, B. B., Di Nardo, P. A., & Cerny, J. A. (1985). The phenomenon of panic. *Journal of Abnormal Psychology, 94*(3), 320–328.

Baron, R. A. (1998). *Psychology* (4th ed.). Boston: Allyn & Bacon.

Başoglu, M., Marks, I. M., Kiliç, C., Swinson, R. P., Noshirvani, H., Kuch, K., & O'Sullivan, G. (1994). Relationship of panic, anticipatory anxiety, agoraphobia and global improvement in panic disorder with agoraphobia treated with alprazolam and exposure. *British Journal of Psychiatry, 164*(5), 647–652.

Baumgarten, F. (1933). *Die Charktereignenschaften [The character traits].* Tubingen, Germany: Francke.

Baune, B. T., Adrian, I., & Jacobi, F. (2007). Medical disorders affect health outcome and general functioning depending on comorbid major depression in the general population. *Journal of Psychosomatic Research, 62*(2), 109–118.

Bayer, R., & Spitzer, R. L. (1985). Neurosis, psychodynamics, and DSM-III: A history of the controversy. *Archives of General Psychiatry, 42*(2), 187–196.

Beard, G. (1869). Neurasthenia, or nervous exhaustion. *Boston Medical and Surgical Journal, 80*(13), 217–221.

Beauchaine, T. P., & McNulty, T. (2013). Comorbidities and continuities as ontogenic processes: Toward a developmental spectrum model of externalizing psychopathology. *Development and Psychopathology, 25*(4, Pt. 2), 1505–1528.

Beck, A. T. (1963). Thinking and depression: Idiosyncratic content and cognitive distortions. *Archives of General Psychiatry, 9*(4), 324–333.

Beck, A. T., & Haigh, E. A. P. (2014). Advances in cognitive theory and therapy: The generic cognitive model. *Annual Review of Clinical Psychology, 10*(1), 1–24.

Beck, A. T., Kovacs, M., & Weissman, A. (1979). Assessment of suicidal intention: The Scale for Suicide Ideation. *Journal of Consulting and Clinical Psychology, 47*(2), 343–352.

Beck, A. T., & Steer, R. A. (1993). *Beck Anxiety Inventory Manual.* San Antonio, TX: Psychological Corporation.

Beck, J. G., & Shipherd, J. C. (1997). Repeated exposure to interoceptive cues: Does habituation of fear occur in panic disorder patients?: A preliminary report. *Behaviour Research and Therapy, 35*(6), 551–557.

Beck, J. G., Shipherd, J. C., & Zebb, B. J. (1997). How does interoceptive exposure for panic disorder work?: An uncontrolled case study. *Journal of Anxiety Disorders, 11*(5), 541–556.

Beck, J. S. (2021). *Cognitive behavior therapy: Basics and beyond* (3rd ed.). New York: Guilford Press.

Belloch, A., Cabedo, E., Carrió, C., Fernández-Alvarez, H., García, F., & Larsson, C. (2011). Group versus individual cognitive treatment for obsessive–compulsive disorder: Changes in non-OCD symptoms and cognitions at post-treatment and one-year follow-up. *Psychiatry Research, 187*(1), 174–179.

Bender, D. S., Morey, L. C., & Skodol, A. E. (2011). Toward a model for assessing level of personality functioning in DSM-5: Part I. A review of theory and methods. *Journal of Personality Assessment, 93*(4), 332–346.

Benet-Martinez, V., & Waller, N. G. (1997). Further evidence for the cross-cultural generality of the big seven factor model: Indigenous and imported Spanish personality constructs. *Journal of Personality and Social Psychology, 65*, 567–598.

Bentley, K. H., Gallagher, M. W., Boswell, J. F., Gorman, J. M., Shear, M. K., Woods, S. W., & Barlow, D. H. (2013). The interactive contributions of perceived control and anxiety sensitivity in panic disorder: A triple vulnerabilities perspective. *Journal of Psychopathology and Behavioral Assessment, 35*(1), 57–64.

Bentley, K. H., Nock, M. K., & Barlow, D. H. (2014). The four-function model of nonsuicidal self-injury. *Clinical Psychological Science, 2*(5), 638–656.

Bentley, K. H., Sauer-Zavala, S., Cassiello-Robbins, C. F., Conklin, L. R., Vento, S., & Homer, D. (2017). Treating suicidal thoughts and behaviors within an emotional disorders framework: Acceptability and feasibility of the Unified Protocol in an inpatient setting. *Behavior Modification, 41*(4), 529–557.

Berking, M., Neacsiu, A., Comtois, K. A., & Linehan, M. M. (2009). The impact of experiential avoidance on the reduction of depression in treatment for borderline personality disorder. *Behaviour Research and Therapy, 47*(8), 663–670.

Bernstein, D. P., Arntz, A., & de Vos, M. (2007). Schema focused therapy in forensic settings: Theoretical model and recommendations for best clinical practice. *International Journal of Forensic Mental Health, 6*(2), 169–183.

Bernstein, D. P., Nijman, H. L. I., Karos, K., Keulen-de Vos, M., de Vogel, V., & Lucker, T. P. (2012). Schema therapy for forensic patients with personality disorders: Design and preliminary findings of a multicenter randomized clinical trial in the Netherlands. *International Journal of Forensic Mental Health, 11*(4), 312–324.

Berridge, K. C., & Robinson, T. E. (1998). What is the role of dopamine in reward: Hedonic impact, reward learning, or incentive salience? *Brain Research: Brain Research Reviews, 28*(3), 309–369.

Biederman, J., Rosenbaum, J. F., Bolduc-Murphy, E. A., Faraone, S. V., Chaloff, J.,

Hirshfeld, D. R., & Kagan, J. (1993). A 3-year follow-up of children with and without behavioral inhibition. *Journal of the American Academy of Child and Adolescent Psychiatry, 32*(4), 814–821.

Biederman, J., Rosenbaum, J. F., Hirshfeld, D. R., Faraone, S. V., Bolduc, E. A., Gersten, M., . . . Reznick, J. S. (1990). Psychiatric correlates of behavioral inhibition in young children of parents with and without psychiatric disorders. *Archives of General Psychiatry, 47*(1), 21–26.

Bijl, R. V., van Zessen, G., Ravelli, A., de Rijk, C., & Langendoen, Y. (1998). The Netherlands Mental Health Survey and Incidence Study (NEMESIS): Objectives and design. *Social Psychiatry and Psychiatric Epidemiology, 33*(12), 581–586.

Bijttebier, P., & Vertommen, H. (1999). Coping strategies in relation to personality disorders. *Personality and Individual Differences, 26*(5), 847–856.

Blair, K., Shaywitz, J., Smith, B. W., Rhodes, R., Geraci, M., Jones, M., . . . Pine, D. S. (2008). Response to emotional expressions in generalized social phobia and generalized anxiety disorder: Evidence for separate disorders. *American Journal of Psychiatry, 165*, 1193–1202.

Blaisdell, K. N., Imhof, A. M., & Fisher, P. A. (2019). Early adversity, child neglect, and stress neurobiology: From observations of impact to empirical evaluations of mechanisms. *International Journal of Developmental Neuroscience, 78*, 139–146.

Blashfield, R. K., Keeley, J. W., Flanagan, E. H., & Miles, S. R. (2014). The cycle of classification: DSM-I through DSM-5. *Annual Review of Clinical Psychology, 10*, 25–51.

Blatt, S. J., Wein, S. J., Chevron, E. S., & Quinlan, D. M. (1979). Parental representations and depression in normal young adults. *Journal of Abnormal Psychology, 88*(4), 388–397.

Bodkin, J. A., Lasser, R. A., Wines, J. D., Gardner, D. M., & Baldessarini, R. J. (1997). Combining serotonin reuptake inhibitors and bupropion in partial responders to antidepressant monotherapy. *Journal of Clinical Psychiatry, 58*(4), 137–145.

Boelen, P. A., & Reijntjes, A. (2009). Intolerance of uncertainty and social anxiety. *Journal of Anxiety Disorders, 23*(1), 130–135.

Boelen, P. A., Vrinssen, I., & van Tulder, F. (2010). Intolerance of uncertainty in adolescents: Correlations with worry, social anxiety, and depression. *Journal of Nervous and Mental Disease, 198*(3), 194–200.

Boeschen, L. E., Koss, M. P., Figueredo, A. J., & Coan, J. A. (2001). Experiential avoidance and post-traumatic stress disorder. *Journal of Aggression, Maltreatment and Trauma, 4*(2), 211–245.

Boettcher, H., & Barlow, D. H. (2019). The unique and conditional effects of interoceptive exposure in the treatment of anxiety: A functional analysis. *Behaviour Research and Therapy, 117*, 65–78.

Boettcher, H., Brake, C. A., & Barlow, D. H. (2016). Origins and outlook of interoceptive exposure. *Journal of Behavior Therapy and Experimental Psychiatry, 53*, 41–51.

Boisseau, C. L., Farchione, T. J., Fairholme, C. P., Ellard, K. K., & Barlow, D. H. (2010). The development of the Unified Protocol for the Transdiagnostic Treatment of Emotional Disorders: A case study. *Cognitive and Behavioral Practice, 17*(1), 102–113.

Bolton, J. M., Robinson, J., & Sareen, J. (2009). Self-medication of mood disorders with alcohol and drugs in the National Epidemiologic Survey on Alcohol and Related Conditions. *Journal of Affective Disorders, 115*(3), 367–375.

Borgatta, E. F. (1964). The structure of personality characteristcs. *Behavioral Science, 9*, 8–17.

Borkovec, T. D. (1994). The nature, functions, and origins of worry. In G. C. Davey & F. Tallis (Eds.), *Worrying: Perspectives on theory, assessment and treatment* (pp. 5–33). New York: Wiley.

Borkovec, T. D., Abel, J. L., & Newman, H. (1995). Effects of psychotherapy on comorbid conditions in generalized anxiety disorder. *Journal of Consulting and Clinical Psychology, 63*(3), 479–483.

Borkovec, T. D., Alcaine, O. M., & Behar, E. (2004). Avoidance theory of worry and generalized anxiety disorder. In R. G. Heimberg, C. L. Turk, & D. S. Mennin (Eds.), *Generalized anxiety disorder: Advances in research and practice* (pp. 77–108). New York: Guilford Press.

Borkovec, T. D., Grayson, J. B., & Cooper, K. M. (1978). Treatment of general tension: Subjective and physiological effects of progressive relaxation. *Journal of Consulting and Clinical Psychology, 46*(3), 518–528.

Borkovec, T. D., & Inz, J. (1990). The nature of worry in generalized anxiety disorder: A predominance of thought activity. *Behaviour Research and Therapy, 28*(2), 153–158.

Borkovec, T. D., & Roemer, L. (1995). Perceived functions of worry among generalized anxiety disorder subjects: Distraction from more emotionally distressing topics? *Journal of Behavior Therapy and Experimental Psychiatry, 26*(1), 25–30.

Bornovalova, M. A., Gratz, K. L., Daughters, S. B., Nick, B., Delany-Brumsey, A., Lynch, T. R., . . . Lejuez, C. W. (2008). A multimodal assessment of the relationship between emotion dysregulation and borderline personality disorder among inner-city substance users in residential treatment. *Journal of Psychiatric Research, 42*(9), 717–726.

Bornstein, R. F. (2004). Integrating cognitive and existential treatment strategies in psychotherapy with dependent patients. *Journal of Contemporary Psychotherapy, 34*(4), 293–309.

Boswell, J. F., Anderson, L. M., & Barlow, D. H. (2014). An idiographic analysis of change processes in the Unified Transdiagnostic Treatment of Depression. *Journal of Consulting and Clinical Psychology, 82*(6), 1060–1071.

Boswell, J. F., Farchione, T. J., Sauer-Zavala, S., Murray, H. W., Fortune, M. R., & Barlow, D. H. (2013a). Anxiety sensitivity and interoceptive exposure: A transdiagnostic construct and change strategy. *Behavior Therapy, 44*(3), 417–431.

Boswell, J. F., Iles, B. R., Gallagher, M. W., & Farchione, T. J. (2017). Behavioral activation strategies in cognitive-behavioral therapy for anxiety disorders. *Psychotherapy, 54*(3), 231–236.

Boswell, J. F., Thompson-Hollands, J., Farchione, T. J., & Barlow, D. H. (2013b). Intolerance of uncertainty: A common factor in the treatment of emotional disorders. *Journal of Clinical Psychology, 69*(6), 630–645.

Botwin, M. D., & Buss, D. M. (1989). Structure of act-report data: Is the five-factor model of personality recaptured? *Journal of Personality and Social Psychology, 56*(6), 988–1001.

Bouchard, T. J., & Loehlin, J. C. (2001). Genes, evolution, and personality. *Behavior Genetics, 31*(3), 243–273.

Bouhuys, A. L., Flentge, F., Oldehinkel, A. J., & van den Berg, M. D. (2004). Potential psychosocial mechanisms linking depression to immune function in elderly subjects. *Psychiatry Research, 127*(3), 237–245.

Bouton, M. E. (1993). Context, time, and memory retrieval in the interference paradigms of Pavlovian learning. *Psychological Bulletin, 114*(1), 80–99.

Bouton, M. E. (2002). Context, ambiguity, and unlearning: Sources of relapse after behavioral extinction. *Biological Psychiatry, 52*(10), 976–986.

Bouton, M. E. (2005). Behavior systems and the contextual control of anxiety, fear, and panic. In L. F. Barrett, P. M. Niedenthal, & P. Winkielman (Eds.), *Emotion and consciousness* (pp. 205–230). New York: Guilford Press.

Bouton, M. E., Mineka, S., & Barlow, D. H. (2001). A modern learning theory perspective on the etiology of panic disorder. *Psychological Review, 108*(1), 4–32.

Bowlby, J. (1969). *Attachment and loss: Vol. 1. Attachment.* New York: Basic Books.

Bowlby, J. (1973). *Attachment and loss: Vol. 2. Separation.* New York: Basic Books.

Bowlby, J. (1980). *Attachment and loss: Vol. 3. Loss, sadness and depression.* New York: Basic Books.

Bowlby, J. (1982). Attachment and loss: Retrospective and prospect. *American Journal of Orthopsychiatry, 52,* 664–678.

Brake, C. A., Sauer-Zavala, S., Boswell, J. F., Gallagher, M. W., Farchione, T. J., & Barlow, D. H. (2016). Mindfulness-based exposure strategies as a transdiagnostic mechanism of change: An exploratory alternating treatment design. *Behavior Therapy, 47*(2), 225–238.

Brandes, C. M., Herzhoff, K., Smack, A. J., & Tackett, J. L. (2019). The *p* factor and the *n* factor: Associations between the general factors of psychopathology and neuroticism in children. *Clinical Psychological Science, 7*(6), 1266–1284.

Brandes, C. M., & Tackett, J. L. (2019). Contextualizing neuroticism in the hierarchical taxonomy of psychopathology. *Journal of Research in Personality, 81,* 238–245.

Brewin, C. R., Gregory, J. D., Lipton, M., & Burgess, N. (2010). Intrusive images in psychological disorders: Characteristics, neural mechanisms, and treatment implications. *Psychological Review, 117*(1), 210–232.

Brickman, A. L., Yount, S. E., Blaney, N. T., Rothberg, S. T., & De-Nour, A. K. (1996). Personality traits and long-term health status: The influence of neuroticism and conscientiousness on renal deterioration in type-1 diabetes. *Psychosomatics, 37*(5), 459–468.

Brockmeyer, T., Skunde, M., Wu, M., Bresslein, E., Rudofsky, G., Herzog, W., & Friederich, H.-C. (2014). Difficulties in emotion regulation across the spectrum of eating disorders. *Comprehensive Psychiatry, 55*(3), 565–571.

Brown, D. B., Bravo, A. J., Roos, C. R., & Pearson, M. R. (2015). Five facets of mindfulness and psychological health: Evaluating a psychological model of the mechanisms of mindfulness. *Mindfulness, 6*(5), 1021–1032.

Brown, M., Robinson, L., Campione, G. C., Wuensch, K., Hildebrandt, T., & Micali, N. (2017). Intolerance of uncertainty in eating disorders: A systematic review and meta-analysis. *European Eating Disorders Review, 25*(5), 329–343.

Brown, T. A. (2007). Temporal course and structural relationships among dimensions of temperament and DSM-IV anxiety and mood disorder constructs. *Journal of Abnormal Psychology, 116*(2), 313–328.

Brown, T. A., Antony, M. M., & Barlow, D. H. (1995). Diagnostic comorbidity in panic disorder: Effect on treatment outcome and course of comorbid diagnoses following treatment. *Journal of Consulting and Clinical Psychology, 63*(3), 408–418.

Brown, T. A., & Barlow, D. H. (2002). Classification of anxiety and mood disorders. In D. H. Barlow (Ed.), *Anxiety and its disorders: The nature and treatment of anxiety and panic* (2nd ed., pp. 292–327). New York: Guilford Press.

Brown, T. A., & Barlow, D. H. (2005). Dimensional versus categorical classification of mental disorders in the fifth edition of the *Diagnostic and Statistical Manual of Mental Disorders* and beyond: Comment on the special section. *Journal of Abnormal Psychology, 114*(4), 551–556.

Brown, T. A., & Barlow, D. H. (2009). A proposal for a dimensional classification system based on the shared features of the DSM-IV anxiety and mood disorders: Implications for assessment and treatment. *Psychological Assessment, 21*(3), 256–271.

Brown, T. A., & Barlow, D. H. (2014). *Anxiety and Related Disorders Interview Schedule for DSM-5 (ADIS-5L): Lifetime Version. Client Interview Schedule.* New York: Oxford University Press.

Brown, T. A., Barlow, D. H., & Di Nardo, P. A. (1994a). *Anxiety Disorders Interview Schedule for DSM-IV (ADIS-IV): Client Interview Schedule.* Boulder, CO: Graywind.

Brown, T. A., Barlow, D. H., & Liebowitz, M. R. (1994b). The empirical basis of generalized anxiety disorder. *American Journal of Psychiatry, 151*(9), 1272–1280.

Brown, T. A., Campbell, L. A., Lehman, C. L., Grisham, J. R., & Mancill, R. B. (2001a). Current and lifetime comorbidity of the DSM-IV anxiety and mood disorders in a large clinical sample. *Journal of Abnormal Psychology, 110*(4), 585–599.

Brown, T. A., Chorpita, B. F., & Barlow, D. H. (1998). Structural relationships among dimensions of the DSM-IV anxiety and mood disorders and dimensions of negative affect, positive affect, and autonomic arousal. *Journal of Abnormal Psychology, 107*(2), 179–192.

Brown, T. A., Di Nardo, P. A., Lehman, C. L., & Campbell, L. A. (2001b). Reliability of DSM-IV anxiety and mood disorders: Implications for the classification of emotional disorders. *Journal of Abnormal Psychology, 110*(1), 49–58.

Brown, T. A., Dowdall, D. J., Côté, G., & Barlow, D. H. (1994c). Worry and obsessions: The distinction between generalized anxiety disorder and obsessive–compulsive disorder. In G. C. Davey & F. Tallis (Eds.), *Worrying: Perspectives on theory, assessment and treatment* (pp. 229–246). Hoboken, NJ: Wiley.

Brown, T. A., & McNiff, J. (2009). Specificity of autonomic arousal to DSM-IV panic disorder and posttraumatic stress disorder. *Behaviour Research and Therapy, 47*(6), 487–493.

Brown, T. A., & Naragon-Gainey, K. (2013). Evaluation of the unique and specific contributions of dimensions of the triple vulnerability model to the prediction of DSM-IV anxiety and mood disorder constructs. *Behavior Therapy, 44*(2), 277–292.

Brown, T. A., & Rosellini, A. J. (2011). The direct and interactive effects of neuroticism and life stress on the severity and longitudinal course of depressive symptoms. *Journal of Abnormal Psychology, 120*(4), 844–856.

Brown, T. A., White, K. S., Forsyth, J. P., & Barlow, D. H. (2004). The structure of perceived emotional control: Psychometric properties of a revised Anxiety Control Questionnaire. *Behavior Therapy, 35*(1), 75–99.

Bruch, M. A., & Heimberg, R. G. (1994). Differences in perceptions of parental and personal characteristics between generalized and nongeneralized social phobics. *Journal of Anxiety Disorders, 8*(2), 155–168.

Bryant, F. B., Smart, C. M., & King, S. P. (2005). Using the past to enhance the present: Boosting happiness through positive reminiscence. *Journal of Happiness Studies, 6*(3), 227–260.

Bryant, F. B., & Veroff, J. (2007). *Savoring: A new model of positive experience.* Mahwah, NJ: Erlbaum.

Bucher, M. A., Suzuki, T., & Samuel, D. B. (2019). A meta-analytic review of personality traits and their associations with mental health treatment outcomes. *Clinical Psychology Review, 70*, 51–63.

Buckner, J. D., Keough, M. E., & Schmidt, N. B. (2007). Problematic alcohol and cannabis use among young adults: The roles of depression and discomfort and distress tolerance. *Addictive Behaviors, 32*(9), 1957–1963.

Bujarski, S. J., Norberg, M. M., & Copeland, J. (2012). The association between distress tolerance and cannabis use-related problems: The mediating and moderating roles of coping motives and gender. *Addictive Behaviors, 37*(10), 1181–1184.

Bullis, J. R., Boettcher, H., Sauer-Zavala, S., Farchione, T. J., & Barlow, D. H. (2019). What is an emotional disorder?: A transdiagnostic mechanistic definition with implications for assessment, treatment, and prevention. *Clinical Psychology: Science and Practice, 26*(2), e12278.

Bullis, J. R., Fortune, M. R., Farchione, T. J., & Barlow, D. H. (2014). A preliminary investigation of the long-term outcome of the Unified Protocol for Transdiagnostic Treatment of Emotional Disorders. *Comprehensive Psychiatry, 55*(8), 1920–1927.

Bullis, J., & Sauer-Zavala, S. (2018). Unified Protocol for Insomnia Disorder. In T. Farchione & D. H. Barlow (Eds.), *Applications of the Unified Protocol for the transdiagnostic treatment of emotional disorders* (pp. 164–178). New York: Oxford University Press.

Bullis, J. R., Sauer-Zavala, S., Bentley, K. H., Thompson-Hollands, J., Carl, J. R., & Barlow, D. H. (2015). The Unified Protocol for Transdiagnostic Treatment of Emotional

Disorders: Preliminary exploration of effectiveness for group delivery. *Behavior Modification, 39*(2), 295–321.

Burghardt, N. S., Sullivan, G. M., McEwen, B. S., Gorman, J. M., & LeDoux, J. E. (2004). The selective serotonin reuptake inhibitor citalopram increases fear after acute treatment but reduces fear with chronic treatment: A comparison with tianeptine. *Biological Psychiatry, 55*(12), 1171–1178.

Burghy, C. A., Stodola, D. E., Ruttle, P. L., Molloy, E. K., Armstrong, J. M., Oler, J. A., . . . Birn, R. M. (2012). Developmental pathways to amygdala-prefrontal function and internalizing symptoms in adolescence. *Nature Neuroscience, 15*(12), 1736–1741.

Buske-Kirschbaum, A., Geiben, A., & Hellhammer, D. (2001). Psychobiological aspects of atopic dermatitis: An overview. *Psychotherapy and Psychosomatics., 70*(1), 6–16.

Buss, A. H., & Durkee, A. (1957). An inventory for assessing different kinds of hostility. *Journal of Consulting Psychology, 21*(4), 343–349.

Buss, A. H., & Plomin, R. (1975). *A temperament theory of personality development.* New York: Wiley-Interscience.

Buss, D. M. (1996). Social adaptation and five major factors of personality. In J. S. Wiggins (Ed.), *The five-factor model of personality: Theoretical perspectives* (pp. 180–207). New York: Guilford Press.

Butler, A. C., Chapman, J. E., Forman, E. M., & Beck, A. T. (2006). The empirical status of cognitive-behavioral therapy: A review of meta-analyses. *Clinical Psychology Review, 26*(1), 17–31.

Cameron, N. M., Champagne, F. A., Parent, C., Fish, E. W., Ozaki-Kuroda, K., & Meaney, M. J. (2005). The programming of individual differences in defensive responses and reproductive strategies in the rat through variations in maternal care. *Neuroscience and Biobehavioral Reviews, 29*(4–5), 843–865.

Campbell-Sills, L., Barlow, D. H., Brown, T. A., & Hofmann, S. G. (2006). Effects of suppression and acceptance on emotional responses of individuals with anxiety and mood disorders. *Behaviour Research and Therapy, 44*(9), 1251–1263.

Campbell-Sills, L., Liverant, G. I., & Brown, T. A. (2004). Psychometric evaluation of the behavioral inhibition/behavioral activation scales in a large sample of outpatients with anxiety and mood disorders. *Psychological Assessment, 16*(3), 244–254.

Campeau, S., Falls, W. A., Cullinan, W. E., Helmreich, D. L., Davis, M., & Watson, S. J. (1997). Elicitation and reduction of fear: Behavioural and neuroendocrine indices and brain induction of the immediate-early gene c-fos. *Neuroscience, 78*(4), 1087–1104.

Canli, T. (2008). Toward a neurogenetic theory of neuroticism. *Annals of the New York Academy of Sciences, 1129*(1), 153–174.

Cannon, W. B. (1929). *Bodily changes in pain, hunger, fear, and rage* (2nd ed.). New York: Appleton-Century-Crofts.

Carl, J. R., Gallagher, M. W., & Barlow, D. H. (2018). Development and preliminary evaluation of a positive emotion regulation augmentation module for anxiety and depression. *Behavior Therapy, 49*(6), 939–950.

Carl, J. R., Soskin, D. P., Kerns, C., & Barlow, D. H. (2013). Positive emotion regulation in emotional disorders: A theoretical review. *Clinical Psychology Review, 33*(3), 343–360.

Carleton, R. N. (2012). The intolerance of uncertainty construct in the context of anxiety disorders: Theoretical and practical perspectives. *Expert Review of Neurotherapeutics, 12*(8), 937–947.

Carleton, R. N. (2016). Into the unknown: A review and synthesis of contemporary models involving uncertainty. *Journal of Anxiety Disorders, 39*, 30–43.

Carpenter, R. W., & Trull, T. J. (2013). Components of emotion dysregulation in borderline personality disorder: A review. *Current Psychiatry Reports, 15*(1), 1–8.

Carr, E. G. (1977). The motivation of self-injurious behavior: A review of some hypotheses. *Psychological Bulletin, 84*(4), 800–816.

Carragher, N., Krueger, R. F., Eaton, N. R., & Slade, T. (2015). Disorders without borders: Current and future directions in the meta-structure of mental disorders. *Social Psychiatry and Psychiatric Epidemiology, 50*(3), 339–350.

Carton, J. S., & Nowicki, S. (1994). Antecedents of individual differences in locus of control of reinforcement: A critical review. *Genetic, Social, and General Psychology Monographs, 120*(1), 31–81.

Carver, C. S. (1997). Adult attachment and personality: Converging evidence and a new measure. *Personality and Social Psychology Bulletin, 23*(8), 865–883.

Caspi, A., Houts, R. M., Belsky, D. W., Goldman-Mellor, S. J., Harrington, H., Israel, S., . . . Moffitt, T. E. (2014). The p factor: One general psychopathology factor in the structure of psychiatric disorders? *Clinical Psychological Science, 2*(2), 119–137.

Caspi, A., Sugden, K., Moffitt, T. E., Taylor, A., Craig, I. W., Harrington, H., . . . Poulton, R. (2003). Influence of life stress on depression: Moderation by a polymorphism in the 5-HTT gene. *Science, 301*(5631), 386–389.

Cassiello-Robbins, C., Sauer-Zavala, S., Wilner, J. G., Bentley, K. H., Conklin, L. R., Farchione, T. J., & Barlow, D. H. (2018). A preliminary examination of the effects of transdiagnostic versus single diagnosis protocols on anger during the treatment of anxiety disorders. *Journal of Nervous and Mental Disease, 206*(7), 549–554.

Cassiello-Robbins, C., Southward, M. W., Tirpak, J. W., & Sauer-Zavala, S. (2020). A systematic review of Unified Protocol applications with adult populations: Facilitating widespread dissemination via adaptability. *Clinical Psychology Review, 78*, 101852.

Cassin, S. E., & von Ranson, K. M. (2005). Personality and eating disorders: A decade in review. *Clinical Psychology Review, 25*(7), 895–916.

Castro, D. C., & Berridge, K. C. (2014). Opioid hedonic hotspot in nucleus accumbens shell: Mu, delta, and kappa maps for enhancement of sweetness "liking" and "wanting." *Journal of Neuroscience, 34*(12), 4239–4250.

Castro-Camacho, L., Rattner, M., Quant, D. M., González, L., Moreno, J. D., & Ametaj, A. (2019). A contextual adaptation of the Unified Protocol for the Transdiagnostic Treatment of Emotional Disorders in victims of the armed conflict in Colombia. *Cognitive and Behavioral Practice, 26*(2), 351–365.

Catalino, L. I., Arenander, J., Epel, E., & Puterman, E. (2017). Trait acceptance predicts fewer daily negative emotions through less stressor-related rumination. *Emotion, 17*(8), 1181–1186.

Cattell, R. B. (1943). The description of personality: Basic traits resolved into clusters. *Journal of Abnormal and Social Psychology, 38*(4), 476–506.

Cattell, R. B. (1962). Advances in the measurement of neuroticism and anxiety in a conceptual framework of unitary-trait theory. *Annals of the New York Academy of Sciences, 93*, 815–839.

Chaplin, W. F., John, O. P., & Goldberg, L. R. (1988). Conceptions of states and traits: Dimensional attributes with ideals as prototypes. *Journal of Personality and Social Psychology, 54*, 541–557.

Chapman, A. L., Gratz, K. L., & Brown, M. Z. (2006). Solving the puzzle of deliberate self-harm: The experiential avoidance model. *Behaviour Research and Therapy, 44*(3), 371–394.

Chapman, A. L., Rosenthal, M. Z., Dixon-Gordon, K. L., Turner, B. J., & Kuppens, P. (2017). Borderline personality disorder and the effects of instructed emotional avoidance or acceptance in daily life. *Journal of Personality Disorders, 31*(4), 483–502.

Chapman, A. L., Rosenthal, M. Z., & Leung, D. W. (2009). Emotion suppression in borderline personality disorder: An experience sampling study. *Journal of Personality Disorders, 23*(1), 29–47.

Chapman, A. L., Specht, M. W., & Cellucci, T. (2005). Borderline personality disorder and deliberate self-harm: Does experiential avoidance play a role? *Suicide and Life-Threatening Behavior, 35*(4), 388–399.

Chapman, A. L., Walters, K. N., & Gordon, K. L. D. (2014). Emotional reactivity to social rejection and negative evaluation among persons with borderline personality features. *Journal of Personality Disorders, 28*(5), 720–733.

Charney, D. S., Deutch, A. Y., Krystal, J. H., Southwick, S. M., & Davis, M. (1993). Psychobiologic mechanisms of posttraumatic stress disorder. *Archives of General Psychiatry, 50*(4), 294–305.

Cheavens, J. S., & Heiy, J. (2011). The differential roles of affect and avoidance in major depressive and borderline personality disorder symptoms. *Journal of Social and Clinical Psychology, 30*(5), 441–457.

Cheavens, J. S., Rosenthal, M. Z., Daughters, S. B., Nowak, J., Kosson, D., Lynch, T. R., & Lejuez, C. W. (2005). An analogue investigation of the relationships among perceived parental criticism, negative affect, and borderline personality disorder features: The role of thought suppression. *Behaviour Research and Therapy, 43*(2), 257–268.

Chien, L. L., Ko, H.-C., & Wu, J. Y. W. (2007). The five-factor model of personality and depressive symptoms: One-year follow-up. *Personality and Individual Differences., 43*, 1013–1023.

Chmielewski, M., Bagby, R. M., Markon, K., Ring, A. J., & Ryder, A. G. (2014). Openness to experience, intellect, schizotypal personality disorder, and psychoticism: Resolving the controversy. *Journal of Personality Disorders, 28*(4), 483–499.

Chorpita, B. F. (2001). Control and the development of negative emotion. In M. W. Vasey & M. R. Dadds, *The developmental psychopathology of anxiety* (pp. 112–142). New York: Oxford University Press.

Chorpita, B. F., Albano, A. M., & Barlow, D. H. (1998a). The structure of negative emotions in a clinical sample of children and adolescents. *Journal of Abnormal Psychology, 107*(1), 74–85.

Chorpita, B. F., & Barlow, D. H. (1998). The development of anxiety: The role of control in the early environment. *Psychological Bulletin, 124*(1), 3–21.

Chorpita, B. F., Brown, T. A., & Barlow, D. H. (1998b). Perceived control as a mediator of family environment in etiological models of childhood anxiety. *Behavior Therapy, 29*(3), 457–476.

Church, A. T., & Katigbak, M. S. (1989). Internal, external, and self-report structure of personality in a non-Western culture: An investigation of cross-language and cross-cultural generalizability. *Journal of Personality and Social Psychology, 57*, 857–872.

Cicchetti, D., & Rogosch, F. A. (2001). Diverse patterns of neuroendocrine activity in maltreated children. *Development and Psychopathology, 13*(3), 677–693.

Ciraulo, D. A., Barlow, D. H., Gulliver, S. B., Farchione, T., Morissette, S. B., Kamholz, B. W., . . . Knapp, C. M. (2013). The effects of venlafaxine and cognitive behavioral therapy alone and combined in the treatment of co-morbid alcohol use–anxiety disorders. *Behaviour Research and Therapy, 51*(11), 729–735.

Cisler, J. M., Olatunji, B. O., Feldner, M. T., & Forsyth, J. P. (2010). Emotion regulation and the anxiety disorders: An integrative review. *Journal of Psychopathology and Behavioral Assessment, 32*(1), 68–82.

Clark, D. M. (1986). A cognitive approach to panic. *Behaviour Research and Therapy, 24*(4), 461–470.

Clark, L. A. (2005). Temperament as a unifying basis for personality and psychopathology. *Journal of Abnormal Psychology, 114*(4), 505–521.

Clark, L. A., Vittengl, J., Kraft, D., & Jarrett, R. B. (2003). Separate personality traits from states to predict depression. *Journal of Personality Disorders, 17*(2), 152–172.

Clark, L. A., & Watson, D. (1991). Tripartite model of anxiety and depression:

Psychometric evidence and taxonomic implications. *Journal of Abnormal Psychology, 100*(3), 316–336.

Clark, L. A., & Watson, D. (2008). Temperament: An organizing paradigm for trait psychology. In O. P. John, R. W. Robins, & L. A. Pervin, *Handbook of personality: Theory and research* (3rd ed., pp. 265–286). New York: Guilford Press.

Clark, L. A., Watson, D., & Mineka, S. (1994). Temperament, personality, and the mood and anxiety disorders. *Journal of Abnormal Psychology, 103*(1), 103–116.

Clarkin, J. F., Hull, J. W., Cantor, J., & Sanderson, C. (1993). Borderline personality disorder and personality traits: A comparison of SCID-II BPD and NEO-PI. *Psychological Assessment, 5*(4), 472–476.

Cole, D. A., Peeke, L. G., Martin, J. M., Truglio, R., & Seroczynski, A. D. (1998). A longitudinal look at the relation between depression and anxiety in children and adolescents. *Journal of Consulting and Clinical Psychology, 66*(3), 451–460.

Cole, D. A., & Turner, J. E. (1993). Models of cognitive mediation and moderation in child depression. *Journal of Abnormal Psychology, 102*(2), 271–281.

Collimore, K. C., McCabe, R. E., Carleton, R. N., & Asmundson, G. J. G. (2008). Media exposure and dimensions of anxiety sensitivity: Differential associations with PTSD symptom clusters. *Journal of Anxiety Disorders, 22*(6), 1021–1028.

Compton, W. M., & Guze, S. B. (1995). The neo-Kraepelinian revolution in psychiatric diagnosis. *European Archives of Psychiatry and Clinical Neuroscience., 245*(4–5), 196–201.

Conley, J. J. (1985). Longitudinal stability of personality traits: A multitrait–multimethod–multioccasion analysis. *Journal of Personality and Social Psychology, 49*(5), 1266–1282.

Conrad, C. D. (2008). Chronic stress-induced hippocampal vulnerability: The glucocorticoid vulnerability hypothesis. *Reviews in the Neurosciences, 19*(6), 395–411.

Conway, C. C., Craske, M. G., Zinbarg, R. E., & Mineka, S. (2016). Pathological personality traits and the naturalistic course of internalizing disorders among high-risk young adults. *Depression and Anxiety, 33*(1), 84–93.

Cook, M., Mineka, S., Wolkenstein, B., & Laitsch, K. (1985). Observational conditioning of snake fear in unrelated rhesus monkeys. *Journal of Abnormal Psychology, 94*(4), 591–610.

Cooper, M. L., Frone, M. R., Russell, M., & Mudar, P. (1995). Drinking to regulate positive and negative emotions: A motivational model of alcohol use. *Journal of Personality and Social Psychology, 69*(5), 990–1005.

Coplan, J. D., Andrews, M. W., Rosenblum, L. A., Owens, M. J., Friedman, S., Gorman, J. M., & Nemeroff, C. B. (1996). Persistent elevations of cerebrospinal fluid concentrations of corticotropin-releasing factor in adult nonhuman primates exposed to early-life stressors: Implications for the pathophysiology of mood and anxiety disorders. *Proceedings of the National Academy of Sciences of the USA, 93*(4), 1619–1623.

Coplan, J. D., Paunica, A. D., & Rosenblum, L. A. (2004). Neuropsychobiology of the variable foraging demand paradigm in nonhuman primates. In J. M. Gorman (Ed.), *Fear and anxiety: The benefits of translational research* (pp. 47–64). Washington, DC: American Psychiatric Association.

Coplan, J. D., Rosenblum, L. A., & Gorman, J. M. (1995). Primate models of anxiety: Longitudinal perspectives. *Psychiatric Clinics of North America, 18*(4), 727–743.

Coplan, J. D., Trost, R. C., Owens, M. J., Cooper, T. B., Gorman, J. M., Nemeroff, C. B., & Rosenblum, L. A. (1998). Cerebrospinal fluid concentrations of somatostatin and biogenic amines in grown primates reared by mothers exposed to manipulated foraging conditions. *Archives of General Psychiatry, 55*(5), 473–477.

Costa, P. T., & McCrae, R. R. (1987). Neuroticism, somatic complaints, and disease: Is the bark worse than the bite? *Journal of Personality, 55*(2), 299–316.

Costa, P. T., & McCrae, R. R. (1992). Normal personality assessment in clinical practice: The NEO Personality Inventory. *Psychological Assessment, 4*(1), 5–13.

Costa, P. T., & Widiger, T. A. (2002). Introduction: Personality disorders and the five-factor model of personality. In P. T. Costa, Jr. & T. A. Widiger (Eds.), *Personality disorders and the five-factor model of personality* (2nd ed., pp. 3–14). Washington, DC: American Psychological Association.

Cowen, P. J. (2010). Not fade away: The HPA axis and depression. *Psychological Medicine, 40*(1), 1–4.

Cox, B. J., Enns, M. W., Walker, J. R., Kjernisted, K., & Pidlubny, S. R. (2001). Psychological vulnerabilities in patients with major depression vs panic disorder. *Behaviour Research and Therapy, 39*(5), 567–573.

Cranston-Cuebas, M. A., & Barlow, D. H. (1990). Cognitive and affective contributions to sexual functioning. *Annual Review of Sex Research, 1,* 119–161.

Craske, M. G., Farchione, T. J., Allen, L. B., Barrios, V., Stoyanova, M., & Rose, R. (2007). Cognitive behavioral therapy for panic disorder and comorbidity: More of the same or less of more? *Behaviour Research and Therapy, 45*(6), 1095–1109.

Craske, M. G., Kircanski, K., Epstein, A., Wittchen, H.-U., Pine, D. S., Lewis-Fernández, R., & Hinton, D. (2010). Panic disorder: A review of DSM-IV panic disorder and proposals for DSM-V. *Depression and Anxiety, 27*(2), 93–112.

Craske, M. G., Meuret, A. E., Ritz, T., Treanor, M., Dour, H., & Rosenfield, D. (2019). Positive affect treatment for depression and anxiety: A randomized clinical trial for a core feature of anhedonia. *Journal of Consulting and Clinical Psychology, 87*(5), 457–471.

Craske, M. G., Miller, P. P., Rotunda, R., & Barlow, D. H. (1990). A descriptive report of features of initial unexpected panic attacks in minimal and extensive avoiders. *Behaviour Research and Therapy, 28*(5), 395–400.

Craske, M. G., Poulton, R., Tsao, J. C., & Plotkin, D. (2001). Paths to panic disorder/agoraphobia: An exploratory analysis from age 3 to 21 in an unselected birth cohort. *Journal of the American Academy of Child and Adolescent Psychiatry, 40*(5), 556–563.

Craske, M. G., Stein, M. B., Eley, T. C., Milad, M. R., Holmes, A., Rapee, R. M., & Wittchen, H. (2017). Anxiety disorders. *Nature Reviews: Disease Primers, 3,* 17024.

Craske, M. G., Treanor, M., Conway, C. C., Zbozinek, T., & Vervliet, B. (2014). Maximizing exposure therapy: An inhibitory learning approach. *Behaviour Research and Therapy, 58,* 10–23.

Crawford, A. M., Pentz, M. A., Chou, C. P., Li, C., & Dwyer, J. H. (2003). Parallel developmental trajectories of sensation seeking and regular substance use in adolescents. *Psychology of Addictive Behaviors, 17*(3), 179–192.

Creswell, K. G., Bachrach, R. L., Wright, A. G. C., Pinto, A., & Ansell, E. (2016). Predicting problematic alcohol use with the DSM-5 alternative model of personality pathology. *Personality Disorders: Theory, Research, and Treatment, 7*(1), 103–111.

Cribb, G., Moulds, M. L., & Carter, S. (2006). Rumination and experiential avoidance in depression. *Behaviour Change, 23*(3), 165–176.

Crittenden, P. M., & Ainsworth, M. D. (1989). 14 child maltreatment and attachment theory. *Child maltreatment: Theory and research on the causes and consequences of child abuse and neglect,* 432–463.

Cross, J. R., & Cross, T. L. (2015). Clinical and mental health issues in counseling the gifted individual. *Journal of Counseling and Development, 93*(2), 163–172.

Crowell, S. E., Beauchaine, T. P., & Linehan, M. M. (2009). A biosocial developmental model of borderline personality: Elaborating and extending linehan's theory. *Psychological Bulletin, 135*(3), 495–510.

Cuijpers, P., Cristea, I. A., Karyotaki, E., Reijnders, M., & Huibers, M. J. H. (2016). How effective are cognitive behavior therapies for major depression and anxiety disorders?: A meta-analytic update of the evidence. *World Psychiatry, 15*(3), 245–258.

Cuijpers, P., Smit, F., Penninx, B. W. J. H., de Graaf, R., ten Have, M., & Beekman, A. T. F. (2010). Economic costs of neuroticism: A population-based study. *Archives of General Psychiatry, 67*(10), 1086–1093.

Currie, S. R., & Wang, J. (2005). More data on major depression as an antecedent risk factor for first onset of chronic back pain. *Psychological Medicine, 35*(9), 1275–1282.

Cuthbert, B. N., & Insel, T. R. (2013). Toward the future of psychiatric diagnosis: The seven pillars of RDoC. *BMC Medicine, 11*(1), 126.

Dan, O., Sagi-Schwartz, A., Bar-haim, Y., & Eshel, Y. (2011). Effects of early relationships on children's perceived control: A longitudinal study. *International Journal of Behavioral Development, 35*(5), 449–456.

Daughters, S. B., Sargeant, M. N., Bornovalova, M. A., Gratz, K. L., & Lejuez, C. W. (2008). The relationship between distress tolerance and antisocial personality disorder among male inner-city treatment seeking substance users. *Journal of Personality Disorders, 22*(5), 509–524.

Davenport, J., Bore, M., & Campbell, J. (2010). Changes in personality in pre- and post-dialectical behaviour therapy borderline personality disorder groups: A question of self-control. *Australian Psychologist, 45*(1), 59–66.

Davis, M. (1986). Pharmacological and anatomical analysis of fear conditioning using the fear-potentiated startle paradigm. *Behavioral Neuroscience, 100*(6), 814–824.

Davis, M. (1992). The role of the amygdala in fear and anxiety. *Annual Review of Neuroscience, 15*(1), 353–375.

Davis, M., Walker, D. L., & Lee, Y. (1997). Roles of the amygdala and bed nucleus of the stria terminalis in fear and anxiety measured with the acoustic startle reflex: Possible relevance to PTSD. In R. Yehuda & A. C. McFarlane (Eds.), *Psychobiology of posttraumatic stress disorder* (pp. 305–331). New York: New York Academy of Sciences.

de Ornelas Maia, A. C. C., Braga, A. A., Nunes, C. A., Nardi, A. E., & Silva, A. C. (2013). Transdiagnostic treatment using a Unified Protocol: Application for patients with a range of comorbid mood and anxiety disorders. *Trends in Psychiatry and Psychotherapy, 35*(2), 134–140.

de Ornelas Maia, A. C. C., Nardi, A. E., & Cardoso, A. (2015). The utilization of unified protocols in behavioral cognitive therapy in transdiagnostic group subjects: A clinical trial. *Journal of Affective Disorders, 172,* 179–183.

de Raad, B., di Blas, L., & Perugini, M. (1998a). Two independently constructed Italian trait taxonomies: Comparisons among Italian and between Italian and Germanic languages. *European Journal of Personality, 12,* 19–41.

de Raad, B., Mulder, E., Kloosterman, K., & Hofstee, W. K. B. (1988). Personality-descriptive verbs. *European Journal of Personality, 2*(2), 81–96.

de Raad, B., Perugini, M., Hrebickova, M., & Szarota, P. (1998b). Lingua franca of personality: Taxonomies and structures based on the psycholexical approach. *Journal of Cross Cultural Psychology, 29,* 212–232.

De Young, K. P., Zander, M., & Anderson, D. A. (2014). Beliefs about the emotional consequences of eating and binge eating frequency. *Eating Behaviors, 15*(1), 31–36.

Deacon, B., & Abramowitz, J. (2006). Anxiety sensitivity and its dimensions across the anxiety disorders. *Journal of Anxiety Disorders, 20*(7), 837–857.

Deal, J. E., Halverson, C. F., Jr., Havill, V., & Martin, R. P. (2005). Temperament factors as longitudinal predictors of young adult personality. *Merrill–Palmer Quarterly, 51*(3), 315–334.

Deaver, C. M., Miltenberger, R. G., Smyth, J., Meidinger, A., & Crosby, R. (2003). An evaluation of affect and binge eating. *Behavior Modification, 27*(4), 578–599.

Delgado, M. R., Nearing, K. I., LeDoux, J. E., & Phelps, E. A. (2008). Neural circuitry underlying the regulation of conditioned fear and its relation to extinction. *Neuron, 59*(5), 829–838.

Deng, W., Aimone, J. B., & Gage, F. H. (2010). New neurons and new memories: How does adult hippocampal neurogenesis affect learning and memory? *Nature Reviews Neuroscience, 11*(5), 339–350.

Dennhardt, A. A., & Murphy, J. G. (2011). Associations between depression, distress tolerance, delay discounting, and alcohol-related problems in European American and African American college students. *Psychology of Addictive Behaviors, 25*(4), 595–604.

Depue, R. A., & Iacono, W. G. (1989). Neurobehavioral aspects of affective disorders. *Annual Review of Psychology, 40,* 457–492.

Der-Avakian, A., & Markou, A. (2012). The neurobiology of anhedonia and other reward-related deficits. *Trends in Neurosciences, 35*(1), 68–77.

DeRubeis, R., Webb, C., Tang, T., & Beck, A. (2010). Cognitive therapy. In K. S. Dobson (Ed.), *Handbook of cognitive-behavioral therapies* (3rd ed., pp. 277–316). New York: Guilford Press.

DeYoung, C. G., Hirsh, J. B., Shane, M. S., Papademetris, X., Rajeevan, N., & Gray, J. R. (2010). Testing predictions from personality neuroscience: Brain structure and the big five. *Psychological Science, 21*(6), 820–828.

DeYoung, C. G., Quilty, L. C., & Peterson, J. B. (2007). Between facets and domains: 10 aspects of the Big Five. *Journal of Personality and Social Psychology, 93*(5), 880–896.

Di Nardo, P., Brown, T. A., & Barlow, D. H. (1994). *Anxiety Disorders Interview Schedule for DSM-IV–Lifetime Version (ADIS-IV-L).* New York: Oxford University Press.

Di Nardo, P. A. D., Moras, K., Barlow, D. H., Rapee, R. M., & Brown, T. A. (1993). Reliability of DSM-III-R anxiety disorder categories: Using the Anxiety Disorders Interview Schedule—Revised (ADIS-R). *Archives of General Psychiatry, 50*(4), 251–256.

Di Nardo, P. A. D., O'Brien, G. T., Barlow, D. H., Waddell, M. T., & Blanchard, E. B. (1983). Reliability of DSM-III anxiety disorder categories using a new structured interview. *Archives of General Psychiatry, 40*(10), 1070–1074.

Di Simplicio, M., Norbury, R., Reinecke, A., & Harmer, C. J. (2014). Paradoxical effects of short-term antidepressant treatment in fMRI emotional processing models in volunteers with high neuroticism. *Psychological Medicine, 44*(2), 241–252.

Dichter, G. S., Tomarken, A. J., Freid, C. M., Addington, S., & Shelton, R. C. (2005). Do venlafaxine XR and paroxetine equally influence negative and positive affect? *Journal of Affective Disorders, 85*(3), 333–339.

Dick, D. M. (2011). Gene–environment interaction in psychological traits and disorders. *Annual Review of Clinical Psychology, 7,* 383–409.

Digman, J. M. (1990). Personality structure: Emergence of the five-factor model. *Annual Review of Psychology, 41*(1), 417–440.

Digman, J. M. (1997). Higher-order factors of the Big Five. *Journal of Personality and Social Psychology, 73*(6), 1246–1256.

Digman, J. M., & Inouye, J. (1986). Further specification of the five robust factors of personality. *Journal of Personality and Social Psychology, 50*(1), 116–123.

Digman, J. M., & Takemoto-Chock, N. K. (1981). Factors in the natural language of personality: Re-analysis and comparison of six major studies. *Multivariate Behavioral Research, 16,* 149–170.

Doane, L. D., Mineka, S., Zinbarg, R. E., Craske, M., Griffith, J. W., & Adam, E. K. (2013). Are flatter diurnal cortisol rhythms associated with major depression and anxiety disorders in late adolescence?: The role of life stress and daily negative emotion. *Development and Psychopathology, 25*(3), 629–642.

Dobson, K. S. (1989). A meta-analysis of the efficacy of cognitive therapy for depression. *Journal of Consulting and Clinical Psychology, 57*(3), 414–419.

Donahue, J. M., Hormes, J. M., Gordis, E. B., & Anderson, D. A. (2019). Attending to the alliance in the application of the Unified Protocol for the Transdiagnostic Treatment of Emotional Disorders: A case study. *Clinical Case Studies, 18*(4), 282–299.

Doos Ali Vand, H., Banafsheh, G., Asghar, A. F. A., Farhad, G. B. M., & Mojtaba, H. (2018a). Investigating the effects of the Unified Protocol on common and specific factors in a comorbid insomniac sample: A single-case experimental design. *Iranian Journal of Psychiatry and Behavioral Sciences, 12*(3), e14452.

Doos Ali Vand, H., Gharraee, B., Asgharnejad Farid, A. A., Ghaleh Bandi, M. F., & Habibi, M. (2018b). The effectiveness of transdiagnostic cognitive behavioral therapy for comorbid insomnia: A case report. *Iranian Journal of Psychiatry, 13*(2), 154–159.

Drabant, E. M., Hariri, A. R., Meyer-Lindenberg, A., Munoz, K. E., Mattay, V. S., Kolachana, B. S., . . . Weinberger, D. R. (2006). Catechol O-methyltransferase val-158met genotype and neural mechanisms related to affective arousal and regulation. *Archives of General Psychiatry, 63*(12), 1396–1406.

Drabant, E. M., Ramel, W., Edge, M. D., Hyde, L. W., Kuo, J. R., Goldin, P. R., . . . Gross, J. J. (2012). Neural mechanisms underlying 5-HTTLPR-related sensitivity to acute stress. *American Journal of Psychiatry, 169*(4), 397–405.

Drvaric, L., Bagby, R. M., Kiang, M., & Mizrahi, R. (2018). Maladaptive personality traits in patients identified at lower-risk and higher-risk for psychosis. *Psychiatry Research, 268*, 348–353.

Du, L., Bakish, D., Ravindran, A. V., & Hrdina, P. D. (2002). Does fluoxetine influence major depression by modifying five-factor personality traits? *Journal of Affective Disorders, 71*(1–3), 235–241.

Dudley, N. M., Orvis, K. A., Lebiecki, J. E., & Cortina, J. M. (2006). A meta-analytic investigation of conscientiousness in the prediction of job performance: Examining the intercorrelations and the incremental validity of narrow traits. *Journal of Applied Psychology, 91*(1), 40–57.

Dugas, M. J., Gagnon, F., Ladouceur, R., & Freeston, M. H. (1998). Generalized anxiety disorder: A preliminary test of a conceptual model. *Behaviour Research and Therapy, 36*(2), 215–226.

Dugas, M. J., & Ladouceur, R. (2000). Treatment of GAD: Targeting intolerance of uncertainty in two types of worry. *Behavior Modification, 24*(5), 635–657.

Duncko, R., Makatsori, A., Fickova, E., Selko, D., & Jezova, D. (2006). Altered coordination of the neuroendocrine response during psychosocial stress in subjects with high trait anxiety. *Progress in Neuro-Psychopharmacology and Biological Psychiatry, 30*(6), 1058–1066.

Duval, E. R., Javanbakht, A., & Liberzon, I. (2015). Neural circuits in anxiety and stress disorders: A focused review. *Therapeutics and Clinical Risk Management, 11*, 115–126.

Eaton, N. R., Krueger, R. F., Keyes, K. M., Skodol, A. E., Markon, K. E., Grant, B. F., & Hasin, D. S. (2011a). Borderline personality disorder co-morbidity: Relationship to the internalizing–externalizing structure of common mental disorders. *Psychological Medicine, 41*(5), 1041–1050.

Eaton, N. R., Krueger, R. F., & Oltmanns, T. F. (2011b). Aging and the structure and long-term stability of the internalizing spectrum of personality and psychopathology. *Psychology and Aging, 26*(4), 987.

Eaves, L. J., Eysenck, H. J., & Martin, N. G. (1989). *Genes, culture and personality: An empirical approach.* New York: Academic Press.

Ebner-Priemer, U. W., Badeck, S., Beckmann, C., Wagner, A., Feige, B., Weiss, I., . . . Bohus, M. (2005). Affective dysregulation and dissociative experience in female patients with borderline personality disorder: A startle response study. *Journal of Psychiatric Research, 39*(1), 85–92.

Ebner-Priemer, U. W., Kuo, J., Kleindienst, N., Welch, S. S., Reisch, T., Reinhard, I., . . . Bohus, M. (2007). State affective instability in borderline personality disorder assessed by ambulatory monitoring. *Psychological Medicine, 37*(7), 961–970.

Eccles, J. (2009). Who am I and what am I going to do with my life?: Personal and collective identities as motivators of action. *Educational Psychologist, 44*(2), 78–89.

Ehlers, A. (1993). Somatic symptoms and panic attacks: A retrospective study of learning experiences. *Behaviour Research and Therapy, 31*(3), 269–278.

Eifert, G. H., & Forsyth, J. P. (2005). *Acceptance and commitment therapy for anxiety disorders: A practitioner's treatment guide to using mindfulness, acceptance, and values-based behavior change.* Oakland, CA: New Harbinger.

Einstein, D. A. (2014). Extension of the transdiagnostic model to focus on intolerance of uncertainty: A review of the literature and implications for treatment. *Clinical Psychology: Science and Practice, 21*(3), 280–300.

Eisenberg, N., Valiente, C., Spinrad, T. L., Cumberland, A., Liew, J., Reiser, M., . . . Losoya, S. H. (2009). Longitudinal relations of children's effortful control, impulsivity, and negative emotionality to their externalizing, internalizing, and co-occurring behavior problems. *Developmental Psychology, 45*(4), 988–1008.

Ellard, K. K. (2013). *An examination of the neural correlates of emotion acceptance versus worry in generalized anxiety disorder.* Unpublished doctoral thesis, Boston University, Boston, MA.

Ellard, K. K., Bernstein, E. E., Hearing, C., Baek, J. H., Sylvia, L. G., Nierenberg, A. A., . . . Deckersbach, T. (2017). Transdiagnostic treatment of bipolar disorder and comorbid anxiety using the Unified Protocol for Emotional Disorders: A pilot feasibility and acceptability trial. *Journal of Affective Disorders, 219,* 209–221.

Ellard, K. K., Deckersbach, T., Sylvia, L. G., Nierenberg, A. A., & Barlow, D. H. (2012). Transdiagnostic treatment of bipolar disorder and comorbid anxiety with the Unified Protocol: A clinical replication series. *Behavior Modification, 36*(4), 482–508.

Ellard, K. K., Fairholme, C. P., Boisseau, C. L., Farchione, T. J., & Barlow, D. H. (2010). Unified Protocol for the Transdiagnostic Treatment of Emotional Disorders: Protocol development and initial outcome data. *Cognitive and Behavioral Practice, 17*(1), 88–101.

Ellickson-Larew, S., Naragon-Gainey, K., & Watson, D. (2013). Pathological eating behaviors, BMI, and facet-level traits: The roles of conscientiousness, neuroticism, and impulsivity. *Eating Behaviors, 14*(4), 428–431.

Elwood, L. S., Mott, J., Williams, N. L., Lohr, J. M., & Schroeder, D. A. (2009). Attributional style and anxiety sensitivity as maintenance factors of posttraumatic stress symptoms: A prospective examination of a diathesis–stress model. *Journal of Behavior Therapy and Experimental Psychiatry, 40*(4), 544–557.

Endicott, J., & Spitzer, R. L. (1978). A diagnostic interview: The schedule for affective disorders and schizophrenia. *Archives of General Psychiatry, 35*(7), 837–844.

Engel, S. G., Wonderlich, S. A., Crosby, R. D., Mitchell, J. E., Crow, S., Peterson, C. B., . . . Gordon, K. H. (2013). The role of affect in the maintenance of anorexia nervosa: Evidence from a naturalistic assessment of momentary behaviors and emotion. *Journal of Abnormal Psychology, 122*(3), 709–719.

Erisman, S. M., & Roemer, L. (2012). A preliminary investigation of the process of mindfulness. *Mindfulness, 3*(1), 30–43.

Essex, M. J., Klein, M. H., Cho, E., & Kalin, N. H. (2002). Maternal stress beginning in infancy may sensitize children to later stress exposure: Effects on cortisol and behavior. *Biological Psychiatry, 52*(8), 776–784.

Essex, M. J., Shirtcliff, E. A., Burk, L. R., Ruttle, P. L., Klein, M. H., Slattery, M. J., . . . Armstrong, J. M. (2011). Influence of early life stress on later hypothalamic–pituitary–adrenal axis functioning and its covariation with mental health symptoms: A study of the allostatic process from childhood into adolescence. *Development and Psychopathology, 23*(4), 1039–1058.

Etkin, A., Prater, K. E., Hoeft, F., Menon, V., & Schatzberg, A. F. (2010). Failure of anterior cingulate activation and connectivity with the amygdala during implicit regulation of emotional processing in generalized anxiety disorder. *American Journal of Psychiatry, 167*(5), 545–554.

Etkin, A., & Wager, T. D. (2007). Functional neuroimaging of anxiety: A meta-analysis of emotional processing in PTSD, social anxiety disorder, and specific phobia. *American Journal of Psychiatry, 164*(10), 1476–1488.

Eun, J. D., Paksarian, D., He, J., & Merikangas, K. R. (2018). Parenting style and mental disorders in a nationally representative sample of U.S. adolescents. *Social Psychiatry and Psychiatric Epidemiology, 53*(1), 11–20.

Eustis, E. H., Cardona, N., Nauphal, M., Sauer-Zavala, S., Rosellini, A. J., Farchione, T. J., & Barlow, D. H. (2020). Experiential avoidance as a mechanism of change across cognitive-behavioral therapy in a sample of participants with heterogeneous anxiety disorders. *Cognitive Therapy and Research, 44*(2), 275–286.

Eustis, E. H., Hayes-Skelton, S. A., Roemer, L., & Orsillo, S. M. (2016). Reductions in experiential avoidance as a mediator of change in symptom outcome and quality of life in acceptance-based behavior therapy and applied relaxation for generalized anxiety disorder. *Behaviour Research and Therapy, 87,* 188–195.

Everaert, J., & Joormann, J. (2019). Emotion regulation difficulties related to depression and anxiety: A network approach to model relations among symptoms, positive reappraisal, and repetitive negative thinking. *Clinical Psychological Science, 7*(6), 1304–1318.

Eysenck, H. J. (1947). *Dimensions of personality.* New Brunswick, NJ: Routledge & Paul.

Eysenck, H. J. (1961). *Handbook of abnormal psychology: An experimental approach.* New York: Basic Books.

Eysenck, H. J. (1967). *The biological bases of personality.* Springfield, IL: Charles C Thomas.

Eysenck, H. J. (1981). *A model for personality.* Berlin: Springer-Verlag.

Eysenck, H. J. (1992). Four ways five factors are not basic. *Personality and Individual Differences, 12,* 773–790.

Eysenck, H. J. (1997). Personality and experimental psychology: The unification of psychology and the possibility of a paradigm. *Journal of Personality and Social Psychology, 73,* 1224–1237.

Eysenck, H. J., & Eysenck, S. B. G. (1975). *Manual of the Eysenck Personality Questionnaire (Adult and Junior).* London: Hodder & Stoughton.

Fairburn, C. G., Cooper, Z., & Shafran, R. (2003). Cognitive behaviour therapy for eating disorders: A "transdiagnostic" theory and treatment. *Behaviour Research and Therapy, 41*(5), 509–528.

Fancher, R. E. (2000). Snapshots of Freud in America, 1899–1999. *American Psychologist, 55*(9), 1025–1028.

Fanselow, M. S. (1994). Neural organization of the defensive behavior system responsible for fear. *Psychonomic Bulletin and Review, 1*(4), 429–438.

Farchione, T. J., Fairholme, C. P., Ellard, K. K., Boisseau, C. L., Thompson-Hollands, J., Carl, J. R., . . . Barlow, D. H. (2012). Unified Protocol for Transdiagnostic Treatment of Emotional Disorders: A randomized controlled trial. *Behavior Therapy, 43*(3), 666–678.

Fava, G. A., & Ruini, C. (2003). Development and characteristics of a well-being enhancing psychotherapeutic strategy: Well-being therapy. *Journal of Behavior Therapy and Experimental Psychiatry, 34*(1), 45–63.

Feighner, J. P., Robins, E., Guze, S. B., Woodruff, R. A., Winokur, G., & Munoz, R. (1972). Diagnostic criteria for use in psychiatric research. *Archives of General Psychiatry, 26*(1), 57–63.

Feldman, G., Dunn, E., Stemke, C., Bell, K., & Greeson, J. (2014). Mindfulness and rumination as predictors of persistence with a distress tolerance task. *Personality and Individual Differences, 56,* 154–158.

Feldner, M. T., Zvolensky, M. J., Eifert, G. H., & Spira, A. P. (2003). Emotional avoidance: An experimental test of individual differences and response suppression using biological challenge. *Behaviour Research and Therapy, 41*(4), 403–411.

Fergusson, D. M., Woodward, L. J., & Horwood, L. J. (2000). Risk factors and life processes associated with the onset of suicidal behaviour during adolescence and early adulthood. *Psychological Medicine, 30*(1), 23–39.

Figueiredo, H. F., Bodie, B. L., Tauchi, M., Dolgas, C. M., & Herman, J. P. (2003). Stress integration after acute and chronic predator stress: Differential activation of central stress circuitry and sensitization of the hypothalamo–pituitary–adrenocortical axis. *Endocrinology, 144*(12), 5249–5258.

Fiske, D. W. (1949). Consistency of the factorial structures of personality ratings from different sources. *Journal of Abnormal and Social Psychology, 44*, 329–344.

Flaskerud, J. (2012). Temperament and personality: From Galen to DSM-5. *Issues in Mental Health Nursing, 33*, 631–634.

Fledderus, M., Bohlmeijer, E. T., & Pieterse, M. E. (2010). Does experiential avoidance mediate the effects of maladaptive coping styles on psychopathology and mental health? *Behavior Modification, 34*(6), 503–519.

Forbes, M. K., Baillie, A. J., Eaton, N. R., & Krueger, R. F. (2017). A place for sexual dysfunctions in an empirical taxonomy of psychopathology. *Journal of Sex Research, 54*(4–5), 465–485.

Forbush, K., & Watson, D. (2006). Emotional inhibition and personality traits: A comparison of women with anorexia, bulimia, and normal controls. *Annals of Clinical Psychiatry, 18*(2), 115–121.

Ford, B. Q., Lam, P., John, O. P., & Mauss, I. B. (2018). The psychological health benefits of accepting negative emotions and thoughts: Laboratory, diary, and longitudinal evidence. *Journal of Personality and Social Psychology, 115*(6), 1075–1092.

Forgas, J. P. (2008). Affect and cognition. *Perspectives on Psychological Science, 3*(2), 94–101.

Forman, E. M., Herbert, J. D., Moitra, E., Yeomans, P. D., & Geller, P. A. (2007). A randomized controlled effectiveness trial of acceptance and commitment therapy and cognitive therapy for anxiety and depression. *Behavior Modification, 31*(6), 772–799.

Forsyth, J. P., Parker, J. D., & Finlay, C. G. (2003). Anxiety sensitivity, controllability, and experiential avoidance and their relation to drug of choice and addiction severity in a residential sample of substance-abusing veterans. *Addictive Behaviors, 28*(5), 851–870.

Fox, J. R., & Froom, K. (2009). Eating disorders: A basic emotion perspective. *Clinical Psychology and Psychotherapy, 16*(4), 328–335.

Fox, N. A., Henderson, H. A., Marshall, P. J., Nichols, K. E., & Ghera, M. M. (2005). Behavioral inhibition: Linking biology and behavior within a developmental framework. *Annual Review of Psychology, 56*(1), 235–262.

Frank, E., Kupfer, D. J., Thase, M. E., Mallinger, A. G., Swartz, H. A., Fagiolini, A. M., . . . Monk, T. (2005). Two-year outcomes for interpersonal and social rhythm therapy in individuals with bipolar I disorder. *Archives of General Psychiatry, 62*(9), 996–1004.

Franzen, P. L., & Buysse, D. J. (2008). Sleep disturbances and depression: Risk relationships for subsequent depression and therapeutic implications. *Dialogues in Clinical Neuroscience, 10*(4), 473–481.

Fredrickson, B. L. (1998). What good are positive emotions? *Review of General Psychology, 2*(3), 300–319.

Fredrickson, B. L. (2001). The role of positive emotions in positive psychology. *American Psychologist, 56*(3), 218–226.

Fredrickson, B. L., & Joiner, T. (2002). Positive emotions trigger upward spirals toward emotional well-being. *Psychological Science, 13*(2), 172–175.

Freud, S. (1953a). The interpretation of dreams. In J. Strachey (Ed. & Trans.), *The standard edition of the complete psychological works of Sigmund Freud* (Vol. 4, pp. 1–338). London: Hogarth Press. (Original work published 1900)

Freud, S. (1953b). Three essays on the theory of sexuality. In J. Strachey (Ed. & Trans.), *The standard complete psychological works of Sigmund Freud* (Vol. 7, pp. 1–138). London: Hogarth Press. (Original work published 1905)

Freud, S. (1964). New introductory lectures on psychoanalysis. In J. Strachey (Ed. & Trans.), *The standard edition of the complete psychological works of Sigmund Freud* (Vol. 22, pp. 1–182). Hogarth Press. (Original work published 1933)

Freud, S. (1968). *Introductory lectures on psychoanalysis.* London: Allen & Unwin. (Original work published 1920)

Frokjaer, V. G., Mortensen, E. L., Nielsen, F. A., Haugbol, S., Pinborg, L. H., Adams, K. H., . . . Knudsen, G. M. (2008). Frontolimbic serotonin 2A receptor binding in healthy subjects is associated with personality risk factors for affective disorder. *Biological Psychiatry, 63*(6), 569–576.

Gaffan, E. A., Tsaousis, J., & Kemp-Wheeler, S. M. (1995). Researcher allegiance and meta-analysis: The case of cognitive therapy for depression. *Journal of Consulting and Clinical Psychology, 63*(6), 966–980.

Galen. (1938). On temperaments. In K. Lamera (Trans.), *The collected works for ancient Greek writers* (Vol. 24). Athens, Greece: Papyros. (Original work written 170 C.E.)

Gallagher, M. W., Bentley, K. H., & Barlow, D. H. (2014). Perceived control and vulnerability to anxiety disorders: A meta-analytic review. *Cognitive Therapy and Research, 38*(6), 571–584.

Gallagher, M. W., Long, L. J., Richardson, A., D'Souza, J., Boswell, J. F., Farchione, T. J., & Barlow, D. H. (2020). Examining hope as a transdiagnostic mechanism of change across anxiety disorders and CBT treatment protocols. *Behavior Therapy, 51*(1), 190–202.

Gantt, W. H. (1942). The origin and development of nervous disturbances experimentally produced. *American Journal of Psychiatry, 98*(4), 475–481.

Garland, E. L., Fredrickson, B., Kring, A. M., Johnson, D. P., Meyer, P. S., & Penn, D. L. (2010). Upward spirals of positive emotions counter downward spirals of negativity: Insights from the broaden-and-build theory and affective neuroscience on the treatment of emotion dysfunctions and deficits in psychopathology. *Clinical Psychology Review, 30*(7), 849–864.

Gelowitz, D. L., & Kokkinidis, L. (1999). Enhanced amygdala kindling after electrical stimulation of the ventral tegmental area: Implications for fear and anxiety. *Journal of Neuroscience, 19*(22), RC41.

Gentes, E. L., & Ruscio, A. M. (2011). A meta-analysis of the relation of intolerance of uncertainty to symptoms of generalized anxiety disorder, major depressive disorder, and obsessive–compulsive disorder. *Clinical Psychology Review, 31*(6), 923–933.

Gershuny, B. S., & Sher, K. J. (1998). The relation between personality and anxiety: Findings from a 3-year prospective study. *Journal of Abnormal Psychology, 107*(2), 252–262.

Gerull, F. C., & Rapee, R. M. (2002). Mother knows best: Effects of maternal modelling on the acquisition of fear and avoidance behaviour in toddlers. *Behaviour Research and Therapy, 40*(3), 279–287.

Gesquiere, L. R., Learn, N. H., Simao, M. C. M., Onyango, P. O., Alberts, S. C., & Altmann, J. (2011). Life at the top: Rank and stress in wild male baboons. *Science, 333*(6040), 357–360.

Ghazwani, J. Y., Khalil, S. N., & Ahmed, R. A. (2016). Social anxiety disorder in Saudi adolescent boys: Prevalence, subtypes, and parenting style as a risk factor. *Journal of Family and Community Medicine, 23*(1), 25–31.

Gibbons, C. J., & DeRubeis, R. J. (2008). Anxiety symptom focus in sessions of cognitive therapy for depression. *Behavior Therapy, 39*(2), 117–125.

Gillespie, C. F., Phifer, J., Bradley, B., & Ressler, K. J. (2009). Risk and resilience: Genetic and environmental influences on development of the stress response. *Depression and Anxiety, 26*(11), 984–992.

Giluk, T. L. (2009). Mindfulness, Big Five personality, and affect: A meta-analysis. *Personality and Individual Differences, 47*(8), 805–811.

Glick, D. M., & Orsillo, S. M. (2011). Relationships among social anxiety, self-focused attention, and experiential distress and avoidance. *Journal of Evidence-Based Psychotherapies, 11*(1), 1.

Gloster, A. T., Wittchen, H.-U., Einsle, F., Lang, T., Helbig-Lang, S., Fydrich, T., . . . Arolt, V. (2011). Psychological treatment for panic disorder with agoraphobia: A randomized controlled trial to examine the role of therapist-guided exposure *in situ* in CBT. *Journal of Consulting and Clinical Psychology, 79*(3), 406–420.

Goldberg, L. R. (1981). Language and individual differences: The search for universals in personality lexicons. *Review of Personality and Social Psychology, 2*(1), 141–165.

Goldberg, L. R. (1990). An alternative "description of personality": The Big-Five factor structure. *Journal of Personality and Social Psychology, 59*(6), 1216–1229.

Goldberg, L. R. (1993). The structure of phenotypic personality traits. *American Psychologist, 48*(1), 26–34.

Goldberg, S. C., Schulz, S. C., Schulz, P. M., Resnick, R. J., Hamer, R. M., & Friedel, R. O. (1986). Borderline and schizotypal personality disorders treated with low-dose thiothixene vs placebo. *Archives of General Psychiatry, 43*(7), 680–686.

Goldman, N., Dugas, M. J., Sexton, K. A., & Gervais, N. J. (2007). The impact of written exposure on worry: A preliminary investigation. *Behavior Modification, 31*(4), 512–538.

Goldsmith, H. H., Buss, A. H., Plomin, R., Rothbart, M. K., Thomas, A., Chess, S., . . . McCall, R. B. (1987). Roundtable: What is temperament?: Four approaches. *Child Development, 58*(2), 505–529.

Goldsmith, H. H., & Campos, J. J. (1982). Toward a theory of infant temperament. In R. N. Emde & R. J. Harmon (Eds.), *The development of attachment and affiliative systems* (pp. 161–193). Boston: Springer.

Goldstein, J. (2002). *One Dharma: The emerging western Buddhism.* New York: Harper Collins.

Goodman, W. K., Price, L. H., Rasmussen, S. A., Mazure, C., Fleischmann, R. L., Hill, C. L., . . . Charney, D. S. (1989). The Yale–Brown Obsessive Compulsive Scale: I. Development, use, and reliability. *Archives of General Psychiatry, 46*(11), 1006–1011.

Goodwin, R. D., & Hamilton, S. P. (2001). Panic attack as a marker of core psychopathological processes. *Psychopathology, 34*(6), 278–288.

Gore, W. L., Presnall, J. R., Miller, J. D., Lynam, D. R., & Widiger, T. A. (2012). A five-factor measure of dependent personality traits. *Journal of Personality Assessment, 94*(5), 488–499.

Gore, W. L., & Widiger, T. A. (2018). Negative emotionality across diagnostic models: RDoC, DSM-5 Section III, and FFM. *Personality Disorders: Theory, Research, and Treatment, 9*(2), 155–164.

Gorka, S. M., Ali, B., & Daughters, S. B. (2012). The role of distress tolerance in the relationship between depressive symptoms and problematic alcohol use. *Psychology of Addictive Behaviors, 26*(3), 621–626.

Gorman, J. M. (2007). *The essential guide to psychiatric drugs* (4th ed.). New York: St. Martin's Griffin.

Goubert, L., Crombez, G., & Van Damme, S. (2004). The role of neuroticism, pain catastrophizing and pain-related fear in vigilance to pain: A structural equations approach. *Pain, 107*(3), 234–241.

Gracious, K. S. (1999). Do SSRIs affect personality traits? *British Journal of Psychiatry, 175,* 287.

Grafton, B., Ang, C., & MacLeod, C. (2012). Always look on the bright side of life: The attentional basis of positive affectivity. *European Journal of Personality, 2*(26), 133–144.

Granger, D. A., Weisz, J. R., & Kauneckis, D. (1994). Neuroendocrine reactivity, internalizing behavior problems, and control-related cognitions in clinic-referred children and adolescents. *Journal of Abnormal Psychology, 103*(2), 267–276.

Grant, B. F., Chou, S. P., Goldstein, R. B., Huang, B., Stinson, F. S., Saha, T. D., . . . Ruan, W. J. (2008). Prevalence, correlates, disability, and comorbidity of DSM-IV borderline personality disorder: Results from the Wave 2 National Epidemiologic Survey on Alcohol and Related Conditions. *Journal of Clinical Psychiatry, 69*(4), 533–545.

Grant, D. M., Beck, J. G., & Davila, J. (2007). Does anxiety sensitivity predict symptoms of panic, depression, and social anxiety? *Behaviour Research and Therapy, 45*(9), 2247–2255.

Gratz, K. L. (2003). Risk factors for and functions of deliberate self-harm: An empirical and conceptual review. *Clinical Psychology: Science and Practice, 10*(2), 192–205.

Gratz, K. L., & Roemer, L. (2004). Multidimensional assessment of emotion regulation and dysregulation: Development, factor structure, and initial validation of the Difficulties in Emotion Regulation Scale. *Journal of Psychopathology and Behavioral Assessment, 26*(1), 41–54.

Gratz, K. L., Tull, M. T., & Gunderson, J. G. (2008). Preliminary data on the relationship between anxiety sensitivity and borderline personality disorder: The role of experiential avoidance. *Journal of Psychiatric Research, 42*(7), 550–559.

Gray, J. A. (1970). The psychophysiological basis of introversion–extraversion. *Behaviour Research and Therapy, 8*(3), 249–266.

Gray, J. A. (1982). *The neuropsychology of anxiety: An enquiry into the functions of the septo-hippocampal system*. London: Clarendon Press/Oxford University Press.

Gray, J. A. (1987). Perspectives on anxiety and impulsivity: A commentary. *Journal of Research in Personality, 21*(4), 493–509.

Gray, J. A. (1991). The neuropsychology of temperament. In J. Strelau & A. Angleitner (Eds.), *Explorations in temperament: International perspectives on theory and measurement* (pp. 105–128). New York: Plenum Press.

Gray, J. A., & McNaughton, N. (1995). The neuropsychology of anxiety: Reprise. In D. A. Hope (Ed.), *Nebraska Symposium on Motivation: Vol. 43. Perspectives on anxiety, panic, and fear* (pp. 61–134). Lincoln: University of Nebraska Press.

Greeley, J., Le, D. A., Poulos, C. X., & Cappell, H. (1984). Alcohol is an effective cue in the conditional control of tolerance to alcohol. *Psychopharmacology, 83*, 159–162.

Greenberg, J. R., & Mitchell, S. A. (1983). *Object relations in psychoanalytic theory*. Cambridge, MA: Harvard University Press.

Griez, E., & van Den Hout, M. A. (1986). CO_2 inhalation in the treatment of panic attacks. *Behaviour Research and Therapy, 24*(2), 145–150.

Griffith, J. W., Zinbarg, R. E., Craske, M. G., Mineka, S., Rose, R. D., Waters, A. M., & Sutton, J. M. (2010). Neuroticism as a common dimension in the internalizing disorders. *Psychological Medicine, 40*(7), 1125–1136.

Grob, G. (1991). Origins of DSM-I: A study in appearance and reality. *American Journal of Psychiatry, 148*(4), 421–431.

Gross, J. J. (2015). The extended process model of emotion regulation: Elaborations, applications, and future directions. *Psychological Inquiry, 26*(1), 130–137.

Gross, J. J., & Levenson, R. W. (1993). Emotional suppression: Physiology, self-report, and expressive behavior. *Journal of Personality and Social Psychology, 64*(6), 970–986.

Grossman, P., Niemann, L., Schmidt, S., & Walach, H. (2004). Mindfulness-based stress reduction and health benefits: A meta-analysis. *Journal of Psychosomatic Research, 57*(1), 35–43.

Gruber, J., Johnson, S. L., Oveis, C., & Keltner, D. (2008). Risk for mania and positive emotional responding: Too much of a good thing? *Emotion, 8*(1), 23–33.

Gunnar, M. R., & Fisher, P. A. (2006). Bringing basic research on early experience and stress neurobiology to bear on preventive interventions for neglected and maltreated children. *Development and Psychopathology, 18*(3), 651–677.

Gunnar, M. R., Larson, M. C., Hertsgaard, L., Harris, M. L., & Brodersen, L. (1992). The stressfulness of separation among nine-month-old infants: Effects of social context variables and infant temperament. *Child Development, 63*(2), 290–303.

Gunnar, M., & Quevedo, K. (2007). The neurobiology of stress and development. *Annual Review of Psychology, 58,* 145–173.

Hague, B., Scott, S., & Kellett, S. (2015). Transdiagnostic CBT treatment of co-morbid anxiety and depression in an older adult: Single case experimental design. *Behavioural and Cognitive Psychotherapy, 43*(1), 119–124.

Hale, N. G. (1971). *Freud and the Americans: The beginnings of psychoanalysis in the United States, 1876–1917.* Oxford, UK: Oxford University Press.

Hallquist, M. N., & Pilkonis, P. A. (2012). Refining the phenotype of borderline personality disorder: Diagnostic criteria and beyond. *Personality Disorders: Theory, Research, and Treatment, 3*(3), 228–246.

Hambrook, D., Oldershaw, A., Rimes, K., Schmidt, U., Tchanturia, K., Treasure, J., . . . Chalder, T. (2011). Emotional expression, self-silencing, and distress tolerance in anorexia nervosa and chronic fatigue syndrome. *British Journal of Clinical Psychology, 50*(3), 310–325.

Hampson, S. E., Edmonds, G. W., Goldberg, L. R., Dubanoski, J. P., & Hillier, T. A. (2013). Childhood conscientiousness relates to objectively measured adult physical health four decades later. *Health Psychology, 32*(8), 925–928.

Hane, A. A., Henderson, H. A., Reeb-Sutherland, B. C., & Fox, N. A. (2010). Ordinary variations in human maternal caregiving in infancy and biobehavioral development in early childhood: A follow-up study. *Developmental Psychobiology, 52*(6), 558–567.

Hanley, A. W., de Vibe, M., Solhaug, I., Gonzalez-Pons, K., & Garland, E. L. (2019). Mindfulness training reduces neuroticism over a 6-year longitudinal randomized control trial in Norwegian medical and psychology students. *Journal of Research in Personality, 82,* 103859.

Hanley, A. W., Garland, E. L., & Tedeschi, R. G. (2017). Relating dispositional mindfulness, contemplative practice, and positive reappraisal with posttraumatic cognitive coping, stress, and growth. *Psychological Trauma: Theory, Research, Practice and Policy, 9*(5), 526–536.

Harmer, C. J., Mackay, C. E., Reid, C. B., Cowen, P. J., & Goodwin, G. M. (2006). Antidepressant drug treatment modifies the neural processing of nonconscious threat cues. *Biological Psychiatry, 59*(9), 816–820.

Harrison, A., Sullivan, S., Tchanturia, K., & Treasure, J. (2009). Emotion recognition and regulation in anorexia nervosa. *Clinical Psychology and Psychotherapy, 16*(4), 348–356.

Harrison, A., Sullivan, S., Tchanturia, K., & Treasure, J. (2010). Emotional functioning in eating disorders: Attentional bias, emotion recognition and emotion regulation. *Psychological Medicine, 40*(11), 1887–1897.

Hayes, S. A., Orsillo, S. M., & Roemer, L. (2010). Changes in proposed mechanisms of action during an acceptance-based behavior therapy for generalized anxiety disorder. *Behaviour Research and Therapy, 48*(3), 238–245.

Hayes, S. C., & Hofmann, S. G. (Eds.). (2018). *Process-based CBT: The science and core clinical competencies of cognitive behavioral therapy.* New York: New Harbinger.

Hayes, S. C., Luoma, J. B., Bond, F. W., Masuda, A., & Lillis, J. (2006). Acceptance and commitment therapy: Model, processes and outcomes. *Behaviour Research and Therapy, 44*(1), 1–25.

Hayes, S. C., Strosahl, K., & Wilson, K. (1999). *Acceptance and commitment therapy: Understanding and treating human suffering.* New York: Guilford Press.

Hayes, S. C., Wilson, K. G., Gifford, E. V., Follette, V. M., & Strosahl, K. (1996). Experiential avoidance and behavioral disorders: A functional dimensional approach to diagnosis and treatment. *Journal of Consulting and Clinical Psychology, 64*(6), 1152–1168.

Hedley, L. M., Hoffart, A., & Sexton, H. (2001). The change process in a cognitive-behavioral therapy: Testing a cognitive, a behavioral, and an integrated model of panic disorder with agoraphobia. *Psychotherapy Research, 11*(4), 401–413.

Hedman, E., Andersson, G., Lindefors, N., Gustavsson, P., Lekander, M., Rück, C., . . . Ljótsson, B. (2014). Personality change following internet-based cognitive behavior therapy for severe health anxiety. *PLOS ONE, 9*(12).

Heim, C., & Nemeroff, C. B. (1999). The impact of early adverse experiences on brain systems involved in the pathophysiology of anxiety and affective disorders. *Biological Psychiatry, 46*(11), 1509–1522.

Heimberg, R. G., Liebowitz, M. R., Hope, D. A., Schneier, F. R., Holt, C. S., Welkowitz, L. A., . . . Klein, D. F. (1998). Cognitive-behavioral group therapy vs phenelzine therapy for social phobia: 12-week outcome. *Archives of General Psychiatry, 55*(12), 1133–1141.

Helson, R., Jones, C., & Kwan, V. S. Y. (2002). Personality change over 40 years of adulthood: Hierarchical linear modeling analyses of two longitudinal samples. *Journal of Personality and Social Psychology, 83*(3), 752–766.

Henriques-Calado, J., Duarte-Silva, M. E., Junqueira, D., Sacoto, C., & Keong, A. M. (2014). Five-factor model personality domains in the prediction of Axis II personality disorders: An exploratory study in late adulthood women non-clinical sample. *Personality and Mental Health, 8*(2), 115–127.

Henry, C., Mitropoulou, V., New, A. S., Koenigsberg, H. W., Silverman, J., & Siever, L. J. (2001). Affective instability and impulsivity in borderline personality and bipolar II disorders: Similarities and differences. *Journal of Psychiatric Research, 35*(6), 307–312.

Hentges, R. F., Graham, S. A., Plamondon, A., Tough, S., & Madigan, S. (2019). A developmental cascade from prenatal stress to child internalizing and externalizing problems. *Journal of Pediatric Psychology, 44*(9), 1057–1067.

Herpertz, S. C., Huprich, S. K., Bohus, M., Chanen, A., Goodman, M., Mehlum, L., . . . Sharp, C. (2017). The challenge of transforming the diagnostic system of personality disorders. *Journal of Personality Disorders, 31*(5), 577–589.

Hershberg, S. G., Carlson, G. A., Cantwell, D. P., & Strober, M. (1982). Anxiety and depressive disorders in psychiatrically disturbed children. *Journal of Clinical Psychiatry, 43*(9), 358–361.

Hertsgaard, L., Gunnar, M., Erickson, M. F., & Nachmias, M. (1995). Adrenocortical responses to the Strange Situation in infants with disorganized/disoriented attachment relationships. *Child Development, 66*(4), 1100–1106.

Hettema, J. M., Neale, M. C., & Kendler, K. S. (2001). A review and meta-analysis of the genetic epidemiology of anxiety disorders. *American Journal of Psychiatry, 158*(10), 1568–1578.

Hezel, D. M., Stewart, S. E., Riemann, B. C., & McNally, R. J. (2019). Standard of proof and intolerance of uncertainty in obsessive–compulsive disorder and social anxiety disorder. *Journal of Behavior Therapy and Experimental Psychiatry, 64*, 36–44.

Hill, P. L., Nickel, L. B., & Roberts, B. W. (2014). Are you in a healthy relationship?: Linking conscientiousness to health via implementing and immunizing behaviors. *Journal of Personality, 82*(6), 485–492.

Hill, P. L., Roberts, B. W., Grogger, J. T., Guryan, J., & Sixkiller, K. (2011). Decreasing delinquency, criminal behavior, and recidivism by intervening on psychological factors other than cognitive ability: A review of the intervention literature. *NBER Working Papers Series, 2011* [online], w16698.

Hill, P. L., Turiano, N. A., Mroczek, D. K., & Roberts, B. W. (2012). Examining concurrent and longitudinal relations between personality traits and social well-being in adulthood. *Social Psychological and Personality Science, 3*(6), 698–705.

Hiller, W., Leibbrand, R., Rief, W., & Fichter, M. M. (2005). Differentiating hypochondriasis from panic disorder. *Journal of Anxiety Disorders, 19*(1), 29–49.

Hippocrates. (1978). On the nature of man. In G. R. Lloyd (Ed.), & J. Chadwick & W. Mann (Trans.), *Hippocratic writings* (pp. 260–271). London: Harmondsworth.

Hirshfeld, D. R., Rosenbaum, J. F., Biederman, J., Bolduc, E. A., Faraone, S. V., Snidman, N., . . . Kagan, J. (1992). Stable behavioral inhibition and its association with anxiety disorder. *Journal of the American Academy of Child and Adolescent Psychiatry, 31*(1), 103–111.

Hirvonen, J., Tuominen, L., Någren, K., & Hietala, J. (2015). Neuroticism and serotonin 5-HT1A receptors in healthy subjects. *Psychiatry Research, 234*(1), 1–6.

Hoehn-Saric, R., Schlund, M. W., & Wong, S. H. Y. (2004). Effects of citalopram on worry and brain activation in patients with generalized anxiety disorder. *Psychiatry Research: Neuroimaging, 131*(1), 11–21.

Hofmann, S. G. (2005). Perception of control over anxiety mediates the relation between catastrophic thinking and social anxiety in social phobia. *Behaviour Research and Therapy, 43*(7), 885–895.

Hofmann, S. G., Heering, S., Sawyer, A. T., & Asnaani, A. (2009). How to handle anxiety: The effects of reappraisal, acceptance, and suppression strategies on anxious arousal. *Behaviour Research and Therapy, 47*(5), 389–394.

Hogan, R. (1982). A socioanalytic theory of personality. In M. Page (Ed.), *Nebraska Symposium on Motivation: Vol. 30. Personality: Current theory and research* (pp. 55–89). Lincoln: University of Nebraska Press.

Holaway, R. M., Heimberg, R. G., & Coles, M. E. (2006). A comparison of intolerance of uncertainty in analogue obsessive–compulsive disorder and generalized anxiety disorder. *Journal of Anxiety Disorders, 20*(2), 158–174.

Hong, R. Y., & Cheung, M. W. L. (2015). The structure of cognitive vulnerabilities to depression and anxiety: Evidence for a common core etiologic process based on a meta-analytic review. *Clinical Psychological Science, 3*(6), 892–912.

Hong, R. Y., Lee, S. S. M., Tsai, F., & Tan, S. H. (2017). Developmental trajectories and origins of a core cognitive vulnerability to internalizing symptoms in middle childhood. *Clinical Psychological Science, 5*(2), 299–315.

Hooker, C. I., Verosky, S. C., Miyakawa, A., Knight, R. T., & D'Esposito, M. (2008). The influence of personality on neural mechanisms of observational fear and reward learning. *Neuropsychologia, 46*(11), 2709–2724.

Hope, D. A., Heimberg, R. G., & Turk, C. L. (2010). *Managing social anxiety: A cognitive-behavioral therapy approach.* New York: Oxford University Press.

Hopko, D. R., Lejuez, C. W., Ruggiero, K. J., & Eifert, G. H. (2003). Contemporary behavioral activation treatments for depression: Procedures, principles, and progress. *Clinical Psychology Review, 23*(5), 699–717.

Hopwood, C. J. (2018). A framework for treating DSM-5 alternative model for personality disorder features. *Personality and Mental Health, 12*(2), 107–125.

Hopwood, C. J., Schade, N., Krueger, R. F., Wright, A. G. C., & Markon, K. E. (2013a). Connecting DSM-5 personality traits and pathological beliefs: Toward a unifying model. *Journal of Psychopathology and Behavioral Assessment, 35*(2), 162–172.

Hopwood, C. J., Thomas, K. M., Markon, K. E., Wright, A. G. C., & Krueger, R. F. (2012). DSM-5 personality traits and DSM-IV personality disorders. *Journal of Abnormal Psychology, 121*(2), 424–432.

Hopwood, C. J., Wright, A. G. C., Ansell, E. B., & Pincus, A. L. (2013b). The interpersonal core of personality pathology. *Journal of Personality Disorders, 27*(3), 270–295.

Horn, C. A. C., Pietrzak, R. H., Corsi-Travali, S., & Neumeister, A. (2014). Linking plasma cortisol levels to phenotypic heterogeneity of posttraumatic stress symptomatology. *Psychoneuroendocrinology, 39*, 88–93.

Hostinar, C. E., Nusslock, R., & Miller, G. E. (2018). Future directions in the study of early-life stress and physical and emotional health: Implications of the neuroimmune network hypothesis. *Journal of Clinical Child and Adolescent Psychology, 47*(1), 142–156.

Howe, A. S., Buttenschøn, H. N., Bani-Fatemi, A., Maron, E., Otowa, T., Erhardt, A., . . . De Luca, V. (2016). Candidate genes in panic disorder: Meta-analyses of 23 common variants in major anxiogenic pathways. *Molecular Psychiatry, 21*(5), 665–679.

Hrebickova, M., & Ostendorf, F. (1995). Lexical approach to personality: 5. Classification of adjectives into categories of personality description. *Ceskoslovenska Psychologie, 39*, 265–276.

Hudson, J. I., & Pope, H. G. (1990). Affective spectrum disorder: Does antidepressant response identify a family of disorders with a common pathophysiology? *American Journal of Psychiatry, 147*(5), 552–564.

Hudson, J. L., & Rapee, R. M. (2002). Parent–child interactions in clinically anxious children and their siblings. *Journal of Clinical Child and Adolescent Psychology, 31*(4), 548–555.

Huovinen, E., Kaprio, J., & Koskenvuo, M. (2001). Asthma in relation to personality traits, life satisfaction, and stress: A prospective study among 11,000 adults. *Allergy, 56*(10), 971–977.

Hutcherson, C. A., Seppala, E. M., & Gross, J. J. (2008). Loving-kindness meditation increases social connectedness. *Emotion, 8*(5), 720–724.

Hy, L. X., & Loevinger, J. (1996). *Measuring ego development* (2nd ed.). Hillsdale, NJ: Erlbaum.

Iacono, W. G., Malone, S. M., & Vrieze, S. I. (2017). Endophenotype best practices. *International Journal of Psychophysiology, 111*, 115–144.

Ilieva, I. (2015). Enhancement of healthy personality through psychiatric medication: The influence of SSRIs on neuroticism and extraversion. *Neuroethics, 8*(2), 127–137.

Ingram, R. E., & Ritter, J. (2000). Vulnerability to depression: Cognitive reactivity and parental bonding in high-risk individuals. *Journal of Abnormal Psychology, 109*(4), 588–596.

Insel, T. R. (2010). The challenge of translation in social neuroscience: A review of oxytocin, vasopressin, and affiliative behavior. *Neuron, 65*(6), 768–779.

Insel, T. R. (2014). The NIMH research domain criteria (RDoC) project: Precision medicine for psychiatry. *American Journal of Psychiatry, 171*(4), 395–397.

Insel, T. R., Cuthbert, B., Garvey, M., Heinssen, R., Pine, D. S., Quinn, K., . . . Wang, P. (2010). Research domain criteria (RDoC): Toward a new classification framework for research on mental disorders. *American Journal of Psychiatry, 167*(7), 748–751.

Insel, T. R., Scanlan, J., Champoux, M., & Suomi, S. J. (1988). Rearing paradigm in a nonhuman primate affects response to !b-CCE challenge. *Psychopharmacology, 96*(1), 81–86.

Ioannou, K., & Fox, J. R. E. (2009). Perception of threat from emotions and its role in poor emotional expression within eating pathology. *Clinical Psychology and Psychotherapy, 16*(4), 336–347.

Ito, M., Horikoshi, M., Kato, N., Oe, Y., Fujisato, H., Nakajima, S., . . . Ono, Y. (2016). Transdiagnostic and transcultural: Pilot study of unified protocol for depressive and anxiety disorders in Japan. *Behavior Therapy, 47*(3), 416–430.

Iverson, K. M., Follette, V. M., Pistorello, J., & Fruzzetti, A. E. (2012). An investigation of experiential avoidance, emotion dysregulation, and distress tolerance in young adult outpatients with borderline personality disorder symptoms. *Personality Disorders, 3*(4), 415–422.

Izard, C. E. (1971). *The face of emotion.* East Norwalk, CT: Appleton-Century-Crofts.

Jacobs, T. L., Shaver, P. R., Epel, E. S., Zanesco, A. P., Aichele, S. R., Bridwell, D. A., . . . Saron, C. D. (2013). Self-reported mindfulness and cortisol during a Shamatha meditation retreat. *Health Psychology, 32*(10), 1104–1109.

Jacobson, N. S., Martell, C. R., & Dimidjian, S. (2001). Behavioral activation treatment for depression. *Clinical Psychology: Science and Practice, 8*(3), 255–270.

Jang, K. L., McCrae, R. R., Angleitner, A., Riemann, R., & Livesley, W. J. (1998).

Heritability of facet-level traits in a cross-cultural twin sample: Support for a hierarchical model of personality. *Journal of Personality and Social Psychology, 74*(6), 1556–1565.

Janiri, D., Moser, D. A., Doucet, G. E., Luber, M. J., Rasgon, A., Lee, W. H., . . . Frangou, S. (2020). Shared neural phenotypes for mood and anxiety disorders: A meta-analysis of 226 task-related functional imaging studies. *JAMA Psychiatry, 77*(2), 172–179.

Jezova, D., Makatsori, A., Duncko, R., Moncek, F., & Jakubek, M. (2004). High trait anxiety in healthy subjects is associated with low neuroendocrine activity during psychosocial stress. *Progress in Neuro-Psychopharmacology and Biological Psychiatry, 28*(8), 1331–1336.

Jimenez, S. S., Niles, B. L., & Park, C. L. (2010). A mindfulness model of affect regulation and depressive symptoms: Positive emotions, mood regulation expectancies, and self-acceptance as regulatory mechanisms. *Personality and Individual Differences, 49*(6), 645–650.

Johari-Fard, R., & Ghafourpour, R. (2015). The effectiveness of unified treatment approach on quality of life and symptoms of patients with irritable bowel syndrome referred to gastrointestinal clinics. *International Journal of Body, Mind and Culture, 2*(2), 85–94.

John, O. P. (1990). The "Big Five" factor taxonomy: Dimensions of personality in the natural language and in questionnaires. In L. A. Pervin (Ed.), *Handbook of personality: Theory and research* (pp. 66–100). New York: Guilford Press.

John, O. P., Naumann, L. P., & Soto, C. J. (2008). Paradigm shift to the integrative big five trait taxonomy: History, measurement, and conceptual issues. In O. P. John, R. W. Robins, & L. A. Pervin (Eds.), *Handbook of personality: Theory and research* (3rd ed., pp. 114–158). New York: Guilford Press.

Johnson, S. L., & Fulford, D. (2009). Preventing mania: A preliminary examination of the GOALS program. *Behavior Therapy, 40*(2), 103–113.

Johnston, J. C. (1927). *Biography: The literature of personality.* New York: Century.

Jylhä, P., & Isometsä, E. (2006). The relationship of neuroticism and extraversion to symptoms of anxiety and depression in the general population. *Depression and Anxiety, 23*(5), 281–289.

Kabat-Zinn, J. (1982). An outpatient program in behavioral medicine for chronic pain patients based on the practice of mindfulness meditation: Theoretical considerations and preliminary results. *General Hospital Psychiatry, 4*(1), 33–47.

Kabat-Zinn, J. (2003). Mindfulness-based interventions in context: Past, present, and future. *Clinical Psychology: Science and Practice, 10*(2), 144–156.

Kaess, M., Whittle, S., O'Brien-Simpson, L., Allen, N. B., & Simmons, J. G. (2018). Childhood maltreatment, pituitary volume and adolescent hypothalamic–pituitary–adrenal axis: Evidence for a maltreatment-related attenuation. *Psychoneuroendocrinology, 98*, 39–45.

Kagan, J. (1989). Temperamental contributions to social behavior. *American Psychologist, 44*(4), 668–674.

Kagan, J. (1994). *Galen's prophecy: Temperament in human nature.* New York: Basic Books.

Kagan, J., Reznick, J. S., & Snidman, N. (1988). Biological bases of childhood shyness. *Science, 240*(4849), 167–171.

Kagan, J., & Snidman, N. (1991). Infant predictors of inhibited and uninhibited profiles. *Psychological Science, 2*(1), 40–44.

Kant, I. (1974). *Anthropology from a pragmatic point of view* (M. J. Gregor, Trans.). Leiden, the Netherlands: Matinus Nijhoff.

Kao, K., Tuladhar, C. T., Meyer, J. S., & Tarullo, A. R. (2019). Emotion regulation moderates the association between parent and child hair cortisol concentrations. *Developmental Psychobiology, 61*(7), 1064–1078.

Karekla, M., Forsyth, J. P., & Kelly, M. M. (2004). Emotional avoidance and panicogenic responding to a biological challenge procedure. *Behavior Therapy, 35*(4), 725–746.

Kasch, K. L., Rottenberg, J., Arnow, B. A., & Gotlib, I. H. (2002). Behavioral activation and inhibition systems and the severity and course of depression. *Journal of Abnormal Psychology, 111*(4), 589–597.

Kawa, S., & Giordano, J. (2012). A brief historicity of the *Diagnostic and Statistical Manual of Mental Disorders:* Issues and implications for the future of psychiatric canon and practice. *Philosophy, Ethics, and Humanities in Medicine, 7*(1), 2.

Keightley, M. L., Seminowicz, D. A., Bagby, R. M., Costa, P. T., Fossati, P., & Mayberg, H. S. (2003). Personality influences limbic-cortical interactions during sad mood induction. *NeuroImage, 4*(20), 2031–2039.

Kenardy, J., Fried, L., Kraemer, H. C., & Taylor, C. B. (1992). Psychological precursors of panic attacks. *British Journal of Psychiatry, 160*(5), 668–673.

Kenardy, J., & Taylor, C. B. (1999). Expected versus unexpected panic attacks: A naturalistic prospective study. *Journal of Anxiety Disorders, 13*(4), 435–445.

Kendler, K. S., Gatz, M., Gardner, C. O., & Pedersen, N. L. (2006). Personality and major depression: A Swedish longitudinal, population-based twin study. *Archives of General Psychiatry, 63*(10), 1113–1120.

Kendler, K. S., & Myers, J. (2010). The genetic and environmental relationship between major depression and the five-factor model of personality. *Psychological Medicine, 40*(5), 801–806.

Kendler, K. S., Neale, M. C., Kessler, R. C., Heath, A. C., & Eaves, L. J. (1993). A longitudinal twin study of personality and major depression in women. *Archives of General Psychiatry, 50*(11), 853–862.

Kendler, K. S., Prescott, C. A., Myers, J., & Neale, M. C. (2003). The structure of genetic and environmental risk factors for common psychiatric and substance use disorders in men and women. *Archives of General Psychiatry, 60*(9), 929–937.

Keng, S.-L., Tan, E. L. Y., Eisenlohr-Moul, T. A., & Smoski, M. J. (2017). Effects of mindfulness, reappraisal, and suppression on sad mood and cognitive resources. *Behaviour Research and Therapy, 91*, 33–42.

Kennedy, S. J., Rapee, R. M., & Edwards, S. L. (2009). A selective intervention program for inhibited preschool-aged children of parents with an anxiety disorder: Effects on current anxiety disorders and temperament. *Journal of the American Academy of Child and Adolescent Psychiatry, 48*(6), 602–609.

Keough, M. E., Riccardi, C. J., Timpano, K. R., Mitchell, M. A., & Schmidt, N. B. (2010). Anxiety symptomatology: The association with distress tolerance and anxiety sensitivity. *Behavior Therapy, 41*(4), 567–574.

Kernberg, O. F. (1975). *Borderline conditions and pathological narcissism.* New York: Jason Aronson.

Kernberg, O. F. (1984). *Severe personality disorders: Psychotherapeutic strategies.* New Haven, CT: Yale University Press.

Kessler, R. C., Berglund, P., Demler, O., Jin, R., Koretz, D., Merikangas, K. R., . . . Wang, P. S. (2003). The epidemiology of major depressive disorder: Results from the National Comorbidity Survey Replication (NCS-R). *Journal of the American Medical Association, 289*(23), 3095–3105.

Kessler, R. C., Chiu, W. T., Demler, O., & Walters, E. E. (2005). Prevalence, severity, and comorbidity of twelve-month DSM-IV disorders in the National Comorbidity Survey Replication (NCS-R). *Archives of General Psychiatry, 62*(6), 617–627.

Kessler, R. C., Cox, B. J., Green, J. G., Ormel, J., McLaughlin, K. A., Merikangas, K. R., . . . Zaslavsky, A. M. (2011). The effects of latent variables in the development of comorbidity among common mental disorders. *Depression and Anxiety, 28*(1), 29–39.

Kessler, R. C., Gruber, M., Hettema, J. M., Hwang, I., Sampson, N., & Yonkers, K. A.

(2008). Co-morbid major depression and generalized anxiety disorders in the National Comorbidity Survey follow-up. *Psychological Medicine, 38*(3), 365–374.

Kessler, R. C., Nelson, C. B., McGonagle, K. A., Liu, J., Swartz, M., & Blazer, D. G. (1996). Comorbidity of DSM-III-R major depressive disorder in the general population: Results from the U.S. National Comorbidity Survey. *British Journal of Psychiatry, 30*(Suppl.), 17–30.

Kessler, R. C., Stang, P. E., Wittchen, H. U., Ustun, T. B., Roy-Burne, P. P., & Walters, E. E. (1998). Lifetime panic–depression comorbidity in the National Comorbidity Survey. *Archives of General Psychiatry, 55*(9), 801–808.

Khakpoor, S., Baytmar, J. M., & Saed, O. (2019). Reductions in transdiagnostic factors as the potential mechanisms of change in treatment outcomes in the Unified Protocol: A randomized clinical trial. *Research in Psychotherapy: Psychopathology, Process and Outcome, 22*(3), 379.

Khalsa, S. S., & Feinstein, J. S. (2018). The somatic error hypothesis of anxiety. In M. Tsakiris & H. De Preester (Eds.), *The interoceptive mind: From homeostasis to awareness* (pp. 144–164). New York: Oxford University Press.

Khan, A. A., Jacobson, K. C., Gardner, C. O., Prescott, C. A., & Kendler, K. S. (2005). Personality and comorbidity of common psychiatric disorders. *British Journal of Psychiatry, 186,* 190–196.

Kheirbek, M. A., Klemenhagen, K. C., Sahay, A., & Hen, R. (2012). Neurogenesis and generalization: A new approach to stratify and treat anxiety disorders. *Nature Neuroscience, 15*(12), 1613–1620.

Kim, B., Lee, S.-H., Kim, Y. W., Choi, T. K., Yook, K., Suh, S. Y., . . . Yook, K.-H. (2010). Effectiveness of a mindfulness-based cognitive therapy program as an adjunct to pharmacotherapy in patients with panic disorder. *Journal of Anxiety Disorders, 24*(6), 590–595.

Kim, Y.-R., Blashfield, R., Tyrer, P., Hwang, S.-T., & Lee, H.-S. (2014). Field trial of a putative research algorithm for diagnosing ICD-11 personality disorders in psychiatric patients: 1. Severity of personality disturbance. *Personality and Mental Health, 8*(1), 67–78.

Kim, Y.-R., Tyrer, P., Lee, H.-S., Kim, S.-G., Hwang, S.-T., Lee, G. Y., & Mulder, R. (2015). Preliminary field trial of a putative research algorithm for diagnosing ICD-11 personality disorders in psychiatric patients: 2. Proposed trait domains. *Personality and Mental Health, 9*(4), 298–307.

King, J. E., & Figueredo, A. J. (1997). The five-factor model plus dominance in chimpanzee personality. *Journal of Research in Personality, 31*(2), 257–271.

Knutson, B., Wolkowitz, O. M., Cole, S. W., Chan, T., Moore, E. A., Johnson, R. C., . . . Reus, V. I. (1998). Selective alteration of personality and social behavior by serotonergic intervention. *American Journal of Psychiatry, 155*(3), 373–379.

Koenigsberg, H. W., Harvey, P. D., Mitropoulou, V., New, A. S., Goodman, M., Silverman, J., . . . Siever, L. J. (2001). Are the interpersonal and identity disturbances in the borderline personality disorder criteria linked to the traits of affective instability and impulsivity? *Journal of Personality Disorders, 15*(4), 358–370.

Koenigsberg, H. W., Harvey, P. D., Mitropoulou, V., Schmeidler, J., New, A. S., Goodman, M., . . . Siever, L. J. (2002). Characterizing affective instability in borderline personality disorder. *American Journal of Psychiatry, 159*(5), 784–788.

Kolar, D. R., Hammerle, F., Jenetzky, E., Huss, M., & Bürger, A. (2016). Aversive tension in female adolescents with anorexia nervosa: A controlled ecological momentary assessment using smartphones. *BMC Psychiatry, 16,* 1–11.

Koolhaas, J. M., Bartolomucci, A., Buwalda, B., de Boer, S. F., Flügge, G., Korte, S. M., . . . Fuchs, E. (2011). Stress revisited: A critical evaluation of the stress concept. *Neuroscience and Biobehavioral Reviews, 35*(5), 1291–1301.

Kornør, H., & Nordvik, H. (2007). Five-factor model personality traits in opioid dependence. *BMC Psychiatry, 7,* 37.

Kotov, R., Gamez, W., Schmidt, F., & Watson, D. (2010). Linking "big" personality traits to anxiety, depressive, and substance use disorders: A meta-analysis. *Psychological Bulletin, 136*(5), 768–821.

Kotov, R., Krueger, R. F., Watson, D., Achenbach, T. M., Althoff, R. R., Bagby, R. M., . . . Zimmerman, M. (2017). The hierarchical taxonomy of psychopathology (HiTOP): A dimensional alternative to traditional nosologies. *Journal of Abnormal Psychology, 126*(4), 454–477.

Kotov, R., Ruggero, C. J., Krueger, R. F., Watson, D., Yuan, Q., & Zimmerman, M. (2011). New dimensions in the quantitative classification of mental illness. *Archives of General Psychiatry, 68*(10), 1003–1011.

Kotov, R., Watson, D., Robles, J. P., & Schmidt, N. B. (2007). Personality traits and anxiety symptoms: The multilevel trait predictor model. *Behaviour Research and Therapy, 45*(7), 1485–1503.

Kovacs, M., & Devlin, B. (1998). Internalizing disorders in childhood. *Journal of Child Psychology and Psychiatry and Allied Disciplines, 39*(1), 47–63.

Kovacs, M., Gatsonis, C., Paulauskas, S. L., & Richards, C. (1989). Depressive disorders in childhood: IV. A longitudinal study of comorbidity with and risk for anxiety disorders. *Archives of General Psychiatry, 46*(9), 776–782.

Krasner, M. S., Epstein, R. M., Beckman, H., Suchman, A. L., Chapman, B., Mooney, C. J., & Quill, T. E. (2009). Association of an educational program in mindful communication with burnout, empathy, and attitudes among primary care physicians. *Journal of the American Medical Association, 302*(12), 1284–1293.

Kring, A. M., Persons, J. B., & Thomas, C. (2007). Changes in affect during treatment for depression and anxiety. *Behaviour Research and Therapy, 45*(8), 1753–1764.

Kristeller, J. L., & Hallett, C. B. (1999). An exploratory study of a meditation-based intervention for binge eating disorder. *Journal of Health Psychology, 4*(3), 357–363.

Kruedelbach, N., McCormick, R. A., Schulz, S. C., & Grueneich, R. (1993). Impulsivity, coping styles, and triggers for craving in substance abusers with borderline personality disorder. *Journal of Personality Disorders, 7*(3), 214–222.

Krueger, R. F. (1999). The structure of common mental disorders. *Archives of General Psychiatry, 56*(10), 921–926.

Krueger, R. F., Derringer, J., Markon, K. E., Watson, D., & Skodol, A. E. (2012). Initial construction of a maladaptive personality trait model and inventory for DSM-5. *Psychological Medicine, 42*(9), 1879–1890.

Krueger, R. F., & Eaton, N. R. (2015). Transdiagnostic factors of mental disorders. *World Psychiatry, 14*(1), 27–29.

Krueger, R. F., Hopwood, C. J., Wright, A. G. C., & Markon, K. E. (2014). DSM-5 and the path toward empirically based and clinically useful conceptualization of personality and psychopathology. *Clinical Psychology: Science and Practice, 21*(3), 245–261.

Krueger, R. F., & Johnson, W. (2008). Behavioral genetics and personality: A new look at the integration of nature and nurture. In O. P. John, R. W. Robins, & L. A. Pervin (Eds.), *Handbook of personality: Theory and research* (2nd ed., pp. 287–310). New York: Guilford Press.

Krueger, R. F., & Markon, K. E. (2006a). Reinterpreting comorbidity: A model-based approach to understanding and classifying psychopathology. *Annual Review of Clinical Psychology, 2*, 111–133.

Krueger, R. F., & Markon, K. E. (2006b). Understanding psychopathology: Melding behavior genetics, personality, and quantitative psychology to develop an empirically based model. *Current Directions in Psychological Science, 15*(3), 113–117.

Krueger, R. F., & Markon, K. E. (2011). A dimensional-spectrum model of psychopathology: Progress and opportunities. *Archives of General Psychiatry, 68*(1), 10–11.

Krueger, R. F., Markon, K. E., Patrick, C. J., Benning, S. D., & Kramer, M. D. (2007a). Linking antisocial behavior, substance use, and personality: An integrative quantitative model of the adult externalizing spectrum. *Journal of Abnormal Psychology, 116*(4), 645–666.

Krueger, R. F., Skodol, A. E., Livesley, W. J., Shrout, P. E., & Huang, Y. (2007b). Synthesizing dimensional and categorical approaches to personality disorders: Refining the research agenda for DSM-V Axis II. *International Journal of Methods in Psychiatric Research, 16*(S1), S65–S73.

Kulkarni, J. (2017). Complex PTSD—a better description for borderline personality disorder? *Australasian Psychiatry, 25*(4), 333–335.

Laceulle, O. M., Ormel, J., Aggen, S. H., Neale, M. C., & Kendler, K. S. (2013). Genetic and environmental influences on the longitudinal structure of neuroticism: A trait–state approach. *Psychological Science, 24*(9), 1780–1790.

Laceulle, O. M., Vollebergh, W. A. M., & Ormel, J. (2015). The structure of psychopathology in adolescence: Replication of a general psychopathology factor in the TRAILS Study. *Clinical Psychological Science, 3*(6), 850–860.

Ladd, C. O., Huot, R. L., Thrivikraman, K. V., Nemeroff, C. B., Meaney, M. J., & Plotsky, P. M. (2000). Long-term behavioral and neuroendocrine adaptations to adverse early experience. *Progress in Brain Research, 122*, 81–103.

Ladouceur, R., Dugas, M. J., Freeston, M. H., Léger, E., Gagnon, F., & Thibodeau, N. (2000). Efficacy of a cognitive–behavioral treatment for generalized anxiety disorder: Evaluation in a controlled clinical trial. *Journal of Consulting and Clinical Psychology, 68*(6), 957–964.

Ladouceur, R., Dugas, M. J., Freeston, M. H., Rhéaume, J., Blais, F., Boisvert, J.-M., . . . Thibodeau, N. (1999). Specificity of generalized anxiety disorder symptoms and processes. *Behavior Therapy, 30*(2), 191–207.

Lahey, B. B. (2009). Public health significance of neuroticism. *American Psychologist, 64*(4), 241–256.

Lahey, B. B., Krueger, R. F., Rathouz, P. J., Waldman, I. D., & Zald, D. H. (2017). A hierarchical causal taxonomy of psychopathology across the life span. *Psychological Bulletin, 143*(2), 142–186.

Lang, A. J., Kennedy, C. M., & Stein, M. B. (2002). Anxiety sensitivity and PTSD among female victims of intimate partner violence. *Depression and Anxiety, 16*(2), 77–83.

Lang, P. J. (1979). A bio-informational theory of emotional imagery. *Psychophysiology, 16*, 495–512.

Lang, P. J. (1985). The cognitive psychophysiology of emotion: Fear and anxiety. In A. H. Tuma & J. D. Maser, *Anxiety and the anxiety disorders* (pp. 131–170). Hillsdale, NJ: Erlbaum.

Lanius, R. A., Frewen, P. A., Vermetten, E., & Yehuda, R. (2010). Fear conditioning and early life vulnerabilities: Two distinct pathways of emotional dysregulation and brain dysfunction in PTSD. *European Journal of Psychotraumatology*. [Epub ahead of print]

Larstone, R. M., Jang, K. L., Livesley, W. J., Vernon, P. A., & Wolf, H. (2002). The relationship between Eysenck's P-E-N model of personality, the five-factor model of personality, and traits delineating personality dysfunction. *Personality and Individual Differences, 33*, 25–37.

Lawson, R., Emanuelli, F., Sines, J., & Waller, G. (2008). Emotional awareness and core beliefs among women with eating disorders. *European Eating Disorders Review, 16*(2), 155–159.

Leahey, T. M., Crowther, J. H., & Irwin, S. R. (2008). A cognitive-behavioral mindfulness group therapy intervention for the treatment of binge eating in bariatric surgery patients. *Cognitive and Behavioral Practice, 15*(4), 364–375.

LeDoux, J. (1996). *The emotional brain: The mysterious underpinnings of emotional life.* New York: Simon & Schuster.

LeDoux, J. E., Iwata, J., Cicchetti, P., & Reis, D. J. (1988). Different projections of the central amygdaloid nucleus mediate autonomic and behavioral correlates of conditioned fear. *Journal of Neuroscience, 8*(7), 2517–2529.

Lee, J. K., Orsillo, S. M., Roemer, L., & Allen, L. B. (2010). Distress and avoidance in generalized anxiety disorder: Exploring the relationships with intolerance of uncertainty and worry. *Cognitive Behaviour Therapy, 39*(2), 126–136.

Lee, S., Ma, Y. L., & Tsang, A. (2011). Psychometric properties of the Chinese 15-item Patient Health Questionnaire in the general population of Hong Kong. *Journal of Psychosomatic Research, 71*(2), 69–73.

Leen-Feldner, E. W., Blumenthal, H., Babson, K., Bunaciu, L., & Feldner, M. T. (2008). Parenting-related childhood learning history and panic vulnerability: A test using a laboratory-based biological challenge procedure. *Behaviour Research and Therapy, 46*(9), 1009–1016.

Leen-Feldner, E. W., Feldner, M. T., Bernstein, A., McCormick, J. T., & Zvolensky, M. J. (2005). Anxiety sensitivity and anxious responding to bodily sensations: A test among adolescents using a voluntary hyperventilation challenge. *Cognitive Therapy and Research, 29*(5), 593–609.

Lesch, K., Bengel, D., Heils, A., Sabol, S. Z., Greenberg, B. D., Petri, S., . . . Murphy, D. L. (1996). Association of anxiety-related traits with a polymorphism in the serotonin transporter gene regulatory region. *Science, 274*(5292), 1527–1531.

Levine, D., Marziali, E., & Hood, J. (1997). Emotion processing in borderline personality disorders. *Journal of Nervous and Mental Disease, 185*(4), 240–246.

Levine, S. (2005). Developmental determinants of sensitivity and resistance to stress. *Psychoneuroendocrinology, 30*(10), 939–946.

Leyro, T. M., Zvolensky, M. J., & Bernstein, A. (2010). Distress tolerance and psychopathological symptoms and disorders: A review of the empirical literature among adults. *Psychological Bulletin, 136*(4), 576–600.

Liddell, H. S. (1949). Adaptation on the threshold of intelligence. In J. Romano (Ed.), *Adaptation* (pp. 53–76). Ithaca, NY: Cornell University Press.

Lieb, R., Wittchen, H. U., Höfler, M., Fuetsch, M., Stein, M. B., & Merikangas, K. R. (2000). Parental psychopathology, parenting styles, and the risk of social phobia in offspring: A prospective-longitudinal community study. *Archives of General Psychiatry, 57*(9), 859–866.

Liebowitz, M. R. (1987). Social phobia. *Modern Problems of Pharmacopsychiatry, 22,* 141–173.

Lilienfeld, S. (1996). Anxiety sensitivity is not distinct from trait anxiety. In R. Rapee (Ed.), *Current controversies in the anxiety disorders* (pp. 228–244). New York: Guilford Press.

Lilienfeld, S. O. (2014). The Research Domain Criteria (RDoC): An analysis of methodological and conceptual challenges. *Behaviour Research and Therapy, 62,* 129–139.

Lilienfeld, S. O. (2020). Microaggression research and application: Clarifications, corrections, and common ground. *Perspectives on Psychological Science, 15*(1), 27–37.

Lilienfeld, S. O., & Penna, S. (2001). Anxiety sensitivity: Relations to psychopathy, DSM-IV personality disorder features, and personality traits. *Journal of Anxiety Disorders, 15*(5), 367–393.

Lilienfeld, S. O., & Treadway, M. T. (2016). Clashing diagnostic approaches: DSM-ICD versus RDoC. *Annual Review of Clinical Psychology, 12*(1), 435–463.

Lilienfeld, S. O., Turner, S. M., & Jacob, R. G. (1993). Anxiety sensitivity: An examination of theoretical and methodological issues. *Advances in Behaviour Research and Therapy, 15*(2), 147–183.

Limburg, K., Watson, H. J., Hagger, M. S., & Egan, S. J. (2017). The relationship between perfectionism and psychopathology: A meta-analysis. *Journal of Clinical Psychology, 73*(10), 1301–1326.

Lindgren, K. P., Kaysen, D., Werntz, A. J., Gasser, M. L., & Teachman, B. A. (2013). Wounds that can't be seen: Implicit trauma associations predict posttraumatic stress disorder symptoms. *Journal of Behavior Therapy and Experimental Psychiatry, 44*(4), 368–375.

Linehan, M. (1993). *Cognitive-behavioral treatment of borderline personality disorder.* New York: Guilford Press.

Linehan, M. M. (2015). *DBT Skills Training Manual* (2nd ed.). New York: Guilford Press.

Linehan, M., & Dexter-Mazza, M. (2008). Dialectical behavior therapy for borderline personality disorder. In D. H. Barlow (Ed.), *Clinical handbook of psychological disorders: A step-by-step treatment manual* (4th ed., pp. 365–420). New York: Guilford Press.

Ling, Y. M. (2018). *A randomized controlled trial with a nine-month follow-up of a transdiagnostic cognitive behavioral therapy (group) for Chinese adults with common mental disorders.* Unpublished doctoral dissertation, Chinese University of Hong Kong.

Livesley, W. J. (2003). *Practical management of personality disorder.* New York: Guilford Press.

Llera, S. J., & Newman, M. G. (2010). Effects of worry on physiological and subjective reactivity to emotional stimuli in generalized anxiety disorder and nonanxious control participants. *Emotion, 10*(5), 640–650.

Llera, S. J., & Newman, M. G. (2014). Rethinking the role of worry in generalized anxiety disorder: Evidence supporting a model of emotional contrast avoidance. *Behavior Therapy, 45*(3), 283–299.

Loehlin, J. C., McCrae, R. R., & Costa, P. T. (1998). Heritabilities of common and measure-specific components of the Big Five personality factors. *Journal of Research in Personality, 32,* 431–453.

Lofti, A., Bakhtiyari, M., Asgharnezhad-Farid, A., & Amini, M. (2014). Comparison of the effect of transdiagnostic therapy and cognitive-behavior therapy on patients with emotional disorders: A randomized clinical trial. *Zahedan Journal of Research in Medical Sciences, 16*(1), 15–18.

Lommen, M. J. J., Engelhard, I. M., & van den Hout, M. A. (2010). Neuroticism and avoidance of ambiguous stimuli: Better safe than sorry? *Personality and Individual Differences, 49*(8), 1001–1006.

Lonsdorf, T. B., Golkar, A., Lindstöm, K. M., Fransson, P., Schalling, M., Öhman, A., & Ingvar, M. (2011). 5-HTTLPR and COMTval158met genotype gate amygdala reactivity and habituation. *Biological Psychology, 87*(1), 106–112.

Lopez, M. E., Stoddard, J. A., Noorollah, A., Zerbi, G., Payne, L. A., Hitchcock, C. A., . . . Ray, D. B. (2015). Examining the efficacy of the Unified Protocol for Transdiagnostic Treatment of Emotional Disorders in the treatment of individuals with borderline personality disorder. *Cognitive and Behavioral Practice, 22*(4), 522–533.

Lopez, M. E., Thorp, S. R., Dekker, M., Noorollah, A., Zerbi, G., Payne, L. A., . . . Stoddard, J. A. (2019). The Unified Protocol for anxiety and depression with comorbid borderline personality disorder: A single case design clinical series. *Cognitive Behaviour Therapist, 12,* E37.

Lorberbaum, J. P., Kose, S., Johnson, M. R., Arana, G. W., Sullivan, L. K., Hamner, M. B., . . . George, M. S. (2004). Neural correlates of speech anticipatory anxiety in generalized social phobia. *NeuroReport, 15*(18), 2701–2705.

Lothmann, C., Holmes, E. A., Chan, S. W., & Lau, J. Y. (2011). Cognitive bias modification training in adolescents: Effects on interpretation biases and mood. *Journal of Child Psychology and Psychiatry, and Allied Disciplines, 52*(1), 24–32.

Lowe, J. R., Edmundson, M., & Widiger, T. A. (2009). Assessment of dependency, agreeableness, and their relationship. *Psychological Assessment, 21*(4), 543–553.

Luten, A. G., Ralph, J. A., & Mineka, S. (1997). Pessimistic attributional style: Is it specific to depression versus anxiety versus negative affect? *Behaviour Research and Therapy, 35*(8), 703–719.

Lykins, E. L. B., & Baer, R. A. (2009). Psychological functioning in a sample of long-term practitioners of mindfulness meditation. *Journal of Cognitive Psychotherapy, 23*(3), 226–241.

Lynch, T. R., Trost, W. T., Salsman, N., & Linehan, M. M. (2007). Dialectical behavior therapy for borderline personality disorder. *Annual Review of Clinical Psychology, 3*(1), 181–205.

Lyubomirsky, S., & Nolen-Hoeksema, S. (1995). Effects of self-focused rumination on negative thinking and interpersonal problem solving. *Journal of Personality and Social Psychology, 69*(1), 176–190.

Lyubomirsky, S., Sheldon, K. M., & Schkade, D. (2005). Pursuing happiness: The architecture of sustainable change. *Review of General Psychology, 9*(2), 111–131.

Lyubomirsky, S., Tucker, K. L., Caldwell, N. D., & Berg, K. (1999). Why ruminators are poor problem solvers: Clues from the phenomenology of dysphoric rumination. *Journal of Personality and Social Psychology, 77*(5), 1041–1060.

Maack, D. J., Tull, M. T., & Gratz, K. L. (2012). Experiential avoidance mediates the association between behavioral inhibition and posttraumatic stress disorder. *Cognitive Therapy and Research, 36*(4), 407–416.

Macdonald, A. W., & Krueger, R. F. (2013). Mapping the country within: A special section on reconceptualizing the classification of mental disorders. *Journal of Abnormal Psychology, 122*(3), 891–893.

MacLeod, C., & Mathews, A. (2012). Cognitive bias modification approaches to anxiety. *Annual Review of Clinical Psychology, 8*, 189–217.

MacPherson, L., Magidson, J. F., Reynolds, E. K., Kahler, C. W., & Lejuez, C. W. (2010). Changes in sensation seeking and risk-taking propensity predict increases in alcohol use among early adolescents. *Alcoholism, Clinical and Experimental Research, 34*(8), 1400–1408.

Magariños, A. M., & McEwen, B. S. (1995). Stress-induced atrophy of apical dendrites of hippocampal CA3c neurons: Involvement of glucocorticoid secretion and excitatory amino acid receptors. *Neuroscience, 69*(1), 89–98.

Magidson, J. F., Roberts, B., Collado-Rodriguez, A., & Lejuez, C. W. (2014). Theory-driven intervention for changing personality: Expectancy value theory, behavioral activation, and conscientiousness. *Developmental Psychology, 50*(5), 1442–1450.

Mahaffey, B. L., Wheaton, M. G., Fabricant, L. E., Berman, N. C., & Abramowitz, J. S. (2013). The contribution of experiential avoidance and social cognitions in the prediction of social anxiety. *Behavioural and Cognitive Psychotherapy, 41*(1), 52–65.

Maier, S. F., & Watkins, L. R. (1998). Cytokines for psychologists: Implications of bidirectional immune-to-brain communication for understanding behavior, mood, and cognition. *Psychological Review, 105*(1), 83–107.

Maller, R. G., & Reiss, S. (1992). Anxiety sensitivity in 1984 and panic attacks in 1987. *Journal of Anxiety Disorders, 6*(3), 241–247.

Malouff, J. M., Thorsteinsson, E. B., Rooke, S. E., & Schutte, N. S. (2007). Alcohol involvement and the Five-Factor Model of personality: A meta-analysis. *Journal of Drug Education, 37*(3), 277–294.

Malouff, J. M., Thorsteinsson, E. B., & Schutte, N. S. (2005). The relationship between the Five-Factor Model of personality and symptoms of clinical disorders: A meta-analysis. *Journal of Psychopathology and Behavioral Assessment, 27*(2), 101–114.

Malouff, J. M., Thorsteinsson, E. B., & Schutte, N. S. (2006). The Five-Factor Model of personality and smoking: A meta-analysis. *Journal of Drug Education, 36*(1), 47–58.

Manos, R. C., Kanter, J. W., & Busch, A. M. (2010). A critical review of assessment strategies to measure the behavioral activation model of depression. *Clinical Psychology Review, 30*(5), 547–561.

Markey, P. M., & Markey, C. N. (2009). A brief assessment of the interpersonal circumplex: The IPIP–IPC. *Assessment, 16*(4), 352–361.

Markon, K. E., Quilty, L. C., Bagby, R. M., & Krueger, R. F. (2013). The development and psychometric properties of an informant-report form of the personality inventory for DSM-5 (PID-5). *Assessment, 20*(3), 370–383.

Marnoch, S. E. (2014). *A pilot randomized controlled trial examining the feasibility, acceptability and potential efficacy of transdiagnostic CBT for depression and anxiety in older people.* Unpublished doctoral dissertation, University of London, King's College.

Marshall-Berenz, E. C., Vujanovic, A. A., Bonn-Miller, M. O., Bernstein, A., & Zvolensky, M. J. (2010). Multimethod study of distress tolerance and PTSD symptom severity in a trauma-exposed community sample. *Journal of Traumatic Stress, 23*(5), 623–630.

Maser, J. D., Norman, S. B., Zisook, S., Everall, I. P., Stein, M. B., Schettler, P. J., & Judd, L. L. (2009). Psychiatric nosology is ready for a paradigm shift in DSM-V. *Clinical Psychology: Science and Practice, 16*(1), 24–40.

Masserman, J. H. (1943). *Behavior and neurosis: An experimental psychoanalytic approach to psychobiologic principles.* Chicago: University of Chicago Press.

Masters, W. H., & Johnson, V. E. (1966). *Human sexual response.* London: Churchill.

Mata, J., Thompson, R. J., Jaeggi, S. M., Buschkuehl, M., Jonides, J., & Gotlib, I. H. (2012). Walk on the bright side: Physical activity and affect in major depressive disorder. *Journal of Abnormal Psychology, 121*(2), 297–308.

Mathews, A., & Mackintosh, B. (2000). Induced emotional interpretation bias and anxiety. *Journal of Abnormal Psychology, 109*(4), 602–615.

Mathews, A., & MacLeod, C. (2005). Cognitive vulnerability to emotional disorders. *Annual Review of Clinical Psychology, 1*, 167–195.

Matthews, G., & Gilliland, K. (1999). The personality theories of H. J. Eysenck and J. A. Gray: A comparative review. *Personality and Individual Differences, 26*(4), 583–626.

Mayberg, H. S., Liotti, M., Brannan, S. K., McGinnis, S., Mahurin, R. K., Jerabek, P. A., . . . Fox, P. T. (1999). Reciprocal limbic-cortical function and negative mood: Converging PET findings in depression and normal sadness. *American Journal of Psychiatry, 156*(5), 675–682.

Mayes, R., & Horwitz, A. V. (2005). DSM-III and the revolution in the classification of mental illness. *Journal of the History of the Behavioral Sciences, 41*(3), 249–267.

McCabe, C., Mishor, Z., Cowen, P. J., & Harmer, C. J. (2010). Diminished neural processing of aversive and rewarding stimuli during selective serotonin reuptake inhibitor treatment. *Biological Psychiatry, 67*(5), 439–445.

McCabe, G. A., & Widiger, T. A. (2020). A comprehensive comparison of the ICD-11 and DSM-5 Section III personality disorder models. *Psychological Assessment, 32*(1), 72–84.

McCaffery, J. M., Frasure-Smith, N., Dubé, M.-P., Théroux, P., Rouleau, G. A., Duan, Q., & Lespérance, F. (2006). Common genetic vulnerability to depressive symptoms and coronary artery disease: A review and development of candidate genes related to inflammation and serotonin. *Psychosomatic Medicine, 68*(2), 187–200.

McCauley, E., Mitchell, J. R., Burke, P. M., & Moss, S. J. (1988). Cognitive attributes of depression in children and adolescents. *Journal of Consulting and Clinical Psychology, 56*(6), 903–908.

McCracken, L. M., & Keogh, E. (2009). Acceptance, mindfulness, and values-based action may counteract fear and avoidance of emotions in chronic pain: An analysis of anxiety sensitivity. *Journal of Pain, 10*(4), 408–415.

McCrae, R. R., & Costa, P. T. (1985). Comparison of EPI and psychoticism scales with measures of the five-factor model of personality. *Personality and Individual Differences, 6*(5), 587–597.

McCrae, R. R., & Costa, P. T. (1987). Validation of the five-factor model of personality across instruments and observers. *Journal of Personality and Social Psychology, 52*(1), 81–90.

McCrae, R. R., & Costa, P. T. (2003). *Personality in adulthood: A five-factor theory perspective*. New York: Guilford Press.

McCrae, R. R., Costa, P. T., Jr., & Martin, T. A. (2005). The NEO-PI-3: A more readable revised NEO personality inventory. *Journal of Personality Assessment, 84*(3), 261–270.

McEvoy, P. M., & Mahoney, A. E. J. (2012). To be sure, to be sure: Intolerance of uncertainty mediates symptoms of various anxiety disorders and depression. *Behavior Therapy, 43*(3), 533–545.

McHugh, R. K., & Barlow, D. H. (2010). The dissemination and implementation of evidence-based psychological treatments: A review of current efforts. *American Psychologist, 65*(2), 73–84.

McHugh, R. K., Murray, H. W., & Barlow, D. H. (2009). Balancing fidelity and adaptation in the dissemination of empirically-supported treatments: The promise of transdiagnostic interventions. *Behaviour Research and Therapy, 47*(11), 946–953.

McLaughlin, K. A., Mennin, D. S., & Farach, F. J. (2007). The contributory role of worry in emotion generation and dysregulation in generalized anxiety disorder. *Behaviour Research and Therapy, 45*(8), 1735–1752.

McLeod, B. D., Wood, J. J., & Weisz, J. R. (2007). Examining the association between parenting and childhood anxiety: A meta-analysis. *Clinical Psychology Review, 27*(2), 155–172.

McNally, R. J. (1996). Methodological controversies in the treatment of panic disorder. *Journal of Consulting and Clinical Psychology, 64*(1), 88–91.

McNally, R. J., & Steketee, G. S. (1985). The etiology and maintenance of severe animal phobias. *Behaviour Research and Therapy, 23*(4), 431–435.

McWilliams, L. A., Stewart, S. H., & MacPherson, P. S. (2000). Does the social concerns component of the anxiety sensitivity index belong to the domain of anxiety sensitivity or the domain of negative evaluation sensitivity? *Behaviour Research and Therapy, 38*(10), 985–992.

Meehl, P. (1962). Schizotaxia, schizotypy, schizophrenia. *American Psychologist, 17*(12), 827–838.

Mennin, D. S., Heimberg, R. G., Turk, C. L., & Fresco, D. M. (2005). Preliminary evidence for an emotion dysregulation model of generalized anxiety disorder. *Behaviour Research and Therapy, 43*(10), 1281–1310.

Merikangas, K. R., Zhang, H., Avenevoli, S., Acharyya, S., Neuenschwander, M., Angst, J., & Zurich Cohort Study. (2003). Longitudinal trajectories of depression and anxiety in a prospective community study: The Zurich Cohort Study. *Archives of General Psychiatry, 60*(10), 993–1000.

Merino, H., Senra, C., & Ferreiro, F. (2016). Are worry and rumination specific pathways linking neuroticism and symptoms of anxiety and depression in patients with generalized anxiety disorder, major depressive disorder and mixed anxiety–depressive disorder? *PLOS ONE, 11*, e0156169.

Merz, E. C., Desai, P. M., Maskus, E. A., Melvin, S. A., Rehman, R., Torres, S. D., . . . Noble, K. G. (2019). Socioeconomic disparities in chronic physiologic stress are associated with brain structure in children. *Biological Psychiatry, 16*(12), 921–929.

Meuret, A. E., Ritz, T., Wilhelm, F. H., & Roth, W. T. (2005). Voluntary hyperventilation in the treatment of panic disorder: Functions of hyperventilation, their implications for breathing training, and recommendations for standardization. *Clinical Psychology Review, 25*(3), 285–306.

Meuret, A. E., Wolitzky-Taylor, K. B., Twohig, M. P., & Craske, M. G. (2012). Coping skills and exposure therapy in panic disorder and agoraphobia: latest advances and future directions. *Behavior Therapy, 43*(2), 271–284.

Meyer, B., Johnson, S. L., & Winters, R. (2001). Responsiveness to threat and incentive in bipolar disorder: Relations of the BIS/BAS scales with symptoms. *Journal of Psychopathology and Behavioral Assessment, 23*(3), 133–143.

Milad, M. R., Wright, C. I., Orr, S. P., Pitman, R. K., Quirk, G. J., & Rauch, S. L. (2007). Recall of fear extinction in humans activates the ventromedial prefrontal cortex and hippocampus in concert. *Biological Psychiatry, 62*(5), 446–454.

Mill, J. (2011). Epigenetic effects on gene function and their role in mediating gene–environment interactions. In K. S. Kendler, S. Jaffee, & D. Romer (Eds.), *The dynamic genome and mental health: The role of genes and environment in youth development* (pp. 145–171). New York: Oxford University Press.

Miller, G. E., Chen, E., & Zhou, E. S. (2007). If it goes up, must it come down?: Chronic stress and the hypothalamic–pituitary–adrenocortical axis in humans. *Psychological Bulletin, 133*(1), 25–45.

Miller, J. D., Lynam, D. R., Hyatt, C. S., & Campbell, W. K. (2017). Controversies in narcissism. *Annual Review of Clinical Psychology, 13*(1), 291–315.

Miller, J. D., Lynam, D., & Leukefeld, C. (2003). Examining antisocial behavior through the lens of the five factor model of personality. *Aggressive Behavior, 29*(6), 497–514.

Millon, T., & Klerman, G. L. (1986). *Contemporary directions in psychopathology: Toward the DSM-IV.* New York: Guilford Press.

Mineka, S., Cook, M., & Miller, S. (1984). Fear conditioned with escapable and inescapable shock: Effects of a feedback stimulus. *Journal of Experimental Psychology: Animal Behavior Processes, 10*(3), 307–323.

Mineka, S., Davidson, M., Cook, M., & Keir, R. (1984). Observational conditioning of snake fear in rhesus monkeys. *Journal of Abnormal Psychology, 93*(4), 355–372.

Mineka, S., Gunnar, M., & Champoux, M. (1986). Control and early socioemotional development: Infant rhesus monkeys reared in controllable versus uncontrollable environments. *Child Development, 57*(5), 1241–1256.

Mineka, S., & Kihlstrom, J. F. (1978). Unpredictable and uncontrollable events: A new perspective on experimental neurosis. *Journal of Abnormal Psychology, 87*(2), 256–271.

Mineka, S., Watson, D., & Clark, L. A. (1998). Comorbidity of anxiety and unipolar mood disorders. *Annual Review of Psychology, 49*, 377–412.

Mischel, W., & Peake, P. (1982). Beyond déjà vu in the search for cross-situational consistency. *Psychological Review, 89*(6), 730–755.

Mitchell, S. A., & Aron, L. (Eds.). (1999). *Relational psychoanalysis: The emergence of a tradition.* Hillsdale, NJ: Analytic Press.

Moehler, E., Kagan, J., Oelkers-Ax, R., Brunner, R., Poustka, L., Haffner, J., & Resch, F. (2008). Infant predictors of behavioural inhibition. *British Journal of Developmental Psychology, 26*(1), 145–150.

Mohajerin, B., Bakhtiyar, M., Olesnycky, O. S., Dolatshahi, B., & Motabi, F. (2019). Application of a transdiagnostic treatment for emotional disorders to body dysmorphic disorder: A randomized controlled trial. *Journal of Affective Disorders, 245*, 637–644.

Mohammadi, F., Bakhtiari, M., Masjedi Arani, A., Dolatshahi, B., & Habibi, M. (2018). The applicability and efficacy of transdiagnostic cognitive behavior therapy on reducing signs and symptoms of borderline personality disorder with co-occurring emotional disorders: A pilot study. *Iranian Journal of Psychiatry and Behavioral Sciences, 12*(1), e9697.

Möhler, E., Parzer, P., Brunner, R., Wiebel, A., & Resch, F. (2006). Emotional stress in pregnancy predicts human infant reactivity. *Early Human Development, 82*(11), 731–737.

Mohsenabadi, H., Zanjani, Z., Shabani, M. J., & Arj, A. (2018). A randomized clinical trial of the Unified Protocol for transdiagnostic treatment of emotional and gastrointestinal symptoms in patients with irritable bowel syndrome: Evaluating efficacy and mechanism of change. *Journal of Psychosomatic Research, 113*, 8–15.

Montag, C., Basten, U., Stelzel, C., Fiebach, C. J., & Reuter, M. (2010). The BDNF Val-66Met polymorphism and anxiety: Support for animal knock-in studies from a genetic association study in humans. *Psychiatry Research, 179*(1), 86–90.

Moore, S. A., Zoellner, L. A., & Mollenholt, N. (2008). Are expressive suppression and cognitive reappraisal associated with stress-related symptoms? *Behaviour Research and Therapy, 46*(9), 993–1000.

Morey, L. C. (1991). *Personality assessment inventory: Professional manual*. Odessa, FL: Psychological Assessment Resources.

Morey, L. C., Skodol, A. E., & Oldham, J. M. (2014). Clinician judgments of clinical utility: A comparison of DSM-IV-TR personality disorders and the alternative model for DSM-5 personality disorders. *Journal of Abnormal Psychology, 123*(2), 398–405.

Mosca, O., Lauriola, M., & Carleton, R. N. (2016). Intolerance of uncertainty: A temporary experimental induction procedure. *PLOS ONE, 11*(6).

Mõttus, R., Johnson, W., & Deary, I. J. (2012). Personality traits in old age: Measurement and rank-order stability and some mean-level change. *Psychology and Aging, 27*(1), 243–249.

Mousavi, E., Hosseini S., Bakhtiyari, M., Mohammadi, A., Isfeedvajani, M. S., Arani, A. M., Sadaat, S. H. (2019). Comparing the effectiveness of the Unified Protocol Transdiagnostic and Mindfulness Based Stress Reduction Program on anxiety and depression in infertile women receiving in vitro fertilization. *Journal of Research in Medical and Dental Science, 7*(2), 44–51.

Mroczek, D. K., & Spiro, A. (2003). Modeling intraindividual change in personality traits: Findings from the normative aging study. *Journals of Gerontology, 58*(3), 153–165.

Mulder, R. T., Horwood, J., Tyrer, P., Carter, J., & Joyce, P. R. (2016). Validating the proposed ICD-11 domains. *Personality and Mental Health, 10*(2), 84–95.

Mullins-Sweatt, S. N., Hopwood, C. J., Chmielewski, M., Meyer, N. A., Min, J., Helle, A. C., & Walgren, M. D. (2020). Treatment of personality pathology through the lens of the hierarchical taxonomy of psychopathology: Developing a research agenda. *Personality and Mental Health, 14*(1), 123–141.

Munafò, M. R., Brown, S. M., & Hariri, A. R. (2008). Serotonin transporter (5-HTTLPR) genotype and amygdala activation: A meta-analysis. *Biological Psychiatry, 63*(9), 852–857.

Murphy, R., Hirsch, C. R., Mathews, A., Smith, K., & Clark, D. M. (2007). Facilitating a benign interpretation bias in a high socially anxious population. *Behaviour Research and Therapy, 45*(7), 1517–1529.

Murphy, S. E., Norbury, R., O'Sullivan, U., Cowen, P. J., & Harmer, C. J. (2009). Effect of a single dose of citalopram on amygdala response to emotional faces. *British Journal of Psychiatry, 194*(6), 535–540.

Murray, H. A. (1943). *Thematic apperception test*. Cambridge, MA: Harvard University Press.

Myin-Germeys, I., & van Os, J. (2007). Stress-reactivity in psychosis: Evidence for an affective pathway to psychosis. *Clinical Psychology Review, 27*(4), 409–424.

Nakaya, N., Hansen, P. E., Schapiro, I. R., Eplov, L. F., Saito-Nakaya, K., Uchitomi, Y., & Johansen, C. (2006). Personality traits and cancer survival: A Danish cohort study. *British Journal of Cancer, 95*(2), 146–152.

Naragon-Gainey, K. (2010). Meta-analysis of the relations of anxiety sensitivity to the depressive and anxiety disorders. *Psychological Bulletin, 136*(1), 128–150.

Naragon-Gainey, K., Gallagher, M. W., & Brown, T. A. (2013). Stable "trait" variance of temperament as a predictor of the temporal course of depression and social phobia. *Journal of Abnormal Psychology, 122*(3), 611–623.

Naragon-Gainey, K., McMahon, T. P., & Park, J. (2018). The contributions of affective traits and emotion regulation to internalizing disorders: Current state of the literature and measurement challenges. *American Psychologist, 73*(9), 1175–1186.

Naragon-Gainey, K., & Watson, D. (2018). What lies beyond neuroticism?: An examination of the unique contributions of social-cognitive vulnerabilities to internalizing disorders. *Assessment, 25*(2), 143–158.

Naragon-Gainey, K., Watson, D., & Markon, K. E. (2009). Differential relations of depression and social anxiety symptoms to the facets of extraversion/positive emotionality. *Journal of Abnormal Psychology, 118*(2), 299–310.

Neisser, U., Boodoo, G., Bouchard, T. J., Jr., Boykin, A. W., Brody, N., Ceci, S. J., . . . Urbina, S. (1996). Intelligence: Knowns and unknowns. *American Psychologist, 51*(2), 77–101.

Nelson, E. A., Abramowitz, J. S., Whiteside, S. P., & Deacon, B. J. (2006). Scrupulosity in patients with obsessive–compulsive disorder: Relationship to clinical and cognitive phenomena. *Journal of Anxiety Disorders, 20*(8), 1071–1086.

Nemeroff, C. B. (2004). Neurobiological consequences of childhood trauma. *Journal of Clinical Psychiatry, 65*, 18–28.

Newman, M. G., & Llera, S. J. (2011). A novel theory of experiential avoidance in generalized anxiety disorder: A review and synthesis of research supporting a contrast avoidance model of worry. *Clinical Psychology Review, 31*(3), 371–382.

Neyer, F. J., & Asendorpf, J. B. (2001). Personality-relationship transaction in young adulthood. *Journal of Personality and Social Psychology, 81*(6), 1190–1204.

Nica, E. I., & Links, P. S. (2009). Affective instability in borderline personality disorder: Experience sampling findings. *Current Psychiatry Reports, 11*(1), 74–81.

Nila, K., Holt, D. V., Ditzen, B., & Aguilar-Raab, C. (2016). Mindfulness-based stress reduction (MBSR) enhances distress tolerance and resilience through changes in mindfulness. *Mental Health and Prevention, 4*(1), 36–41.

Nolen-Hoeksema, S. (1991). Responses to depression and their effects on the duration of depressive episodes. *Journal of Abnormal Psychology, 100*(4), 569–582.

Nolen-Hoeksema, S., Girgus, J. S., & Seligman, M. E. (1992). Predictors and consequences of childhood depressive symptoms: A 5-year longitudinal study. *Journal of Abnormal Psychology, 101*(3), 405–422.

Nolen-Hoeksema, S., & Watkins, E. R. (2011). A heuristic for developing transdiagnostic models of psychopathology: Explaining multifinality and divergent trajectories. *Perspectives on Psychological Science, 6*(6), 589–609.

Nolen-Hoeksema, S., Wisco, B. E., & Lyubomirsky, S. (2008). Rethinking rumination. *Perspectives on Psychological Science, 3*(5), 400–424.

Norman, W. T. (1963). Toward an adequate taxonomy of personality attributes: Replicated factor structure in peer nomination personality ratings. *Journal of Personality and Social Psychology, 66*, 574–583.

Norr, A. M., Oglesby, M. E., Capron, D. W., Raines, A. M., Korte, K. J., & Schmidt, N. B. (2013). Evaluating the unique contribution of intolerance of uncertainty relative to other cognitive vulnerability factors in anxiety psychopathology. *Journal of Affective Disorders, 151*(1), 136–142.

Norton, G. R., Cox, B. J., Hewitt, P. L., & McLeod, L. (1997). Personality factors associated with generalized and non-generalized social anxiety. *Personality and Individual Differences, 22*(5), 655–660.

Norton, G. R., Cox, B. J., & Malan, J. (1992). Nonclinical panickers: A critical review. *Clinical Psychology Review, 12*(2), 121–139.

Nowicki, S., & Strickland, B. R. (1973). A locus of control scale for children. *Journal of Consulting and Clinical Psychology, 40*(1), 148–154.

Nunn, G. D. (1988). Concurrent validity between the Nowicki–Strickland locus of control scale and the State–Trait Anxiety Inventory for Children. *Educational and Psychological Measurement, 48*(2), 435–438.

Ochsner, K. N., Bunge, S. A., Gross, J. J., & Gabrieli, J. D. E. (2002). Rethinking feelings: An fMRI study of the cognitive regulation of emotion. *Journal of Cognitive Neuroscience, 14*(8), 1215–1229.

Ochsner, K. N., Ray, R. D., Cooper, J. C., Robertson, E. R., Chopra, S., Gabrieli, J. D. E., & Gross, J. J. (2004). For better or for worse: Neural systems supporting the cognitive down- and up-regulation of negative emotion. *NeuroImage, 23*(2), 483–499.

Öhman, A., Flykt, A., & Lundqvist, D. (2000). Unconscious emotion: Evolutionary perspectives, psychophysiological data and neuropsychological mechanisms. In R. D. Lane & L. Nadel (Eds.), *Cognitive neuroscience of emotion* (pp. 296–327). New York: Oxford University Press.

Olajide, K., Munjiza, J., Moran, P., O'Connell, L., Newton-Howes, G., Bassett, P., . . . Crawford, M. J. (2018). Development and psychometric properties of the standardized assessment of severity of personality disorder (SASPD). *Journal of Personality Disorders, 32*(1), 44–56.

Oldershaw, A., DeJong, H., Hambrook, D., Broadbent, H., Tchanturia, K., Treasure, J., & Schmidt, U. (2012). Emotional processing following recovery from anorexia nervosa. *European Eating Disorders Review, 20*(6), 502–509.

Olino, T. M., Dougherty, L. R., Bufferd, S. J., Carlson, G. A., & Klein, D. N. (2014). Testing models of psychopathology in preschool-aged children using a structured interview-based assessment. *Journal of Abnormal Child Psychology, 42*(7), 1201–1211.

Ollendick, T. H., & King, N. J. (1991). Origins of childhood fears: An evaluation of Rachman's theory of fear acquisition. *Behaviour Research and Therapy, 29*(2), 117–123.

Oltmanns, J. R., Smith, G. T., Oltmanns, T. F., & Widiger, T. A. (2018). General factors of psychopathology, personality, and personality disorder: Across domain comparisons. *Clinical Psychological Science, 6*(4), 581–589.

Oltmanns, J. R., & Widiger, T. A. (2019). Evaluating the assessment of the ICD-11 personality disorder diagnostic system. *Psychological Assessment, 31*(5), 674–684.

O'Neil Rodriguez, K. A., & Kendall, P. C. (2014). Suicidal ideation in anxiety-disordered youth: Identifying predictors of risk. *Journal of Clinical Child and Adolescent Psychology, 43*(1), 51–62.

Opbroek, A., Delgado, P. L., Laukes, C., McGahuey, C., Katsanis, J., Moreno, F. A., & Manber, R. (2002). Emotional blunting associated with SSRI-induced sexual dysfunction: Do SSRIs inhibit emotional responses? *International Journal of Neuropsychopharmacology, 5*(2), 147–151.

Orcutt, H. K., Pickett, S. M., & Pope, E. B. (2005). Experiential avoidance and forgiveness as mediators in the relation between traumatic interpersonal events and post-traumatic stress disorder symptoms. *Journal of Social and Clinical Psychology, 24*(7), 1003–1029.

Orvaschel, H., Lewinsohn, P. M., & Seeley, J. R. (1995). Continuity of psychopathology in a community sample of adolescents. *Journal of the American Academy of Child and Adolescent Psychiatry, 34*(11), 1525–1535.

Osma, J., Castellano, C., Crespo, E., & García-Palacios, A. (2015). The Unified Protocol for Transdiagnostic Treatment of Emotional Disorders in group format in a Spanish public mental health setting. *Behavioral Psychology, 23*(3), 447–466.

Osma, J., Sánchez-Gómez, A., & Peris-Baquero, Ó. (2018). Applying the Unified Protocol to a single case of major depression with schizoid and depressive personality traits. *Psicothema, 30*(4), 364–369.

Öst, L. G., & Hugdahl, K. (1983). Acquisition of agoraphobia, mode of onset and anxiety response patterns. *Behaviour Research and Therapy, 21*(6), 623–631.

Ostafin, B. D., Brooks, J. J., & Laitem, M. (2014). Affective reactivity mediates an inverse relation between mindfulness and anxiety. *Mindfulness, 5*(5), 520–528.

Ostendorf, F. (1990). *Sprache und peroenlichkeitsstruktur: Zur validitaet des fuenffaktoren-modells der persoenlichkeit [Language and personality structure: On the validity of the five factor model of personality]*. Regensburg, Germany: Roederer Verlag.

Oswald, L. M., Zandi, P., Nestadt, G., Potash, J. B., Kalaydjian, A. E., & Wand, G. S. (2006). Relationship between cortisol responses to stress and personality. *Neuropsychopharmacology, 31*(7), 1583–1591.

Overton, S. M., & Menzies, R. G. (2005). Cognitive change during treatment of compulsive checking. *Behaviour Change, 22*(3), 172–184.

Owens, M., Stevenson, J., Hadwin, J. A., & Norgate, R. (2012). Anxiety and depression in academic performance: An exploration of the mediating factors of worry and working memory. *School Psychology International, 33*(4), 433–449.

Pabian, S., & Vandebosch, H. (2016). An investigation of short-term longitudinal associations between social anxiety and victimization and perpetration of traditional bullying and cyberbullying. *Journal of Youth and Adolescence, 45*(2), 328–339.

Pace, T. W. W., Mletzko, T. C., Alagbe, O., Musselman, D. L., Nemeroff, C. B., Miller, A. H., & Heim, C. M. (2006). Increased stress-induced inflammatory responses in male patients with major depression and increased early life stress. *American Journal of Psychiatry, 163*(9), 1630–1633.

Pachankis, J. E., Hatzenbuehler, M. L., Rendina, H. J., Safren, S. A., & Parsons, J. T. (2015). LGB-affirmative cognitive-behavioral therapy for young adult gay and bisexual men: A randomized controlled trial of a transdiagnostic minority stress approach. *Journal of Consulting and Clinical Psychology, 83*(5), 875–889.

Paquette, V., Lévesque, J., Mensour, B., Leroux, J. M., Beaudoin, G., Bourgouin, P., & Beauregard, M. (2003). "Change the mind and you change the brain": Effects of cognitive-behavioral therapy on the neural correlates of spider phobia. *NeuroImage, 18*(2), 401–409.

Parkinson, L., & Rachman, S. (1981). Part II. The nature of intrusive thoughts. *Advances in Behaviour Research and Therapy, 3*(3), 101–110.

Parsons, J. T., Rendina, H. J., Moody, R. L., Gurung, S., Starks, T. J., & Pachankis, J. E. (2017). Feasibility of an emotion regulation intervention to improve mental health and reduce HIV transmission risk behaviors for HIV-positive gay and bisexual men with sexual compulsivity. *AIDS and Behavior, 21*(6), 1540–1549.

Paulesu, E., Sambugaro, E., Torti, T., Danelli, L., Ferri, F., Scialfa, G., . . . Sassaroli, S. (2010). Neural correlates of worry in generalized anxiety disorder and in normal controls: A functional MRI study. *Psychological Medicine, 40*(1), 117–124.

Paulus, D. J., Talkovsky, A. M., Heggeness, L. F., & Norton, P. J. (2015). Beyond negative affectivity: A hierarchical model of global and transdiagnostic vulnerabilities for emotional disorders. *Cognitive Behaviour Therapy, 44*(5), 389–405.

Pavlov, I. P. (1927). *Conditional reflexes: An investigation of the physiological activity of the cerebral cortex.* London: Oxford University Press.

Paxton, S. J., & Diggens, J. (1997). Avoidance coping, binge eating, and depression: An examination of the escape theory of binge eating. *International Journal of Eating Disorders, 22*(1), 83–87.

Payne, L. A., Ellard, K. K., Farchione, T. J., Fairholme, C. P., & Barlow, D. H. (2014). Emotional disorders: A unified transdiagnostic protocol. In D. H. Barlow (Ed.), *Clinical handbook of psychological disorders: A step-by-step treatment manual* (5th ed., pp. 237–274). New York: Guilford Press.

Penninx, B. W. J., Beekman, A. T. F., Honig, A., Deeg, D. J. H., Schoevers, R. A., van Eijk, J. T. M., & van Tilburg, W. (2001). Depression and cardiac mortality. *Archives of General Psychiatry, 58*(3), 221.

Pérez-Cadahía, B., Drobic, B., & Davie, J. R. (2011). Activation and function of immediate-early genes in the nervous system. *Biochemistry and Cell Biology, 89*(1), 61–73.

Persson, B. N. (2019). Current directions in psychiatric classification: From the DSM to RDoC. In D. Garcia, T. Archer, & R. M. Kostrzewa (Eds.), *Personality and brain disorders: Associations and interventions* (pp. 253–268). Cham, Switzerland: Springer International.

Pervin, L. A. (1982). The stasis and flow of behavior: Toward a theory of goals. In M. M. Page (Ed.), *Nebraska Symposium on Motivation: Vol. 30. Personality: Current theory and research* (pp. 10–32). Lincoln: University of Nebraska Press.

Pezawas, L., Meyer-Lindenberg, A., Drabant, E. M., Verchinski, B. A., Munoz, K. E., Kolachana, B. S., . . . Weinberger, D. R. (2005). 5-HTTLPR polymorphism impacts human cingulate-amygdala interactions: A genetic susceptibility mechanism for depression. *Nature Neuroscience, 8*(6), 828–834.

Phan, K. L., Fitzgerald, D. A., Nathan, P. J., & Tancer, M. E. (2006). Association between amygdala hyperactivity to harsh faces and severity of social anxiety in generalized social phobia. *Biological Psychiatry, 59*(5), 424–429.

Phelps, E. A., Delgado, M. R., Nearing, K. I., & LeDoux, J. E. (2004). Extinction learning in humans: Role of the amygdala and vmPFC. *Neuron, 43*(6), 897–905.

Pickett, S. M., Lodis, C. S., Parkhill, M. R., & Orcutt, H. K. (2012). Personality and experiential avoidance: A model of anxiety sensitivity. *Personality and Individual Differences, 53*(3), 246–250.

Pincus, A. L. (2011). Some comments on nomology, diagnostic process, and narcissistic personality disorder in the DSM-5 proposal for personality and personality disorders. *Personality Disorders: Theory, Research, and Treatment, 2*(1), 41–53.

Pizzagalli, D. A. (2014). Depression, stress, and anhedonia: Toward a synthesis and integrated model. *Annual Review of Clinical Psychology, 10*, 393–423.

Plumb, J. C., Orsillo, S. M., & Luterek, J. A. (2004). A preliminary test of the role of experiential avoidance in post-event functioning. *Journal of Behavior Therapy and Experimental Psychiatry, 35*(3), 245–257.

Pole, N. (2007). The psychophysiology of posttraumatic stress disorder: A meta-analysis. *Psychological Bulletin, 133*(5), 725–746.

Poropat, A. E. (2009). A meta-analysis of the five-factor model of personality and academic performance. *Psychological Bulletin, 135*(2), 322–338.

Porto, P. R., Oliveira, L., Mari, J., Volchan, E., Figueira, I., & Ventura, P. (2009). Does cognitive behavioral therapy change the brain?: A systematic review of neuroimaging in anxiety disorders. *Journal of Neuropsychiatry and Clinical Neurosciences, 21*(2), 114–125.

Prenoveau, J. M., Craske, M. G., Zinbarg, R. E., Mineka, S., Rose, R. D., & Griffith, J. W. (2011). Are anxiety and depression just as stable as personality during late adolescence?: Results from a three-year longitudinal latent variable study. *Journal of Abnormal Psychology, 120*, 832–843.

Price, J., Cole, V., & Goodwin, G. M. (2009). Emotional side-effects of selective serotonin reuptake inhibitors: Qualitative study. *British Journal of Psychiatry, 195*(3), 211–217.

Purdon, C. (1999). Thought suppression and psychopathology. *Behaviour Research and Therapy, 37*(11), 1029–1054.

Putnam, K. M., & Silk, K. R. (2005). Emotion dysregulation and the development of borderline personality disorder. *Development and Psychopathology, 17*(4), 899–925.

Quilty, L. C., Meusel, L.-A. C., & Bagby, R. M. (2008). Neuroticism as a mediator of treatment response to SSRIs in major depressive disorder. *Journal of Affective Disorders, 111*(1), 67–73.

Quilty, L. C., Sellbom, M., Tackett, J. L., & Bagby, R. M. (2009). Personality trait predictors of bipolar disorder symptoms. *Psychiatry Research, 169*(2), 159–163.

Quinn, E., Brandon, T., & Copeland, A. (1996). Is task persistence related to smoking and substance abuse?: The application of learned industriousness theory to addictive behaviors. *Experimental and Clinical Psychopharmacology, 4*(2), 186–190.

Rachman, S., & de Silva, P. (1978). Abnormal and normal obsessions. *Behaviour Research and Therapy, 16*(4), 233–248.

Racine, S. E., & Wildes, J. E. (2015). Dynamic longitudinal relations between emotion regulation difficulties and anorexia nervosa symptoms over the year following intensive treatment. *Journal of Consulting and Clinical Psychology, 83*(4), 785–795.

Radley, A. (2012). *The body and social psychology.* New York: Springer-Verlag.

Rapee, R. M., Brown, T. A., Antony, M. M., & Barlow, D. H. (1992). Response to hyperventilation and inhalation of 5.5% carbon dioxide–enriched air across the DSM-III-R anxiety disorders. *Journal of Abnormal Psychology, 101*(3), 538–552.

Rapee, R. M., Craske, M. G., Brown, T. A., & Barlow, D. H. (1996). Measurement of perceived control over anxiety-related events. *Behavior Therapy, 27*(2), 279–293.

Rapee, R. M., & Heimberg, R. G. (1997). A cognitive-behavioral model of anxiety in social phobia. *Behaviour Research and Therapy, 35*(8), 741–756.

Rapee, R. M., & Jacobs, D. (2002). The reduction of temperamental risk for anxiety in withdrawn preschoolers: A pilot study. *Behavioural and Cognitive Psychotherapy, 30*(2), 211–215.

Rapee, R. M., Kennedy, S., Ingram, M., Edwards, S., & Sweeney, L. (2005). Prevention and early intervention of anxiety disorders in inhibited preschool children. *Journal of Consulting and Clinical Psychology, 73*(3), 488–497.

Rapee, R. M., Kennedy, S. J., Ingram, M., Edwards, S. L., & Sweeney, L. (2010). Altering the trajectory of anxiety in at-risk young children. *American Journal of Psychiatry, 167*(12), 1518–1525.

Rapee, R. M., & Melville, L. F. (1997). Recall of family factors in social phobia and panic disorder: Comparison of mother and offspring reports. *Depression and Anxiety, 5*(1), 7–11.

Rassin, E., & Koster, E. (2003). The correlation between thought–action fusion and religiosity in a normal sample. *Behaviour Research and Therapy, 41*(3), 361–368.

Rassin, E., Merckelbach, H., & Muris, P. (2000a). Paradoxical and less paradoxical effects of thought suppression: A critical review. *Clinical Psychology Review, 20*(8), 973–995.

Rassin, E., Muris, P., Schmidt, H., & Merckelbach, H. (2000b). Relationships between thought–action fusion, thought suppression and obsessive–compulsive symptoms: A structural equation modeling approach. *Behaviour Research and Therapy, 38*(9), 889–897.

Razran, G. (1961). The observable and the inferable conscious in current Soviet psychophysiology: Interoceptive conditioning, semantic conditioning, and the orienting reflex. *Psychological Review, 68*(2), 81–147.

Reardon, J. M., & Williams, N. L. (2007). The specificity of cognitive vulnerabilities to emotional disorders: Anxiety sensitivity, looming vulnerability and explanatory style. *Journal of Anxiety Disorders, 21*(5), 625–643.

Reck, C., Müller, M., Tietz, A., & Möhler, E. (2013). Infant distress to novelty is associated with maternal anxiety disorder and especially with maternal avoidance behavior. *Journal of Anxiety Disorders, 27*(4), 404–412.

Redlich, F., & Kellert, S. R. (1978). Trends in American mental health. *American Journal of Psychiatry, 135*(1), 22–28.

Reinholt, N., Aharoni, R., Winding, C., Rosenberg, N., Rosenbaum, B., & Arnfred, S. (2017). Transdiagnostic group CBT for anxiety disorders: The Unified Protocol in mental health services. *Cognitive Behaviour Therapy, 46*(1), 29–43.

Reiss, D., Hetherington, M., Plomin, R., Howe, G. W., Simmens, S. J., Henderson, S. H., . . . Law, T. (1995). Genetic questions for environmental studies: Differential parenting and psychopathology in adolescence. *Archives of General Psychiatry, 52*(11), 925–936.

Reiss, S. (1991). Expectancy model of fear, anxiety, and panic. *Clinical Psychology Review, 11*(2), 141–153.

Reiss, S., & McNally, R. J. (1985). Expectancy model of fear. In S. Reiss & R. R. Bootzin (Eds.), *Theoretical issues in behaviour therapy* (pp. 107–121). New York: Academic Press.

Reiss, S., Peterson, R. A., Gursky, D. M., & McNally, R. J. (1986). Anxiety sensitivity, anxiety frequency and the prediction of fearfulness. *Behaviour Research and Therapy, 24*(1), 1–8.

Renton, J. C., & Mankiewicz, P. D. (2015). Paranoid, schizotypal, and schizoid personality disorder. In A. T. Beck, D. D. Davis, & A. Freeman (Eds.), *Cognitive therapy of personality disorders* (pp. 244–275). New York: Guilford Press.

Rescorla, R. A., & Furrow, D. R. (1977). Stimulus similarity as a determinant of Pavlovian conditioning. *Journal of Experimental Psychology: Animal Behavior Processes, 3*(3), 203–215.

Rescorla, R. A., & Gillan, D. J. (1980). An analysis of the facilitative effect of similarity on second-order conditioning. *Journal of Experimental Psychology: Animal Behavior Processes, 6*(4), 339–351.

Reynolds, G. O., Saint-Hilaire, M., Thomas, C. A., Barlow, D. H., & Cronin-Golomb, A. (2019). Cognitive-behavioral therapy for anxiety in Parkinson's disease. *Behavior Modification, 44*(4), 552–579.

Reynolds, W. M. (1993). Self-report methods. In T. H. Ollendick & M. Hersen (Eds.), *Handbook of child and adolescent assessment.* New York: Plenum Press.

Riemann, R., Angleitner, A., & Strelau, J. (1997). Genetic and environmental influences on personality: A study of twins reared together using the self- and peer report NEO-FFI scales. *Journal of Personality, 65*(3), 449–475.

Rizvi, S. L., & Linehan, M. M. (2005). The treatment of maladaptive shame in borderline personality disorder: A pilot study of "opposite action." *Cognitive and Behavioral Practice, 12*(4), 437–447.

Roberts, B. W., & DelVecchio, W. F. (2000). The rank-order consistency of personality traits from childhood to old age: A quantitative review of longitudinal studies. *Psychological Bulletin, 126*(1), 3–25.

Roberts, B. W., Hill, P. L., & Davis, J. P. (2017a). How to change conscientiousness: The sociogenomic trait intervention model. *Personality Disorders: Theory, Research, and Treatment, 8*(3), 199–205.

Roberts, B. W., Lejuez, C., Krueger, R. F., Richards, J. M., & Hill, P. L. (2014). What is conscientiousness and how can it be assessed? *Developmental Psychology, 50*(5), 1315–1330.

Roberts, B. W., Luo, J., Briley, D. A., Chow, P. I., Su, R., & Hill, P. L. (2017b). A systematic review of personality trait change through intervention. *Psychological Bulletin, 143*(2), 117–141.

Roberts, B. W., & Mroczek, D. (2008). Personality trait change in adulthood. *Current Directions in Psychological Science, 17*(1), 31–35.

Roberts, B. W., Walton, K. E., & Viechtbauer, W. (2006). Patterns of mean-level change in personality traits across the life course: A meta-analysis of longitudinal studies. *Psychological Bulletin, 132*(1), 1–25.

Robins, C. J., & Chapman, A. L. (2004). Dialectical behavior therapy: Current status, recent developments, and future directions. *Journal of Personality Disorders, 18*(1), 73–89.

Robinson, J. A., Sareen, J., Cox, B. J., & Bolton, J. M. (2009). Correlates of self-medication for anxiety disorders: Results from the National Epidemiolgic Survey on Alcohol and Related Conditions. *Journal of Nervous and Mental Disease, 197*(12), 873–878.

Robinson, J. L., Kagan, J., Reznick, J. S., & Corley, R. (1992). The heritability of inhibited and uninhibited behavior: A twin study. *Developmental Psychology, 28*(6), 1030–1037.

Robles, T. F., Glaser, R., & Kiecolt-Glaser, J. K. (2005). Out of balance. *Current Directions in Psychological Science, 14*(2), 111–115.

Rodriguez, B. F., Bruce, S. E., Pagano, M. E., Spencer, M. A., & Keller, M. B. (2004). Factor structure and stability of the Anxiety Sensitivity Index in a longitudinal study of anxiety disorder patients. *Behaviour Research and Therapy, 42*(1), 79–91.

Roemer, L., Salters, K., Raffa, S. D., & Orsillo, S. M. (2005). Fear and avoidance of internal experiences in GAD: Preliminary tests of a conceptual model. *Cognitive Therapy and Research, 29*(1), 71–88.

Rogers, A. H., Kauffman, B. Y., Bakhshaie, J., McHugh, R. K., Ditre, J. W., Zvolensky, M. J., . . . Zvolensky, M. J. (2019). Anxiety sensitivity and opioid misuse among opioid-using adults with chronic pain. *American Journal of Drug and Alcohol Abuse, 45*(5), 470–478.

Rogosch, F. A., Dackis, M. N., & Cicchetti, D. (2011). Child maltreatment and allostatic load: Consequences for physical and mental health in children from low-income families. *Development and Psychopathology, 23*(4), 1107–1124.

Roma, P. G., Champoux, M., & Suomi, S. J. (2006). Environmental control, social context, and individual differences in behavioral and cortisol responses to novelty in infant rhesus monkeys. *Child Development, 77*(1), 118–131.

Rorschach, H. (1942). *Psychodiagnostics.* New York: Grune & Stratton.

Rosellini, A. J., & Brown, T. A. (2019). The Multidimensional Emotional Disorder Inventory (MEDI): Assessing transdiagnostic dimensions to validate a profile approach to emotional disorder classification. *Psychological Assessment, 31*(1), 59–72.

Rosellini, A. J., Lawrence, A. E., Meyer, J. F., & Brown, T. A. (2010). The effects of extraverted temperament on agoraphobia in panic disorder. *Journal of Abnormal Psychology, 119*(2), 420–426.

Rosen, J. B., & Schulkin, J. (1998). From normal fear to pathological anxiety. *Psychological Review, 105*(2), 325–350.

Rosenthal, M. Z., Cheavens, J., Lejuez, C., & Lynch, T. (2005). Thought suppression mediates the relationship between negative affect and borderline personality disorder symptoms. *Behaviour Research and Therapy, 43*(9), 1173–1185.

Rothbart, M. K. (2011). *Becoming who we are: Temperament and personality in development.* New York: Guilford Press.

Rothbart, M. K., Ahadi, S. A., & Evans, D. E. (2000). Temperament and personality: Origins and outcomes. *Journal of Personality and Social Psychology, 78*(1), 122–135.

Rothbart, M. K., & Derryberry, D. (1981). Theoretical issues in temperament. In M. Lewis & L. T. Taft (Eds.), *Developmental disabilities: Theory, assessment, and intervention* (pp. 383–400). Leiden, the Netherlands: Springer.

Rotter, J. B. (1966). Generalized expectancies for internal versus external control of reinforcement. *Psychological Monographs: General and Applied, 80*(1), 1–28.

Rowsell, M., MacDonald, D. E., & Carter, J. C. (2016). Emotion regulation difficulties in anorexia nervosa: Associations with improvements in eating psychopathology. *Journal of Eating Disorders, 4*(1), 17.

Roxbury, A. (2017). *Does adding mantra-based meditation training improve the efficacy of the Unified Protocol for individuals with generalized anxiety disorder?* (Publication No. 10253550) [Doctoral dissertation, Hofstra University]. ProQuest Dissertations and Theses Global.

Rubin, K. H., Coplan, R. J., & Bowker, J. C. (2009). Social withdrawal in childhood. *Annual Review of Psychology, 60,* 141–171.

Rudaz, M., Craske, M. G., Becker, E. S., Ledermann, T., & Margraf, J. (2010). Health anxiety and fear of fear in panic disorder and agoraphobia vs. social phobia: A prospective longitudinal study. *Depression and Anxiety, 27*(4), 404–411.

Ruiz, F. J. (2012). Acceptance and commitment therapy versus traditional cognitive behavioral therapy: A systematic review and meta-analysis of current empirical evidence. *International Journal of Psychology, 12*(3), 333–357.

Ruiz, M. A., Pincus, A. L., & Schinka, J. A. (2008). Externalizing pathology and the five-factor model: A meta-analysis of personality traits associated with antisocial personality disorder, substance use disorder, and their co-occurrence. *Journal of Personality Disorders, 22*(4), 365–388.

Ruscio, A. M., Gentes, E. L., Jones, J. D., Hallion, L. S., Coleman, E. S., & Swendsen, J. (2015). Rumination predicts heightened responding to stressful life events in major depressive disorder and generalized anxiety disorder. *Journal of Abnormal Psychology, 124*(1), 17–26.

Rush, A. J., & Weissenburger, J. E. (1994). Melancholic symptom features and DSM-IV. *American Journal of Psychiatry, 151*(4), 489–498.

Russo, J., Katon, W., Lin, E., Von Korff, M., Bush, T., Simon, G., & Walker, E. (1997). Neuroticism and extraversion as predictors of health outcomes in depressed primary care patients. *Psychosomatics, 38*(4), 339–348.

Rutter, M. (2010). Gene–environment interplay. *Depression and Anxiety, 27*(1), 1–4.

Rutter, M., Moffitt, T. E., & Caspi, A. (2006). Gene–environment interplay and psychopathology: Multiple varieties but real effects. *Journal of Child Psychology and Psychiatry, 47*(3–4), 226–261.

Sackett, D., Strauss, S., Richardson, W., Rosenberg, W., & Haynes, R. (2000). *Evidence-based medicine: How to practice and teach EBM* (2nd ed.). London: Churchill Livingstone.

Sahay, A., Scobie, K. N., Hill, A. S., O'Carroll, C. M., Kheirbek, M. A., Burghardt, N. S., . . . Hen, R. (2011). Increasing adult hippocampal neurogenesis is sufficient to improve pattern separation. *Nature, 472*(7344), 466–470.

Sakiris, N., & Berle, D. (2019). A systematic review and meta-analysis of the Unified Protocol as a transdiagnostic emotion regulation–based intervention. *Clinical Psychology Review, 72*, 101751.

Salkovskis, P. M., & Campbell, P. (1994). Thought suppression induces intrusion in naturally occurring negative intrusive thoughts. *Behaviour Research and Therapy, 32*(1), 1–8.

Salkovskis, P., Shafran, R., Rachman, S., & Freeston, M. H. (1999). Multiple pathways to inflated responsibility beliefs in obsessional problems: Possible origins and implications for therapy and research. *Behaviour Research and Therapy, 37*(11), 1055–1072.

Samuel, D. B., & Gore, W. L. (2012). Maladaptive variants of conscientiousness and agreeableness. *Journal of Personality, 80*(6), 1669–1696.

Samuel, D. B., & Widiger, T. A. (2006). Clinicians' judgments of clinical utility: A comparison of the DSM-IV and five-factor models. *Journal of Abnormal Psychology, 115*(2), 298–308.

Samuel, D., & Widiger, T. (2008). A meta-analytic review of the relationships between the five-factor model and DSM-IV-TR personality disorders: A facet level analysis. *Clinical Psychology Review, 28*(8), 1326–1342.

Sanderson, W. C., Rapee, R. M., & Barlow, D. H. (1989). The influence of an illusion of control on panic attacks induced via inhalation of 5.5% carbon dioxide-enriched air. *Archives of General Psychiatry, 46*(2), 157–162.

Sandler, J., & Sandler, A. (1978). On the development of object relationships and affects. *International Journal of Psycho-Analysis, 59*(2–3), 285–296.

Santanello, A. W., & Gardner, F. L. (2007). The role of experiential avoidance in the relationship between maladaptive perfectionism and worry. *Cognitive Therapy and Research, 31*(3), 319–332.

Sapolsky, R. M. (1990). Adrenocortical function, social rank, and personality among wild baboons. *Biological Psychiatry, 28*(10), 862–878.

Sapolsky, R. M. (1992). *Stress, the aging brain, and the mechanisms of neuron death.* Cambridge, MA: MIT Press.

Sapolsky, R. M. (2005). The influence of social hierarchy on primate health. *Science, 308*(5722), 648–652.

Sapolsky, R. M., Alberts, S. C., & Altmann, J. (1997). Hypercortisolism associated with social subordinance or social isolation among wild baboons. *Archives of General Psychiatry, 54*(12), 1137–1143.

Sapolsky, R. M., & Ray, J. C. (1989). Styles of dominance and their endocrine correlates among wild olive baboons (*Papio anubis*). *American Journal of Primatology, 18*(1), 1–13.

Sapolsky, R. M., Romero, L. M., & Munck, A. U. (2000). How do glucocorticoids influence stress responses?: Integrating permissive, suppressive, stimulatory, and preparative actions. *Endocrine Reviews, 21*(1), 55–89.

Sareen, J., Cox, B. J., Clara, I., & Asmundson, G. J. (2005). The relationship between anxiety disorders and physical disorders in the U.S. National Comorbidity Survey. *Depression and Anxiety, 21*(4), 193–202.

Saucier, G., Georgiades, S., Tsouasis, I., & Goldberg, L. R. (2005). Factor structure of Greek personaity-descriptive adjectives. *Journal of Personality and Social Psychology, 88*, 856–875.

Sauer, S. E., & Baer, R. A. (2009a). Relationships between thought suppression and symptoms of borderline personality disorder. *Journal of Personality Disorders, 23*(1), 48–61.

Sauer, S. E., & Baer, R. A. (2009b). Responding to negative internal experience: Relationships between acceptance and change-based approaches and psychological adjustment. *Journal of Psychopathology and Behavioral Assessment, 31*(4), 378–386.

Sauer, S. E., & Baer, R. A. (2009c). Mindfulness and decentering as mechanisms of change in mindfulness- and acceptance-based interventions. In R. A. Baer (Ed.), *Assessing mindfulness and acceptance processes in clients: Illuminating the theory and practice of change* (pp. 25–50). Oakland, CA: New Harbinger

Sauer, S. E., & Baer, R. A. (2012). Ruminative and mindful self-focused attention in borderline personality disorder. *Personality Disorders: Theory, Research, and Treatment, 3*(4), 433–441.

Sauer-Zavala, S., Ametaj, A. A., Wilner, J. G., Bentley, K. H., Marquez, S., Patrick, K. A., . . . Marques, L. (2019a). Evaluating transdiagnostic, evidence-based mental health care in a safety-net setting serving homeless individuals. *Psychotherapy, 56*(1), 100–114.

Sauer-Zavala, S., & Barlow, D. H. (2014). The case for borderline personality disorder as an emotional disorder: Implications for treatment. *Clinical Psychology: Science and Practice, 21*(2), 118–138.

Sauer-Zavala, S., Bentley, K. H., & Wilner, J. G. (2016). Transdiagnostic treatment of borderline personality disorder and comorbid disorders: A clinical replication series. *Journal of Personality Disorders, 30*(1), 35–51.

Sauer-Zavala, S., Boswell, J. F., Gallagher, M. W., Bentley, K. H., Ametaj, A., & Barlow, D. H. (2012). The role of negative affectivity and negative reactivity to emotions in predicting outcomes in the Unified Protocol for the Transdiagnostic Treatment of Emotional Disorders. *Behaviour Research and Therapy, 50*(9), 551–557.

Sauer-Zavala, S., Cassiello-Robbins, C., Ametaj, A. A., Wilner, J. G., & Pagan, D. (2019b). Transdiagnostic treatment personalization: The feasibility of ordering Unified Protocol modules according to patient strengths and weaknesses. *Behavior Modification, 43*(4), 518–543.

Sauer-Zavala, S., Cassiello-Robbins, C., Woods, B. K., Curreri, A., Wilner Tirpak, J., & Rassaby, M. (2020). Countering emotional behaviors in the treatment of borderline personality disorder. *Personality Disorders: Theory, Research, and Treatment, 11*(5), 328–338.

Sauer-Zavala, S., Fournier, J. C., Steele, S. J., Woods, B. K., Wang, M., Farchione, T. J., & Barlow, D. H. (2020). Does the Unified Protocol really change neuroticism?: Results from a randomized trial. *Psychological Medicine.* [Epub ahead of print]

Sauer-Zavala, S., Wilner, J. G., Cassiello-Robbins, C., Saraff, P., & Pagan, D. (2019c). Isolating the effect of opposite action in borderline personality disorder: A laboratory-based alternating treatment design. *Behaviour Research and Therapy, 117*, 79–86.

Saulsman, L. M., & Page, A. C. (2004). The five-factor model and personality disorder empirical literature: A meta-analytic review. *Clinical Psychology Review, 23*(8), 1055–1085.

Scharf, J. S., & Scharf, D. (1998). *Object relations individual therapy.* Northvale, NJ: Jason Aronson.

Schmidt, N. B., Keough, M. E., Timpano, K. R., & Richey, J. A. (2008). Anxiety sensitivity profile: Predictive and incremental validity. *Journal of Anxiety Disorders, 22*(7), 1180–1189.

Schmidt, N. B., Lerew, D. R., & Jackson, R. J. (1997). The role of anxiety sensitivity in the pathogenesis of panic: Prospective evaluation of spontaneous panic attacks during acute stress. *Journal of Abnormal Psychology, 106*(3), 355–364.

Schmidt, N. B., Lerew, D. R., & Joiner, T. E. (1998). Anxiety sensitivity and the pathogenesis of anxiety and depression: Evidence for symptom specificity. *Behaviour Research and Therapy, 36*(2), 165–177.

Schmidt, N. B., Zvolensky, M. J., & Maner, J. K. (2006). Anxiety sensitivity: Prospective prediction of panic attacks and Axis I pathology. *Journal of Psychiatric Research, 40*(8), 691–699.

Schneewind, K. A. (1995). Impact of family processes on control beliefs. In A. Bandura (Ed.), *Self-efficacy in changing societies* (pp. 114–148). Cambridge, UK: Cambridge University Press.

Segal, Z. V., Teasdale, J. D., Williams, J. M., & Gemar, M. C. (2002). The Mindfulness-Based Cognitive Therapy Adherence Scale: Inter-rater reliability, adherence to protocol and treatment distinctiveness. *Clinical Psychology and Psychotherapy, 9*(2), 131–138.

Segerstrom, S. C., Tsao, J. C. I., Alden, L. E., & Craske, M. G. (2000). Worry and rumination: Repetitive thought as a concomitant and predictor of negative mood. *Cognitive Therapy and Research, 24*(6), 671–688.

Selby, E. A., Anestis, M. D., Bender, T. W., & Joiner, T. E., Jr. (2009). An exploration of the emotional cascade model in borderline personality disorder. *Journal of Abnormal Psychology, 118*(2), 375–387.

Selby, E. A., Anestis, M. D., & Joiner, T. E. (2008). Understanding the relationship between emotional and behavioral dysregulation: Emotional cascades. *Behaviour Research and Therapy, 46*(5), 593–611.

Seligman, M. E. P. (1975). *Helplessness: On depression, development, and death.* New York: Freeman.

Seligman, M. E. P., Steen, T. A., Park, N., & Peterson, C. (2005). Positive psychology progress: Empirical validation of interventions. *American Psychologist, 60*(5), 410–421.

Shackman, A. J., Tromp, D. P. M., Stockbridge, M. D., Kaplan, C. M., Tillman, R. M., & Fox, A. S. (2016). Dispositional negativity: An integrative psychological and neurobiological perspective. *Psychological Bulletin, 142*(12), 1275–1314.

Shafran, R., Thordarson, D. S., & Rachman, S. (1996). Thought–action fusion in obsessive compulsive disorder. *Journal of Anxiety Disorders, 10*(5), 379–391.

Shahar, B., & Herr, N. R. (2011). Depressive symptoms predict inflexibly high levels of experiential avoidance in response to daily negative affect: A daily diary study. *Behaviour Research and Therapy, 49*(10), 676–681.

Shapiro, S. L. (2009). The integration of mindfulness and psychology. *Journal of Clinical Psychology, 65*(6), 555–560.

Shear, K., Belnap, B. H., Mazumdar, S., Houck, P., & Rollman, B. L. (2006). Generalized anxiety disorder severity scale (GADSS): A preliminary validation study. *Depression and Anxiety, 23*(2), 77–82.

Shear, M. K. (1991). The concept of uncontrollability. *Psychological Inquiry, 2*(1), 88–93.

Shear, M. K., Brown, T. A., Barlow, D. H., Money, R., Sholomskas, D. E., Woods, S. W., . . . Papp, L. A. (1997). Multicenter Collaborative Panic Disorder Severity Scale. *American Journal of Psychiatry, 154*(11), 1571–1575.

Sheng, M., & Greenberg, M. E. (1990). The regulation and function of c-fos and other immediate early genes in the nervous system. *Neuron, 4*(4), 477–485.

Sher, K. J., & Trull, T. J. (1994). Personality and disinhibitory psychopathology: Alcoholism and antisocial personality disorder. *Journal of Abnormal Psychology, 103*(1), 92–102.

Shihata, S., McEvoy, P. M., & Mullan, B. A. (2017). Pathways from uncertainty to anxiety: An evaluation of a hierarchical model of trait- and disorder-specific intolerance of uncertainty on anxiety disorder symptoms. *Journal of Anxiety Disorders, 45,* 72–79.

Shin, C., McNamara, J. O., Morgan, J. I., Curran, T., & Cohen, D. R. (1990). Induction of c-fos mRNA expression by afterdischarge in the hippocampus of naive and kindled rats. *Journal of Neurochemistry, 55*(3), 1050–1055.

Shin, L. M., & Liberzon, I. (2010). The neurocircuitry of fear, stress, and anxiety disorders. *Neuropsychopharmacology, 35*(1), 169–191.

Shin, L. M., Wright, C. I., Cannistraro, P. A., Wedig, M. M., McMullin, K., Martis, B., . . . Rauch, S. L. (2005). A functional magnetic resonance imaging study of amygdala and medial prefrontal cortex responses to overtly presented fearful faces in post-traumatic stress disorder. *Archives of General Psychiatry, 62*(3), 273–281.

Shiner, R. L., Buss, K. A., McClowry, S. G., Putnam, S. P., Saudino, K. J., & Zentner, M. (2012). What is temperament now?: Assessing progress in temperament research on the twenty-fifth anniversary of Goldsmith et al. *Child Development Perspectives, 6*(4), 436–444.

Shipley, B. A., Weiss, A., Der, G., Taylor, M. D., & Deary, I. J. (2007). Neuroticism, extraversion, and mortality in the UK Health and Lifestyle Survey: A 21-year prospective cohort study. *Psychosomatic Medicine, 69*(9), 923–931.

Shmelyov, A., & Pokhil'ko, V. I. (1993). A taxonomy-oriented study of Russian personality-trait names. *European Journal of Personality, 7*(1), 1–17.

Shorey, R. C., Elmquist, J., Wolford-Clevenger, C., Gawrysiak, M. J., Anderson, S., & Stuart, G. L. (2016). The relationship between dispositional mindfulness, borderline personality features, and suicidal ideation in a sample of women in residential substance use treatment. *Psychiatry Research, 238,* 122–128.

Siegel, L. J., & Griffin, N. J. (1984). Correlates of depressive symptoms in adolescents. *Journal of Youth and Adolescence, 13*(6), 475–487.

Siegel, R. E. (1973). *Galen on psychology, psychopathology, and function and diseases of the nervous system: An analysis of his doctrines, observations, and experiments.* Basel, Switzerland: Karger.

Simon, N. M., Otto, M. W., Fischmann, D., Racette, S., Nierenberg, A. A., Pollack, M. H., & Smoller, J. W. (2005). Panic disorder and bipolar disorder: Anxiety sensitivity as a potential mediator of panic during manic states. *Journal of Affective Disorders, 87*(1), 101–105.

Simon, N. M., Smoller, J. W., Fava, M., Sachs, G., Racette, S. R., Perlis, R., . . . Rosenbaum, J. F. (2003). Comparing anxiety disorders and anxiety-related traits in bipolar disorder and unipolar depression. *Journal of Psychiatric Research, 37*(3), 187–192.

Simons, J. S., & Gaher, R. M. (2005). The Distress Tolerance Scale: Development and validation of a self-report measure. *Motivation and Emotion, 29*(2), 83–102.

Siqueland, L., Kendall, P. C., & Steinberg, L. (1996). Anxiety in children: Perceived family environments and observed family interaction. *Journal of Clinical Child Psychology, 25*(2), 225–237.

Sirois, F. M., Molnar, D. S., & Hirsch, J. K. (2017). A meta-analytic and conceptual update on the associations between procrastination and multidimensional perfectionism. *European Journal of Personality, 31*(2), 137–159.

Skinner, E. A., Chapman, M., & Baltes, P. B. (1988). Control, means–ends, and agency beliefs: A new conceptualization and its measurement during childhood. *Journal of Personality and Social Psychology, 54*(1), 117–133.

Skre, I., Onstad, S., Torgersen, S., Lygren, S., & Kringlen, E. (1993). A twin study of DSM-III-R anxiety disorders. *Acta Psychiatrica Scandinavica, 88*(2), 85–92.

Sloan, D. M. (2004). Emotion regulation in action: Emotional reactivity in experiential avoidance. *Behaviour Research and Therapy, 42*(11), 1257–1270.

Small, B. J., Hertzog, C., Hultsch, D. F., & Dixon, R. A. (2003). Stability and change in adult personality over 6 years: Findings from the Victoria Longitudinal Study. *Journals of Gerontology, 58*(3), 166–176.

Smith, D. J., Escott-Price, V., Davies, G., Bailey, M. E. S., Colodro-Conde, L., Ward, J., . . . O'Donovan, M. C. (2016). Genome-wide analysis of over 106,000 individuals identifies 9 neuroticism-associated loci. *Molecular Psychiatry, 21*(6), 749–757.

Smith, J. M., Grandin, L. D., Alloy, L. B., & Abramson, L. Y. (2006). Cognitive vulnerability to depression and Axis II personality dysfunction. *Cognitive Therapy and Research, 30*(5), 609–621.

Smith, N. S., Albanese, B. J., Schmidt, N. B., & Capron, D. W. (2019). Intolerance of uncertainty and responsibility for harm predict nocturnal panic attacks. *Psychiatry Research, 273*, 82–88.

Smith, T. W., & MacKenzie, J. (2006). Personality and risk of physical illness. *Annual Review of Clinical Psychology, 2*(1), 435–467.

Smits, J. A., Berry, A. C., Tart, C. D., & Powers, M. B. (2008). The efficacy of cognitive-behavioral interventions for reducing anxiety sensitivity: A meta-analytic review. *Behaviour Research and Therapy, 46*(9), 1047–1054.

Somer, O., & Goldberg, L. R. (1999). The structure of Turkish trait-descriptive adjectives. *Journal of Personality and Social Psychology, 76*(3), 431–450.

Soskin, D. P., Carl, J. R., Alpert, J., & Fava, M. (2012). Antidepressant effects on emotional temperament: Toward a biobehavioral research paradigm for major depressive disorder. *CNS Neuroscience and Therapeutics, 18*(6), 441–451.

Spijker, J., de Graaf, R., Oldehinkel, A. J., Nolen, W. A., & Ormel, J. (2007). Are the vulnerability effects of personality and psychosocial functioning on depression accounted for by subthreshold symptoms? *Depression and Anxiety, 24*(7), 472–478.

Spiller, R. C. (2007). Role of infection in irritable bowel syndrome. *Journal of Gastroenterology, 42*(17), 41–47.

Spinhoven, P., Drost, J., de Rooij, M., van Hemert, A. M., & Penninx, B. W. (2016). Is experiential avoidance a mediating, moderating, independent, overlapping, or proxy risk factor in the onset, relapse and maintenance of depressive disorders? *Cognitive Therapy and Research, 40*(2), 150–163.

Spitzer, R. L., Endicott, J., & Robins, E. (1978). Research diagnostic criteria: Rationale and reliability. *Archives of General Psychiatry, 35*(6), 773–782.

Spitzer, R. L., & Wilson, P. T. (1968). A guide to the American Psychiatric Association's new diagnostic nomenclature. *American Journal of Psychiatry, 124*(12), 1619–1629.

Stassen, H. H., Angst, J., & Delini-Stula, A. (1996). Delayed onset of action of antidepressant drugs?: Survey of results of Zurich meta-analyses. *Pharmacopsychiatry, 29*(3), 87–96.

Steele, S. J., Farchione, T. J., Cassiello-Robbins, C., Ametaj, A., Sbi, S., Sauer-Zavala, S., & Barlow, D. H. (2018). Efficacy of the Unified Protocol for transdiagnostic treatment of comorbid psychopathology accompanying emotional disorders compared to treatments targeting single disorders. *Journal of Psychiatric Research, 104*, 211–216.

Stein, M. B., Campbell-Sills, L., & Gelernter, J. (2009). Genetic variation in 5HTTLPR is associated with emotional resilience. *American Journal of Medical Genetics Part B: Neuropsychiatric Genetics, 150*(7), 900–906.

Stein, M. B., Simmons, A. N., Feinstein, J. S., & Paulus, M. P. (2007). Increased amygdala and insula activation during emotion processing in anxiety-prone subjects. *American Journal of Psychiatry, 164*(2), 318–327.

Steketee, G., Chambless, D. L., & Tran, G. Q. (2001). Effects of axis I and II comorbidity on behavior therapy outcome for obsessive–compulsive disorder and agoraphobia. *Comprehensive Psychiatry, 42*(1), 76–86.

Steketee, G., Quay, S., & White, K. (1991). Religion and guilt in OCD patients. *Journal of Anxiety Disorders, 5*(4), 359–367.

Stelmack, R., & Stalikas, R. (1991). Galen and the humor theory of temperament. *Personality and Individual Differences, 12*(3), 255–263.

Stewart, S. H., Zvolensky, M. J., & Eifert, G. H. (2002). The relations of anxiety sensitivity, experiential avoidance, and alexithymic coping to young adults' motivations for drinking. *Behavior Modification, 26*(2), 271–296.

Stice, E., & Shaw, H. E. (2002). Role of body dissatisfaction in the onset and maintenance of eating pathology: A synthesis of research findings. *Journal of Psychosomatic Research, 53*(5), 985–993.

Straub, T., Mentzel, H. J., & Miltner, W. H. (2006). Neural mechanisms of automatic and direct processing of phobogenic stimuli in specific phobia. *Biological Psychiatry, 59*(2), 162–170.

Strelau, J., Angleitner, A., Bantelmann, J., & Ruch, W. (1990). The Strelau Temperament Inventory—Revised (STI-R): Theoretical considerations and scale development. *European Journal of Personality, 4*(3), 209–235.

Strelau, J., & Zawadzki, B. (1995). The formal characteristics of Behaviour–Temperament Inventory (FCB-TI): Validity studies. *European Journal of Personality, 9*(3), 207–229.

Strupp, H. H. (1973). *Psychotherapy: Clinical, research, and theoretical issues.* New York: Jason Aronson.

Suárez, L., Bennett, S., Goldstein, C., & Barlow, D. H. (2009). Understanding anxiety disorders from a "triple vulnerability" framework. In M. M. Antony & M. B. Stein (Eds.), *Oxford handbook of anxiety and related disorders* (pp. 153–172). New York: Oxford University Press.

Suls, J., & Bunde, J. (2005). Anger, anxiety, and depression as risk factors for cardiovascular disease: The problems and implications of overlapping affective dispositions. *Psychological Bulletin, 131*(2), 260–300.

Suomi, S. J. (1986). Anxiety-like disorders in young nonhuman primates. In R. Gittelman (Ed.), *Anxiety disorders of childhood* (pp. 1–23). New York: Guilford Press.

Suomi, S. J. (1999). Attachment in rhesus monkeys. In J. Cassidy & P. R. Shaver (Eds.), *Handbook of attachment: Theory, research, and clinical applications* (pp. 181–197). New York: Guilford Press.

Suomi, S. J. (2000). A biobehavioral perspective on developmental psychopathology. In A. J. Sameroff, M. Lewis, & S. M. Miller (Eds.), *Handbook of developmental psychopathology* (pp. 237–256). Boston: Springer.

Susman, W. (1979). Personality and the making of the twentieth-century culture. In P. Conklin (Ed.), *New directions in American intellectual history* (pp. 212–226). Baltimore: Johns Hopkins University Press.

Svaldi, J., Griepenstroh, J., Tuschen-Caffier, B., & Ehring, T. (2012). Emotion regulation deficits in eating disorders: A marker of eating pathology or general psychopathology? *Psychiatry Research, 197*(1–2), 103–111.

Swendsen, J. D., Conway, K. P., Rounsaville, B. J., & Merikangas, K. R. (2002). Are personality traits familial risk factors for substance use disorders?: Results of a controlled family study. *American Journal of Psychiatry, 159*(10), 1760–1766.

Syzdek, M. R., Addis, M. E., & Martell, C. R. (2009). Working with emotion and emotion regulation in behavioral activation treatment for depressed mood. In A. M. Kring & D. M. Sloan (Eds.), *Emotion regulation and psychopathology: A transdiagnostic approach to etiology and treatment* (pp. 405–426). New York: Guilford Press.

Szarota, P. (1995). Polska Lista Przymiotnikowa (PLP): Narzedzie do diagnozy Pieciu Wielkich czynnikow osobowsci [Polish Adjective List: An instrument to assess the five-factor model of personality]. *Studia Psychologiczne, 33*(1–2), 227–256.

Szirmak, Z., & de Raad, B. (1994). Taxonomy and structure of Hungarian personality traits. *European Journal of Personality, 8*(2), 95–117.

Tackett, J. L., & Lahey, B. B. (2017). Neuroticism. In T. A. Widiger (Ed.), *Oxford handbook of the five factor model* (pp. 39–56). New York: Oxford University Press.

Tackett, J. L., Lahey, B. B., Van Hulle, C., Waldman, I., Krueger, R. F., & Rathouz, P. J.

(2013). Common genetic influences on negative emotionality and a general psychopathology factor in childhood and adolescence. *Journal of Abnormal Psychology, 122*(4), 1142–1153.

Tafet, G. E., & Bernardini, R. (2003). Psychoneuroendocrinological links between chronic stress and depression. *Progress in Neuro-Psychopharmacology and Biological Psychiatry, 27*(6), 893–903.

Tamir, M., & Robinson, M. D. (2007). The happy spotlight: Positive mood and selective attention to rewarding information. *Personality and Social Psychology Bulletin, 33*(8), 1124–1136.

Tang, A. C., Reeb-Sutherland, B. C., Romeo, R. D., & McEwen, B. S. (2012). Reducing behavioral inhibition to novelty via systematic neonatal novelty exposure: The influence of maternal hypothalamic–pituitary–adrenal regulation. *Biological Psychiatry, 72*(2), 150–156.

Tang, T. Z., DeRubeis, R. J., Hollon, S. D., Amsterdam, J., Shelton, R., & Schalet, B. (2009). A placebo-controlled test of the effects of paroxetine and cognitive therapy on personality risk factors in depression. *Archives of General Psychiatry, 66*(12), 1322–1330.

Tarullo, A. R., St. John, A. M., & Meyer, J. S. (2017). Chronic stress in the mother–infant dyad: Maternal hair cortisol, infant salivary cortisol and interactional synchrony. *Infant Behavior and Development, 47*, 92–102.

Taylor, S. (Ed.). (1999). *Anxiety sensitivity: Theory, research, and treatment of the fear of anxiety.* Mahwah, NJ: Erlbaum.

Taylor, S. (2003). Anxiety sensitivity and its implications for understanding and treating PTSD. *Journal of Cognitive Psychotherapy, 17*(2), 179–186.

Taylor, S., Woody, S., Koch, W. J., McLean, P. D., & Anderson, K. W. (1996). Suffocation false alarms and efficacy of cognitive-behavioral therapy for panic disorder. *Behavior Therapy, 27*(1), 115–126.

Tellegen, A. (1985). Structures of mood and personality and their relevance to assessing anxiety, with an emphasis on self-report. In A. H. Tuma & J. D. Maser (Eds.), *Anxiety and the anxiety disorders* (pp. 681–706). Mahwah, NJ: Erlbaum.

ten Have, M., Oldehinkel, A., Vollebergh, W., & Ormel, J. (2005). Does neuroticism explain variations in care service use for mental health problems in the general population?: Results from the Netherlands Mental Health Survey and Incidence Study (NEMESIS). *Social Psychiatry and Psychiatric Epidemiology, 40*(6), 425–431.

Terracciano, A., Balaci, L., Thayer, J., Scally, M., Kokinos, S., Ferrucci, L., . . . Costa, P. T. (2009a). Variants of the serotonin transporter gene and NEO-PI-R neuroticism. *American Journal of Medical Genetics: Part B. Neuropsychiatric Genetics, 150*(8), 1070–1077.

Terracciano, A., Sutin, A. R., McCrae, R. R., Deiana, B., Ferrucci, L., Schlessinger, D., . . . Costa, P. T. (2009b). Facets of personality linked to underweight and overweight. *Psychosomatic Medicine, 71*(6), 682–689.

Thayer, J. F., Friedman, B. H., & Borkovec, T. D. (1996). Autonomic characteristics of generalized anxiety disorder and worry. *Biological Psychiatry, 39*(4), 255–266.

Thomas, A., & Chess, S. (1977). *Temperament and development.* London: Brunner/Mazel.

Thompson, J. K., & Stice, E. (2001). Thin-ideal internalization: Mounting evidence for a new risk factor for body-image disturbance and eating pathology. *Current Directions in Psychological Science, 10*(5), 181–183.

Thompson, R. A. (1998). Early sociopersonality development. In W. Damon & N. Eisenberg (Eds.), *Handbook of child psychology: Social, emotional, and personality development* (pp. 25–104). New York: Wiley.

Thompson, R. J., Kuppens, P., Mata, J., Jaeggi, S. M., Buschkuehl, M., Jonides, J., & Gotlib, I. H. (2015). Emotional clarity as a function of neuroticism and major depressive disorder. *Emotion, 15*(5), 615–624.

Thompson-Brenner, H., Boswell, J. F., Espel-Huynh, H., Brooks, G., & Lowe, M. R.

(2018a). Implementation of transdiagnostic treatment for emotional disorders in residential eating disorder programs: A preliminary pre–post evaluation. *Psychotherapy Research, 29*(8), 1045–1061.

Thompson-Brenner, H., Brooks, G. E., Boswell, J. F., Espel-Huynh, H., Dore, R., Franklin, D. R., . . . Lowe, M. R. (2018b). Evidence-based implementation practices applied to the intensive treatment of eating disorders: Summary of research and illustration of principles using a case example. *Clinical Psychology: Science and Practice, 25*(1), e12221.

Tillfors, M., Furmark, T., Marteinsdottir, I., & Fredrikson, M. (2002). Cerebral blood flow during anticipation of public speaking in social phobia: A PET study. *Biological Psychiatry, 52*(11), 1113–1119.

Tolin, D. F., Abramowitz, J. S., Brigidi, B. D., & Foa, E. B. (2003). Intolerance of uncertainty in obsessive–compulsive disorder. *Journal of Anxiety Disorders, 17*(2), 233–242.

Tomkins, S. (1962). *Affect, imagery, consciousness: Vol. 1. The positive affects.* New York: Springer.

Topper, M., Molenaar, D., Emmelkamp, P. M. G., & Ehring, T. (2014). Are rumination and worry two sides of the same coin?: A structural equation modelling approach. *Journal of Experimental Psychopathology, 5*(3), 363–381.

Treadway, M. T., Buckholtz, J. W., Schwartzman, A. N., Lambert, W. E., & Zald, D. H. (2009). Worth the 'EEfRT'? The effort expenditure for rewards task as an objective measure of motivation and anhedonia. *PloS One, 4*(8), e6598.

Treadway, M. T., & Zald, D. H. (2011). Reconsidering anhedonia in depression: Lessons from translational neuroscience. *Neuroscience and Biobehavioral Reviews, 35*(3), 537–555.

Tronel, S., Belnoue, L., Grosjean, N., Revest, J., Piazza, P., Koehl, M., & Abrous, D. N. (2012). Adult-born neurons are necessary for extended contextual discrimination. *Hippocampus, 22*(2), 292–298.

Troy, A. S., Shallcross, A. J., Brunner, A., Friedman, R., & Jones, M. C. (2018). Cognitive reappraisal and acceptance: Effects on emotion, physiology, and perceived cognitive costs. *Emotion, 18*(1), 58–74.

Trull, T. J., & Sher, K. J. (1994). Relationship between the five-factor model of personality and Axis I disorders in a nonclinical sample. *Journal of Abnormal Psychology, 103*(2), 350–360.

Trull, T. J., Sher, K. J., Minks-Brown, C., Durbin, J., & Burr, R. (2000). Borderline personality disorder and substance use disorders: A review and integration. *Clinical Psychology Review, 20*(2), 235–253.

Tsao, J. C. I., Lewin, M. R., & Craske, M. G. (1998). The effects of cognitive-behavior therapy for panic disorder on comorbid conditions. *Journal of Anxiety Disorders, 12*(4), 357–371.

Tsao, J. C. I., Mystkowski, J. L., Zucker, B. G., & Craske, M. G. (2002). Effects of cognitive-behavioral therapy for panic disorder on comorbid conditions: Replication and extension. *Behavior Therapy, 33*(4), 493–509.

Tull, M. T., Gratz, K. L., Salters, K., & Roemer, L. (2004). The role of experiential avoidance in posttraumatic stress symptoms and symptoms of depression, anxiety, and somatization. *Journal of Nervous and Mental Disease, 192*(11), 754–761.

Tull, M. T., & Roemer, L. (2007). Emotion regulation difficulties associated with the experience of uncued panic attacks: Evidence of experiential avoidance, emotional nonacceptance, and decreased emotional clarity. *Behavior Therapy, 38*(4), 378–391.

Tupes, E. C., & Christal, R. C. (1961). *Recurrent personality factors based on trait ratings.* Washington, DC: U.S. Air Force.

Turk, C. L., Heimberg, R. G., Luterek, J. A., Mennin, D. S., & Fresco, D. M. (2005). Emotion dysregulation in generalized anxiety disorder: A comparison with social anxiety disorder. *Cognitive Therapy and Research, 29*(1), 89–106.

Turkheimer, E. (2000). Three laws of behavior genetics and what they mean. *Current Directions in Psychological Science, 9*(5), 160–164.

Tyrer, P. (Ed.). (1989). *Classification of neurosis.* New York: Wiley.

Tyrer, P. (2014). A comparison of DSM and ICD classifications of mental disorder. *Advances in Psychiatric Treatment, 20*(4), 280–285.

Tyrer, P., Mulder, K., & Crawford, M. J. (2019). The development of ICD-11 classification of personality disorders: An amalgam of science, pragmatism, and politics. *Annual Review of Clinical Psychology, 15,* 481–502.

Tyrer, P., Reed, G. M., & Crawford, M. J. (2015). Classification, assessment, prevalence, and effect of personality disorder. *Lancet, 385*(9969), 717–726.

Tyrer, P., Tyrer, H., Yang, M., & Guo, B. (2016). Long-term impact of temporary and persistent personality disorder on anxiety and depressive disorders. *Personality and Mental Health, 10*(2), 76–83.

Uliaszek, A. A., Al-Dajani, N., & Bagby, R. M. (2015). The relationship between psychopathology and a hierarchical model of normal personality traits: Evidence from a psychiatric patient sample. *Journal of Personality Disorders, 29*(6), 719–734.

Van Apeldoorn, F. J., Van Hout, W. J. P. J., Mersch, P. P. A., Huisman, M., Slaap, B. R., Hale, W. W., . . . Den Boer, J. A. (2008). Is a combined therapy more effective than either CBT or SSRI alone?: Results of a multicenter trial on panic disorder with or without agoraphobia. *Acta Psychiatrica Scandinavica, 117*(4), 260–270.

van den Hurk, P. A. M., Wingens, T., Giommi, F., Barendregt, H. P., Speckens, A. E. M., & van Schie, H. T. (2011). On the relationship between the practice of mindfulness meditation and personality: An exploratory analysis of the mediating role of mindfulness skills. *Mindfulness, 2*(3), 194–200.

van der Bruggen, C. O., Stams, G. J. J. M., & Bögels, S. M. (2008). Research review: The relation between child and parent anxiety and parental control: A meta-analytic review. *Journal of Child Psychology and Psychiatry, 49*(12), 1257–1269.

van der Kaap-Deeder, J., Soenens, B., Boone, L., Vandenkerckhove, B., Stemgée, E., & Vansteenkiste, M. (2016). Evaluative concerns perfectionism and coping with failure: Effects on rumination, avoidance, and acceptance. *Personality and Individual Differences, 101,* 114–119.

Van Deusen, E. H. (1869). Observations on a form of nervous prostration (neurasthenia), culminating in insanity. *American Journal of Psychiatry, 25*(4), 445–461.

Varkovitzky, R. L., Sherrill, A. M., & Reger, G. M. (2018). Effectiveness of the Unified Protocol for Transdiagnostic Treatment of Emotional Disorders among veterans with posttraumatic stress disorder: A pilot study. *Behavior Modification, 42*(2), 210–230.

Viana, A. G., & Rabian, B. (2009). Fears of cognitive dyscontrol and publicly observable anxiety symptoms: Depression predictors in moderate-to-high worriers. *Journal of Anxiety Disorders, 23*(8), 1126–1131.

Vujanovic, A. A., Zvolensky, M. J., & Bernstein, A. (2008). Incremental associations between facets of anxiety sensitivity and posttraumatic stress and panic symptoms among trauma-exposed adults. *Cognitive Behaviour Therapy, 37*(2), 76–89.

Vujanovic, A. A., Zvolensky, M. J., Gibson, L. E., Lynch, T. R., Leen-Feldner, E. W., Feldner, M. T., & Bernstein, A. (2006). Affect intensity: Association with anxious and fearful responding to bodily sensations. *Journal of Anxiety Disorders, 20*(2), 192–206.

Wadlinger, H. A., & Isaacowitz, D. M. (2008). Looking happy: The experimental manipulation of a positive visual attention bias. *Emotion, 8*(1), 121–126.

Wagner, A. W., & Linehan, M. M. (1998). Dissociative behavior. In V. M. Follette, J. I. Ruzek, & F. R. Abueg (Eds.), *Cognitive-behavioral therapies for trauma* (pp. 191–225). New York: Guilford Press.

Wald, J., Taylor, S., Chiri, L. R., & Sica, C. (2010). Posttraumatic stress disorder and chronic pain arising from motor vehicle accidents: Efficacy of interoceptive exposure plus trauma-related exposure therapy. *Cognitive Behaviour Therapy*, 39(2), 104–113.

Walton, K. E., Pantoja, G., & McDermut, W. (2018). Associations between lower order facets of personality and dimensions of mental disorder. *Journal of Psychopathology and Behavioral Assessment*, 40(3), 465–475.

Waszczuk, M. A., Kotov, R., Ruggero, C., Gamez, W., & Watson, D. (2017). Hierarchical structure of emotional disorders: From individual symptoms to the spectrum. *Journal of Abnormal Psychology*, 126(5), 613–634.

Watkins, L. L., Blumenthal, J. A., Davidson, J. R. T., Babyak, M. A., McCants, C. B., & Sketch, M. H. (2006). Phobic anxiety, depression, and risk of ventricular arrhythmias in patients with coronary heart disease. *Psychosomatic Medicine*, 68(5), 651–656.

Watson, D. (2005). Rethinking the mood and anxiety disorders: A quantitative hierarchical model for DSM-V. *Journal of Abnormal Psychology*, 114(4), 522–536.

Watson, D., & Clark, L. A. (1984). Negative affectivity: The disposition to experience aversive emotional states. *Psychological Bulletin*, 96(3), 465–490.

Watson, D., & Clark, L. A. (1993). Behavioral disinhibition versus constraint: A dispositional perspective. In D. M. Wegner & J. W. Pennebaker (Eds.), *Handbook of mental control* (pp. 506–527). New York: Prentice Hall.

Watson, D., & Clark, L. A. (1994a). *The PANAS-X: Manual for the Positive and Negative Affect Schedule—Expanded Form*. Ames: University of Iowa.

Watson, D., & Clark, L. A. (1994b). Introduction to the special issue on personality and psychopathology. *Journal of Abnormal Psychology*, 103(1), 3–5.

Watson, D., Clark, L. A., & Carey, G. (1988). Positive and negative affectivity and their relation to anxiety and depressive disorders. *Journal of Abnormal Psychology*, 97(3), 346–353.

Watson, D., Clark, L. A., Weber, K., Assenheimer, J. S., Strauss, M. E., & McCormick, R. A. (1995). Testing a tripartite model: II. Exploring the symptom structure of anxiety and depression in student, adult, and patient samples. *Journal of Abnormal Psychology*, 104(1), 15–25.

Watson, D., O'Hara, M. W., Simms, L. J., Kotov, R., Chmielewski, M., McDade-Montez, E. A., . . . Stuart, S. (2007). Development and validation of the Inventory of Depression and Anxiety Symptoms (IDAS). *Psychological Assessment*, 19(3), 253–268.

Watson, D., & Tellegen, A. (1985). Toward a consensual structure of mood. *Psychological Bulletin*, 98(2), 219–235.

Watt, M. C., Stewart, S. H., & Cox, B. J. (1998). A retrospective study of the learning history origins of anxiety sensitivity. *Behaviour Research and Therapy*, 36(5), 505–525.

Watters, C. A., Bagby, R. M., & Sellbom, M. (2019). Meta-analysis to derive an empirically based set of personality facet criteria for the alternative DSM-5 model for personality disorders. *Personality Disorders: Theory, Research, and Treatment*, 10(2), 97–104.

Waugh, M. H., Hopwood, C. J., Krueger, R. F., Morey, L. C., Pincus, A. L., & Wright, A. G. C. (2017). Psychological assessment with the DSM-5 alternative model for personality disorders: Tradition and innovation. *Professional Psychology: Research and Practice*, 48(2), 79–89.

Weber, H., Richter, J., Straube, B., Lueken, U., Domschke, K., Schartner, C., . . . Reif, A. (2016). Allelic variation in CRHR1 predisposes to panic disorder: Evidence for biased fear processing. *Molecular Psychiatry*, 21(6), 813–822.

Wegner, D. M. (1987). Transactive memory: A contemporary analysis of the group mind. In B. Mullen & G. R. Goethals (Eds.), *Theories of group behavior* (pp. 185–208). New York: Springer.

Wegner, D. M., Schneider, D. J., Carter, S. R., & White, T. L. (1987). Paradoxical effects of thought suppression. *Journal of Personality and Social Psychology*, 53(1), 5–13.

Weinstock, L. M., & Whisman, M. A. (2006). Neuroticism as a common feature of the depressive and anxiety disorders: A test of the revised integrative hierarchical model in a national sample. *Journal of Abnormal Psychology, 115*(1), 68–74.

Weisz, J. R., & Stipek, D. J. (1982). Competence, contingency, and the development of perceived control. *Human Development, 25*(4), 250–281.

Wells, A., Clark, D. M., Salkovskis, P., Ludgate, J., Hackmann, A., & Gelder, M. (1995). Social phobia: The role of in-situation safety behaviors in maintaining anxiety and negative beliefs. *Behavior Therapy, 26*(1), 153–161.

Wen, D. J., Soe, N. N., Sim, L. W., Sanmugam, S., Kwek, K., Chong, Y.-S., . . . Qiu, A. (2017). Infant frontal EEG asymmetry in relation with postnatal maternal depression and parenting behavior. *Translational Psychiatry, 7*(3), e1057.

Westen, D., Weinberger, J., & Bradley, R. (2007). Motivation, decision making, and consciousness: From psychodynamics to subliminal priming and emotional constraint satisfaction. In D. Zelazo, M. Moscovitch, & E. Thompson (Eds.), *The Cambridge handbook of consciousness* (pp. 673–702). Cambridge, UK: Cambridge University Press.

Westlye, L. T., Bjørnebekk, A., Grydeland, H., Fjell, A. M., & Walhovd, K. B. (2011). Linking an anxiety-related personality trait to brain white matter microstructure: Diffusion tensor imaging and harm avoidance. *Archives of General Psychiatry, 68*(4), 369–377.

White, K. S., Brown, T. A., Somers, T. J., & Barlow, D. H. (2006). Avoidance behavior in panic disorder: The moderating influence of perceived control. *Behaviour Research and Therapy, 44*(1), 147–157.

Widiger, T. A., Lynam, D. R., Miller, J. D., & Oltmanns, T. F. (2012). Measures to assess maladaptive variants of the five-factor model. *Journal of Personality Assessment, 94*(5), 450–455.

Widiger, T. A., & Presnall, J. R. (2013). Clinical application of the five-factor model. *Journal of Personality, 81*(6), 515–527.

Widiger, T. A., & Trull, T. J. (2007). Plate tectonics in the classification of personality disorder: Shifting to a dimensional model. *American Psychologist, 62*(2), 71–83.

Widiger, T. A., Verheul, R., & van den Brink, W. (1999). Personality and psychopathology. In L. A. Pervin & O. P. John (Eds.), *Handbook of personality: Theory and research* (pp. 347–366). New York: Guilford Press.

Wiegel, M., Scepkowski, L. A., & Barlow, D. H. (2007). Cognitive-affective processes in sexual arousal and sexual dysfunction. In E. Janssen (Ed.), *The psychophysiology of sex* (pp. 143–165). Bloomington: Indiana University Press.

Wiers, R. W., & Stacy, A. W. (2013). Implicit and associative processes in addiction. In P. M. Miller, S. A. Ball, M. E. Bates, A. W. Blume, K. M. Kampman, D. J. Kavanagh, . . . P. De Witte (Eds.), *Principles of addiction* (pp. 405–412). San Diego, CA: Academic Press.

Wiersma, J. E., van Oppen, P., van Schaik, D. J. F., van der Does, A. J. W., Beekman, A. T. F., & Penninx, B. W. J. H. (2011). Psychological characteristics of chronic depression: A longitudinal cohort study. *Journal of Clinical Psychiatry, 72*(3), 288–294.

Wiggins, J. S. (2003). *Paradigms of personality assessment.* New York: Guilford Press.

Wildes, J. E., Ringham, R. M., & Marcus, M. D. (2010). Emotion avoidance in patients with anorexia nervosa: Initial test of a functional model. *International Journal of Eating Disorders, 43*(5), 398–404.

Williams, A. D., Thompson, J., & Andrews, G. (2013). The impact of psychological distress tolerance in the treatment of depression. *Behaviour Research and Therapy, 51*(8), 469–475.

Williams, J. B. (1988). A structured interview guide for the Hamilton Depression Rating Scale. *Archives of General Psychiatry, 45*(8), 742–747.

Williams, J. B. W., Gibbon, M., First, M. B., Spitzer, R. L., Davies, M., Borus, J., . . .

Wittchen, H.-U. (1992). The Structured Clinical Interview for DSM-III-R (SCID): II. Multisite test–retest reliability. *Archives of General Psychiatry, 49*(8), 630–636.

Williams, L. R., Degnan, K. A., Perez-Edgar, K. E., Henderson, H. A., Rubin, K. H., Pine, D. S., . . . Fox, N. A. (2009). Impact of behavioral inhibition and parenting style on internalizing and externalizing problems from early childhood through adolescence. *Journal of Abnormal Child Psychology, 37*(8), 1063–1075.

Williams, T. F., & Simms, L. J. (2018). Personality traits and maladaptivity: Unipolarity versus bipolarity. *Journal of Personality, 86*(5), 888–901.

Wilner Tirpak, J., Cassiello-Robbins, C., Ametaj, A., Olesnycky, O. S., Sauer-Zavala, S., Farchione, T. J., & Barlow, D. H. (2019). Changes in positive affect in cognitive-behavioral treatment of anxiety disorders. *General Hospital Psychiatry, 61,* 111–115.

Wilson, M. (1993). DSM-III and the transformation of American psychiatry: A history. *American Journal of Psychiatry, 150*(3), 399–410.

Wilson, R. S., de Leon, C. F. M., Bennett, D. A., Bienias, J. L., & Evans, D. A. (2004). Depressive symptoms and cognitive decline in a community population of older persons. *Journal of Neurology, Neurosurgery and Psychiatry, 75*(1), 126–129.

Wilson, R. S., Krueger, K. R., Gu, L., Bienias, J. L., Mendes de Leon, C. F., & Evans, D. A. (2005). Neuroticism, extraversion, and mortality in a defined population of older persons. *Psychosomatic Medicine, 67*(6), 841–845.

Witkiewitz, K., Marlatt, G. A., & Walker, D. (2005). Mindfulness-based relapse prevention for alcohol and substance use disorders. *Journal of Cognitive Psychotherapy, 19*(3), 211–228.

World Health Organization. (1979). *The ICD-9 classification of mental and behavioural disorders.* Geneva: Author.

World Health Organization. (1999). *The ICD-10 classification of mental and behavioural disorders.* Geneva: Author.

World Health Organization. (2019). *The ICD-11 classification of mental and behavioural disorders.* Geneva: Author.

Wright, A. G. C., Calabrese, W. R., Rudick, M. M., Yam, W. H., Zelazny, K., Williams, T. F., . . . Simms, L. J. (2015). Stability of the DSM-5 Section III pathological personality traits and their longitudinal associations with psychosocial functioning in personality disordered individuals. *Journal of Abnormal Psychology, 124*(1), 199–207.

Wright, A. G. C., Pincus, A. L., Thomas, K. M., Hopwood, C. J., Markon, K. E., & Krueger, R. F. (2013). Conceptions of narcissism and the DSM-5 pathological personality traits. *Assessment, 20*(3), 339–352.

Wright, A. G. C., & Simms, L. J. (2015). A metastructural model of mental disorders and pathological personality traits. *Psychological Medicine, 45*(11), 2309–2319.

Wright, A. G. C., Thomas, K. M., Hopwood, C. J., Markon, K. E., Pincus, A. L., & Krueger, R. F. (2012). The hierarchical structure of DSM-5 pathological personality traits. *Journal of Abnormal Psychology, 121*(4), 951–957.

Wundt, W. (1886). *Elements du psychologie physiologique.* Paris: Ancienne Librairie Germer Bailliere et Cie.

Wupperman, P., Neumann, C. S., & Axelrod, S. R. (2008). Do deficits in mindfulness underlie borderline personality features and core difficulties? *Journal of Personality Disorders, 22*(5), 466–482.

Wupperman, P., Neumann, C. S., Whitman, J. B., & Axelrod, S. R. (2009). The role of mindfulness in borderline personality disorder features. *Journal of Nervous and Mental Disease, 197*(10), 766–771.

Wurm, M., Klein Strandberg, E., Lorenz, C., Tillfors, M., Buhrman, M., Holländare, F., & Boersma, K. (2017). Internet-delivered transdiagnostic treatment with telephone support for pain patients with emotional comorbidity: A replicated single case study. *Internet Interventions, 10,* 54–64.

Yang, K. S., & Bond, M. H. (1990). Exploring implicit personality theories with indigenous or imported constructs: The Chinese case. *Journal of Personality and Social Psychology, 58*(6), 1087–1095.

Yen, S., Zlotnick, C., & Costello, E. (2002). Affect regulation in women with borderline personality disorder traits. *Journal of Nervous and Mental Disease, 190*(10), 693–696.

Young, J. E., Klosko, J. S., & Weishaar, M. E. (2003). *Schema therapy: A practitioner's guide.* New York: Guilford Press.

Young, K. (1928). The measurement of personal and social traits. *Journal of Abnormal and Social Psychology, 22*(4), 431–442.

Zachar, P., & First, M. B. (2015). Transitioning to a dimensional model of personality disorder in DSM 5.1 and beyond. *Current Opinion in Psychiatry, 28*(1), 66–72.

Zeev-Wolf, M., Levy, J., Goldstein, A., Zagoory-Sharon, O., & Feldman, R. (2019). Chronic early stress impairs default mode network connectivity in preadolescents and their mothers. *Biological Psychiatry: Cognitive Neuroscience and Neuroimaging, 4*(1), 72–80.

Zemestani, M., Imani, M., & Ottaviani, C. (2017). A preliminary investigation on the effectiveness of unified and transdiagnostic cognitive behavior therapy for patients with comorbid depression and anxiety. *International Journal of Cognitive Therapy, 10*(2), 175–185.

Zinbarg, R. E., & Barlow, D. H. (1996). Structure of anxiety and the anxiety disorders: A hierarchical model. *Journal of Abnormal Psychology, 105*(2), 181–193.

Zinbarg, R. E., Barlow, D. H., & Brown, T. A. (1997). Hierarchical structure and general factor saturation of the Anxiety Sensitivity Index: Evidence and implications. *Psychological Assessment, 9*(3), 277–284.

Zinbarg, R. E., Brown, T. A., Barlow, D. H., & Rapee, R. M. (2001). Anxiety sensitivity, panic, and depressed mood: A reanalysis teasing apart the contributions of the two levels in the hierarchial structure of the Anxiety Sensitivity Index. *Journal of Abnormal Psychology, 110*(3), 372–377.

Zinbarg, R. E., Craske, M. G., & Barlow, D. H. (2006). *Mastery of your anxiety and worry: Therapist guide.* New York: Oxford University Press.

Zinbarg, R. E., Mineka, S., Bobova, L., Craske, M. G., Vrshek-Schallhorn, S., Griffith, J. W., . . . Anand, D. (2016). Testing a hierarchical model of neuroticism and its cognitive facets: Latent structure and prospective prediction of first onsets of anxiety and unipolar mood disorders during 3 years in late adolescence. *Clinical Psychological Science, 4*(5), 805–824.

Zvolensky, M. J., Feldner, M. T., Eifert, G. H., & Stewart, S. H. (2001). Evaluating differential predictions of emotional reactivity during repeated 20% carbon dioxide-enriched air challenge. *Cognition and Emotion, 15*(6), 767–786.

Index

Note. *f* or *t* following a page number indicates a figure or table.